SUICIDE PREVENTION AFTER NEURODISABILITY

Suicide Prevention after Neurodisability

AN EVIDENCE-INFORMED APPROACH

Grahame K. Simpson
INGHAM INSTITUTE OF APPLIED MEDICAL RESEARCH,
LIVERPOOL, SYDNEY, AUSTRALIA

Lisa A. Brenner
UNIVERSITY OF COLORADO, ANSCHUTZ MEDICAL CAMPUS,
COLORADO, USA

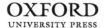
OXFORD
UNIVERSITY PRESS

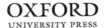

OXFORD
UNIVERSITY PRESS

Oxford University Press is a department of the University of Oxford. It furthers
the University's objective of excellence in research, scholarship, and education
by publishing worldwide. Oxford is a registered trade mark of Oxford University
Press in the UK and certain other countries.

Published in the United States of America by Oxford University Press
198 Madison Avenue, New York, NY 10016, United States of America.

Library of Congress Cataloging-in-Publication Data
Names: Simpson, Grahame K., author. | Brenner, Lisa A., author.
Title: Suicide prevention after neurodisability /
Grahame K. Simpson, Lisa A. Brenner.
Description: New York, NY : Oxford University Press, [2019]
Identifiers: LCCN 2018044927 | ISBN 9780199928415
Subjects: LCSH: Suicide—Prevention. | Suicidal behavior.
Classification: LCC RC569.S563 2019 | DDC 616.85/8445—dc23
LC record available at https://lccn.loc.gov/2018044927

9 8 7 6 5 4 3 2 1

Printed by Webcom, Inc., Canada

To my beloved wife Teresa Simpson, my father Geoffrey Simpson (1923–2015), my mother Margaret, and my sister Catherine, and to Abbey and Hayley; you all have brought such love and happiness into my life.
—Grahame K. Simpson

To my grandmother, Kathryn Brenner, whose stories inspired me to seek out those of others.
—Lisa A. Brenner

Contents

List of Tables

List of Figures

List of Boxes

Acknowledgments

THIS BOOK COMES out of 30 years of clinical practice and research at the Liverpool Brain Injury Rehabilitation Unit (LBIRU), located in South Western Sydney. It was in providing long-term support as a practitioner to clients of the LBIRU community rehabilitation team that I first encountered the clinical challenge of suicidality. Without the service model and compassionate person-centered culture of the LBIRU, this book may never have been written. I want to acknowledge the unswerving support of the LBIRU Director, Dr. Adeline Hodgkinson; Professor Robyn Tate, my valued mentor and collaborator on much of the early research; Professor Elsebeth Stenager, the international pioneer in neurodisability and suicide research; Ms. Barbara Strettles; and my other colleagues in the Brain Injury Rehabilitation Research Group at the Ingham Institute of Applied Medical Research. Collaborating with Professor Lisa Brenner has been inspiring, providing new opportunities to advance the science and clinical practice in suicide prevention after brain injury. Finally, I want to thank my family for their support; in particular my wife Teresa Simpson, whose encouragement, patience, and understanding made the book possible.

—Grahame K. Simpson

People, places, and events shape one's path toward a project such as this book. Time spent among those living with traumatic brain injury, as well as other chronic health conditions, has been my greatest teacher. I am forever grateful for the willingness of these individuals to share their challenges and triumphs. Many of these teachers have been veterans, some of whom were injured overseas. Their determination to find new ways of being in the world is one of the many sparks that motivates me to search for answers. My colleagues at the Department of Veterans Affairs have provided me with a clinical and academic home, and for this I am truly grateful. Many thanks to Dr. Grahame Simpson for both the inspiration and collaboration. Finally, I would like to acknowledge my friends and the three men in my life, Patrick, Benjamin, and Jacob, who keep loving and laughing.

—Lisa A. Brenner

List of Abbreviations

AOR	adjusted odds ratio
ALS	amyotrophic lateral sclerosis
ASIA	American Spinal Injury Association
BHS	Beck Hopelessness Scale
BSS	Beck Scale for Suicide Ideation
CBT	cognitive behavior therapy
CDC	Centers for Disease Control
CVA	cerebral vascular accident
DBT	dialectic behavior therapy
HD	Huntington's disease
LSARS	Lethality of Suicide Attempts Rating Scale
L-SASI	Lifetime Suicide Attempt Self-Injury Interview
MBT	mentalization-based treatment
MIRECC	Mental Illness Research Education and Clinical Center
MDD	major depressive disorder
MS	multiple sclerosis
OEF	Operation Enduring Freedom
OIF	Operation Iraqi Freedom
OR	odds ratio
PD	Parkinson's disease
PST	Problem-Solving Therapy
RCT	randomized controlled trial
RLI	Reasons for Living Inventory
RR	relative risk
SCI	spinal cord injury
SDV	self-directed violence
SDVCS	Self-Directed Violence Classification System
SMR	standardized mortality ratio
TBI	traumatic brain injury
VHA	Veterans Health Administration
WHO	World Health Organization

I Understanding Suicide after Neurodisability

1 Introduction

SUICIDE IS A significant public health problem. It is among the top 10 causes of death in many Western and developing countries and is commonly the leading cause of death among young adults. Across the globe, an estimated 800,000 suicides occur every year, which is higher than fatalities from motor vehicle accidents and wars combined (World Health Organization, 2006a). Moreover, deaths by suicide are only the tip of the iceberg. For every death, there are much larger numbers of suicide attempts and even greater numbers of people who report suicidal ideation. Furthermore, suicidal thoughts and behaviors have a ripple effect, impacting family members, broader social networks, health and human service systems, and society at large.

People with neurodisability have a significantly increased risk of death by suicide. Early work regarding the relationship between psychiatric complications and suicide risk associated with different types of neurodisability were reported in the second half of the nineteenth century, including multiple sclerosis (MS; Charcot, 1879), epilepsy (Gowers, 1901), and Huntington's disease (HD; Huntington, 1872). In the mid-twentieth century, ground-breaking findings regarding suicide after traumatic brain injury (TBI; Hillbom, 1960; Vaukhonen, 1959), epilepsy (Prudhomme, 1941), and spinal cord injury (SCI; Damanski & Gibbon, 1956) were also published. The first decade of the twenty-first century has seen a continued increase of research into suicide across groups of individuals living with neurodisability (e.g., TBI; Simpson & Brenner, 2011).

The descriptor "neurodisability" is used throughout the book rather than the term "neurological disorders." Implicit in the term "neurological disorders" is an orientation which primarily focuses on disease processes underlying neurological conditions (World Health Organization, 2006b). In contrast, the term "neurodisability" emphasizes the disabling consequences (functional and psychosocial) of neurological conditions (Morris, Janssens, Tomlinson, Williams, & Logan, 2013).

Despite the growing evidence of elevated suicide risk associated with neurodisability, there have been few published overviews of this issue. Whitlock (1982) documented research and clinical data about affective disorders and suicide across neurological syndromes (infections, head injuries, cerebrovascular disease, cerebral tumors, disease of the basal ganglia, multiple sclerosis, epilepsy). In a highly cited review published a decade later, Stenager and Stenager (1992) found strong evidence for an increased risk of suicide among people with MS, SCI, and some subcategories of epilepsy, as well as accounts of suicide among people with other types of neurodisability. In 2002, Arciniegas and Anderson updated the growing evidence for the link between suicide and neurodisability. The long interval since this last review, the continued publication of research regarding suicide among people living with different types of neurodisability, and a greater focus on suicide prevention at international and national levels provide the context for this book.

The previous three reviews each focused on overlapping but different sets of neurological disorders. In this book, we focus on the eight that have been most commonly addressed in the previous reviews. Focusing on eight types of neurodisability at once can be unwieldy. Therefore, to aid readability, the eight types have been grouped into nonprogressive (cerebrovascular accident [CVA], SCI, TBI) and progressive conditions (amyotrophic lateral sclerosis [ALS], epilepsy, HD, MS, Parkinson's disease [PD]). Arguments could be made that CVA or TBI are in fact progressive or that epilepsy is nonprogressive. However, the convenience groupings are a useful device to assist in communication and do not presuppose the existence of a formal classification of neurological conditions.

The authors' shared value of suicide prevention provides the foundation for this book. The World Health Organization (2006a) has asserted that suicide is often preventable. Authors in neurodisability have echoed this sentiment. In addressing neurological disorders in general, Faber (2003) has stated that "suicide is an avoidable tragedy" (p. 103). More specifically, Achte, Lonnqvist, and Hillborm (1971) observed that suicide after TBI was the "endpoint of an unsuccessful adaptation process" (p. 80). Implicit in both of these assertions is a belief that intervention can reduce the likelihood of suicide after neurodisability. Further impetus for the development of effective approaches to suicide prevention is the concern that while advances are being made in addressing the physical health needs of those with neurodisability, there is a lag in effectively addressing their mental health needs. For example, it has been found that the standardized mortality ratios for most causes of death after SCI have declined except for suicide (Hartkopp et al., 1997; Kewman & Tate, 1998).

The second driver is the belief that suicide prevention is everyone's business. The US 2012 National Strategy for Suicide Prevention states that government, business, academics, the healthcare industry, communities, and individuals all have a role in helping to prevent suicide (US Department of Health and Human Services [USDHHS], 2012, p. 23). In concordance with such an inclusive approach, this book aims to be informative for clinicians, students, researchers, service managers, and policymakers and relevant to disciplines within psychology, allied health, and medicine.

Our aim is to provide clinically useful information underpinned by the best available evidence while at the same time noting where limited evidence exists. In understanding the risk and rates for suicidal thoughts and behaviors, we have given emphasis where possible to methodologically robust studies based on population-based registries for neurological disorders (e.g., regional, national) with well-defined diagnostic criteria and compared to the underlying population using age- and sex-matched standardized mortality ratios (Stenager & Stenager, 2009). In terms of intervention and prevention, neurologically focused evidence-based guidelines are sparse, and so it has been necessary to form "a synthesis of current scientific knowledge and rational practice" (Department of Veterans Affairs [DVA/DoD], 2013, p. 7). In undertaking this task, our approach is consistent with key national and international policy statements outlining approaches to suicide prevention. These include the US 2012 National Strategy for Suicide Prevention (USDHHS, 2012); the Veterans Affairs (VA)/Department of Defense (DoD) *Clinical Practice Guideline for Assessment and Management of Patients at Risk for Suicide* (2013); and *Self-Harm: Longer-Term Management* (National Institute for Health and Clinical Excellence, 2011).

The great majority of studies published in English about suicide and neurodisability address epidemiology and risk factors. These studies are situated across North America, the United Kingdom, Northern Europe and Australasia, and as many as could be identified have been included. However, there are far fewer works on the clinical aspects of suicide prevention, meaning that the clinical management section of the book relies much more heavily on the broader suicide literature. To make this a manageable task, the information on clinical care is primarily focused on the United States, although many of the principles, insights, and strategies will be applicable to a broader international audience.

In addressing the subject material, a thematic rather than diagnostic-specific approach has been taken. Therefore, the reader will not find chapters addressing each of the various types of neurodisability. This thematic approach provides an opportunity to compare and contrast the features of suicidal thoughts and behaviors across the various conditions, thereby generating invaluable insights into the features of suicide spanning neurodisability. For the latter sections of the book, it reduces repetition and enables the aggregation of the limited work available to produce the most comprehensive clinical resource to date in addressing the assessment and management of suicide.

The book is divided into two parts. Part I, Understanding Suicide after Neurodisability, comprises six chapters. In Chapter 1, a general introduction to the key elements and underlying principles of the book is outlined. In Chapter 2, information is provided about the causes and prevalence; survival, life expectancy, and mortality; common impairments; and functional and psychiatric consequences for the eight types of neurodisability. Chapter 3 then describes the general epidemiology of suicidal behavior, a framework of definitions, and key clinical concepts including the *Diagnostic and Statistical Manual of Mental Disorders* (DSM-5) Suicide Behavior Disorder (DSM-5; American Psychiatric Association, 2013).

Chapter 4 introduces a range of theoretical models for suicide and examines which theoretical constructs have been applied to the field of neurodisability to help account for the elevated suicide risk. Chapter 5 addresses the neuroanatomy, neurobiology, and neuropsychological processes that help explain suicidal thoughts and behaviors after neurodisability. Chapter 6 then details the epidemiology and associated risk factors for suicide, suicide attempts, and suicide ideation after neurodisability.

Part II, Suicide Prevention after Neurodisability, comprising a further eight chapters, turns the focus onto suicide prevention. Chapter 7 addresses possible approaches to screening for suicide risk, and Chapter 8 describes the clinical content and therapeutic processes involved in undertaking a suicide risk assessment. Chapter 9 outlines current knowledge about evidence-based approaches to suicide prevention more broadly and the available evidence in neurodisability. This knowledge is complemented by a broader range of clinical management options outlined in Chapter 10. Chapter 11 then examines the application of these approaches in a cross-cultural context. Chapter 12 addresses the public health and organizational dimensions of suicide prevention and how they can be applied to neurodisability, followed by Chapter 13, within which the legal issues relating to clinical practice in suicide prevention are outlined, as well as the ethical issues that arise around wishing to hasten death. Chapter 14 then provides the conclusion, highlighting major themes that were developed throughout the book as well as potential next steps in both clinical practice and research.

To aid the clinical relevance of the book, each chapter will conclude with a section addressing key clinical implications. To further the clinical emphasis, all the furnished case examples are either previously published or derived from clinical practice. A number of checklists and/or decision trees are provided as aids for clinicians. In addition, references are made to useful assessment tools and validated measures. Finally, the Appendix provides a series of snapshots of disability-specific suicide prevalence and risk data for each of the eight types of neurodisability.

We hope that *Suicide Prevention after Neurodisability* will both inform and stimulate the reader in considering the issue of suicide prevention after neurodisability. We believe that the information presented here will better equip staff in the detection, assessment, treatment, management, and support of clients with suicidal thoughts and behaviors. As we increase our knowledge to better assess and effectively intervene, we can realize the goal of reducing suicide-related thoughts and behaviors among all people with neurodisability.

Implications for Clinicians

1. Suicide is often preventable.
2. Suicide prevention is everyone's business.
3. The association between some types of neurodisability and suicide were flagged as early as the nineteenth century.
4. Suicidal thoughts and behaviors arising from neurological impairment may have a similar presentation across various neurological conditions.
5. A good understanding of suicide across different types of neurodisability will be invaluable in shaping prevention.

References

Achte, K. A., Lonnqvist, J., & Hillbom, E. (1971). Suicides following war brain-injuries. *Acta Psychiatrica Scandinavica, 47*, Supplemen 225, 1–94.

American Psychiatric Association. (2013). *Diagnostic and statistical manual of mental disorders* (5th ed.). Arlington, VA: American Psychiatric Publishing.

Arciniegas, D. B., & Anderson, C. A. (2002). Suicide in neurologic illness. *Current Treatment Options in Neurology, 4*, 457–468.

Charcot, J. M. (1879). *Lectures on the diseases of the nervous system delivered at la Salpetriere.* Philadelphia, PA: Henry C. Lea.

Damanski, M., & Gibbon, N. (1956). The upper urinary tracts in the paraplegic: A long-term survey. *British Journal Urology, 28*, 24–36.

Department of Veterans Affairs/Department of Defense (DVA/DoD). *Clinical Practice Guideline for Assessment and Management of Patients at Risk for Suicide 2013 version 1.0*. Retrieved from http://www.guideline.gov/content.aspxid=47023.

Faber, R. A. (2003). Suicide in neurological disorders. *Neuroepidemiology, 22*, 103–105.

Gowers, W. R. (1901). *Epilepsy and other chronic convulsive diseases* (2nd ed.). London: J & A Churchill.

Hartkopp, A., Brønnum-Hansen, H., Seidenschnur, A-M., & Biering-Sørensen, F. (1997). Survival and cause of death after traumatic spinal cord injury: A long-term epidemiological survey from Denmark. *Spinal Cord, 35*, 76–85.

Hillbom, E. (1960). After-effect of brain injuries. *Acta Psychiatrica Scandinavica, 35*, Supplement 142, 5–135.

Huntington, G. (1872). On chorea. *Medical-Surgical Reports of Philadelphia, 26*, 317–321.

Kewman, D. G., & Tate, D. G. (1998). Suicide in spinal cord injury: A psychological autopsy. *Rehabilitation Psychology, 43*, 143–151.

Morris, C., Janssens, A., Tomlinson, R., Williams, J., & Logan, S. (2013). Towards a definition of neurodisability: A Delphi survey. *Developmental Medicine & Child Neurology, 55*, 1103–1108.

National Institute for Health and Clinical Excellence. (2011). *Self-harm: Longer-term management. NICE Clinical Guideline 133*. London: Author.

Prudhomme, C. (1941). Epilepsy and suicide. *Journal of Nervous and Mental Disease, 94*, 722–731.

Simpson, G. K., & Brenner, L. (2011). Perspectives on suicide and traumatic brain injury. *Journal of Head Trauma Rehabilitation, 26*, 241–243.

Stenager, E., & Stenager, E. (2009). Somatic diseases and suicidal behaviour. In D. Wasserman & C. Wasserman (Eds.), *Oxford textbook of suicidology and suicide prevention: A global perspective* (pp. 293–299). New York: Oxford University Press.

Stenager, E. N., & Stenager, E. (1992). Suicide and patients with neurologic diseases: Methodologic problems. *Archives of Neurology, 49*, 1296–1303.

US Department of Health and Human Services (USDHHS), Office of the Surgeon General and National Action Alliance for Suicide Prevention. (2012). *2012 National strategy for suicide prevention: Goals and objectives for action*. Washington, DC: HHS.

Vaukhonen, K. (1959). Suicide among the male disabled with war injuries to the brain. *Acta Psychiatrica et Neurologica Scandinavica, 34*, Supplement 137, 90–91.

Whitlock, F. A. (1982). The neurology of affective disorder and suicide. *Australian and New Zealand Journal of Psychiatry, 16*, 1–12.

World Health Organization. (2006a). *Suicide Prevention (SUPRE)*. Retrieved from www.who.int/mental_health/prevention/suicide/suicideprevent/en/. Accessed December 31, 2013.

World Health Organization. (2006b). *Neurological disorders: Public health challenges*. Geneva: Author.

2   Understanding Neurodisability

Introduction

The purpose of this chapter is to provide a broad overview regarding the epidemiology of neurodisability, with the goal of highlighting challenges faced by individuals living with diseases or injuries that may lead to increased suicidal thoughts and/or behaviors. As outlined in the Chapter 1, the eight types of neurodisability that are the focus of this book include nonprogressive (cerebrovascular accident [CVA], spinal cord injury [SCI], traumatic brain injury [TBI]) and progressive (amyotrophic lateral sclerosis [ALS], epilepsy, Huntington's disease [HD], multiple sclerosis [MS], and Parkinson's disease [PD]) conditions. For each type of neurodisability, a brief description and epidemiology will be provided, followed by information regarding survival/life-expectancy post-onset/mortality (albeit that data on all these three aspects of longevity were not available across all eight conditions). This will be followed by a brief overview of the impairments and disabilities associated with motor-sensory, cognitive, communication, and behavioral changes, as well as psychiatric sequelae associated with each condition (see Table 2.1 for definitions of impairment and disability). The final section of the chapter will highlight notable

TABLE 2.1

Key terms with definition

Key term	Definition
Impairment	Loss or abnormality in body structure or physiological function (including mental functions), where abnormality means significant variation from established statistical norms (WHO, 2011, p. 305).
Disability	An umbrella term for impairments, activity limitations, and participation restrictions, referring to the negative aspects of the interaction between an individual (with a health condition) and that individual's contextual factors (environmental and personal factors). Defining disability as an interaction means that "disability" is not an attribute of the person (WHO, 2011).

similarities and differences among the conditions which influence the respective patterns of suicidal thoughts and behaviors.

Nonprogressive Conditions

CEREBRAL VASCULAR ACCIDENT/STROKE

Description and Epidemiology

A CVA or stroke is the "sudden occurrence of a non-convulsive, focal neurological deficit," due to cerebral vascular disease (CVD) (Ropper & Brown, 2005a, p. 662). The number of new or recurrent stroke cases per year is approximately 795,000 (610,000 first and 185,000 recurrent attacks) (Go et al., 2013). In the United States, risk factors for stroke include age (risk for stroke doubles in each decade between 55 and 85), gender (men), race (e.g., for African Americans, strokes are more common and lethal), and family history of stroke (National Institute for Neurological Disorders and Stroke [NINDS], 2016a). Eighty-seven percent of CVAs are ischemic, 10% are intracerebral hemorrhagic, and 3% are subarachnoid hemorrhagic (Go et al., 2013). On average, the age of onset for women is higher than for men (≈75 years vs. 71 years) (Roger et al., 2012).

Survival/Life Expectancy Post-Onset/Mortality

Many strokes are fatal, with approximately one death in the United States every 4 minutes (Mozzafarian et al., 2015). Among those living in the United States, stroke rated fifth among all causes of death (CDC, 2016e); worldwide, in 2012, 6.7 million deaths were attributed to stroke (World Health Organization [WHO], 2016b). Among those 65 and older, the US 1-month case fatality rate was 12.6% for all strokes, 8.1% for ischemic strokes, and 44.6% for hemorrhagic strokes, with the most consistent predictor of 30-day mortality being stroke severity (Hankey, 2003). Boysen, Marott, Gronbaek, Hassanpour, and Truelsen (2009) looked at long-term survival after first stroke and found that of the 2,051 patients in their cohort, 1,801 died during the follow-up period. Causes of death included cerebrovascular disease (37%), cardiovascular disease (28%), cancer (12%), and other (23%). Age at the time of first stroke was found to be the most important determinant. In comparing survival rates at 15 years, 11% of those between the ages of 65 and 72 versus 28% among those younger than 65 were found to be alive.

Impairments, Disability, and Psychiatric Sequelae

Impairment and disability associated with CVA varies and is associated with a number of factors including the location and severity of the bleed, the individual's overall health, and the availability of social and physical resources. Impairments in cognition, speech, and physical functioning are common, particularly in older adults with more severe disease (Ropper & Brown, 2005a). In fact, stroke is the most common cause of disability among those living in the United States (NINDS, 2016a).

Among 220 individuals who received care at four centers in Europe, the prevalence and predictors of anxiety and depression at 2, 4, and 6 months and 5 years post-event was evaluated (Lincoln et al., 2013). Five years post-CVA, the prevalence of anxiety and depression was 29% and 33%, respectively. The severity of symptoms significantly increased between month 6 and year 5. Moreover, there is emerging evidence to suggest that among the elderly, the relationship between depression and stroke is bidirectional, with depression contributing to risk for CVA and vice versa (Göthe et al., 2012). A history of post-CVA depression has also been associated with poorer functional outcomes and higher mortality. Due to challenges associated with such impairments, international guidelines recommend post-stroke assessment for cognitive and mood-related symptoms (Lees, Fearon, Harrison, Broomfield, & Quinn, 2012).

SPINAL CORD INJURY

Description and Epidemiology

An SCI involves a lesion to the spinal cord. Such lesions can be complete or incomplete, and the severity of the injury is classified by the level (cervical, thoracic, lumbar, sacral) at which in the injury occurred. It is estimated that 282,0000 people in the United States are living with SCI, with 17,000 new cases of injury each year (National Spinal Cord Injury [SCI] Statistical Center, 2016). Over the past 50 years, the average age of injury has increased from 29 to 42 (National SCI Statistical Center, 2016). Frequently noted mechanisms of civilian injury include motor vehicle accidents, falls, gunshot or stab wounds, crushing industrial injury, or birth injury (Ropper & Brown, 2005c). For a small proportion of individuals with SCI, a previous suicide attempt is the cause of injury.

Survival/Life Expectancy Post-Onset/Mortality

According to work by Strauss, Devivo, Paculdo, and Shavelle (2006), over the past 30 years there has been a 40% decline in mortality during the first 2 years post-injury. Nevertheless, work by the same group suggests that, between 1973 and 2004, the decline in mortality after the first 2 years of SCI is small (Strauss et al., 2006). That is, despite advances in the long-term care of patients with SCI, life span, when measured from the second year post-injury, has not been significantly lengthened. However, it should be noted that work exploring life expectancy among those living with SCI is complicated by the heterogeneity of those injured, as well as of the injuries sustained (e.g., mechanism of injury, race, age, time since injury, and injury level and American Spinal Injury Association [ASIA] grade). To illustrate, Strauss et al. (2006) present sample life expectancies for a 25-year-old white male, 3 years post-SCI (nonviolent) by level and ASIA grade. Life expectancies (years) presented range from 25.4 (C1–C3, grade A) to 44.7 (all grade D). Causes of death that appear to have the greatest impact on reduced life expectancy include pneumonia and septicemia (National SCI Center, 2016).

Impairment, Disability, and Psychiatric Sequelae

Depending on the severity of the injury, individuals can experience a wide range of impairments and disability. Those associated with physical functioning are common (e.g., mobility, continence, sexual function, fertility, pain; Gill, 1999; Kennedy, Evans, & Sandhu, 2009) and impact on psychosocial functioning (e.g., feelings of grief and loss, isolation, depression, anxiety; Chan, 2000; Kennedy & Rogers, 2000; Dryden et al., 2005). Anderson, Vogel, Chlan, Betz, and McDonald (2007) conducted follow-up telephone interviews among adults (age ≥24) who had sustained an SCI at age 18 or younger and found that among the 864 individuals interviewed, 27% reported having depressive thoughts which ranged from mild to severe, and 3% endorsed symptoms consistent with major depressive disorder (MDD). Mean time post-injury in this sample was 16 years. One-year post-injury, Bombardier, Richards, Krause, Tulsky, and Tatke (2004) assessed individuals for depression and found that 11% met criteria for MDD.

TRAUMATIC BRAIN INJURY

Description and Epidemiology

TBI occurs as the result of an external force ("a bump, blow, or jolt to the head or a penetrating brain injury") that impacts brain functioning (CDC, 2016b). In the United States, TBI is the leading cause of death and disability among children and young adults. It is estimated that that there are 2.8 million TBI-related Emergency Department visits per year, with the vast majority of injuries being concussions (i.e., mild TBI) (CDC, 2016b). Those at greatest risk for sustaining a TBI are children aged 0–4 years, older adolescents aged 15–19 years, and adults aged 65 years and over. Although motor vehicle accidents (e.g., autos, trucks, motorcycles, bicycles, and pedestrians hit by vehicles) are the leading cause of injury, mechanism varies by age (i.e., falls among those over 65 and transportation for those under the age of 65). An estimated 300,000 injuries per year are associated with sports (Thurman, Branche, & Sniezke, 1998). Moreover, individuals serving in the military are sustaining injuries (including blast injuries) associated with combat and service (Terrio et al., 2009). Injury severity (mild, moderate, severe) is determined based on brain functioning and/or damage post-injury versus associated sequelae (see Table 2.2). There are at least 5.3 million Americans (2% of the US population) living with disabilities associated with TBI (CDC, 2016d).

Survival/Life Expectancy Post-Injury/Mortality

In the United States, TBI is thought to be a contributing factor in around a third of all injury-related deaths (CDC, n.d.). In terms of decreased life expectancy post-injury, Colorado residents with TBI discharged alive from acute hospitalization between 1998 and 2003 were found to be at 2.5 times the risk of death when compared with the general population (Ventura et al., 2010). Harrison-Felix et al. (2009) explored mortality and life expectancy among persons with TBI ($n = 1,678$) who survived to the first anniversary of their injury and found that those with a TBI were 1.5 times more likely to die than persons in the general population of similar age, sex, and race. Despite this, resulting average life expectancy was largely preserved, with an estimated reduction of only 4 years.

TABLE 2.2

Departments of Defense and Veterans Affairs consensus-based classification of closed traumatic brain injury (TBI) severity[a]

Criteria	TBI severity		
	Mild	Moderate	Severe
Structural Imaging	Normal	Normal or abnormal	Normal or abnormal
Loss of consciousness	0–30 minutes	>30 min and <24 hours	>24 hours
Alteration of consciousness/ mental state[b]	Up to 24 hours	>24 hours; severity based on other criteria	
Posttraumatic amnesia	0–1 day	>1 day and <7 days	>7 days
Glasgow Coma Score (best available score in first 24 hours)	13–15	9–12	<9

[a]See Department of Veterans Affairs & Department of Defense (2009).

[b]Alteration of mental status must be immediately related to the trauma to the head. Typical symptoms would be looking and feeling dazed and uncertain of what is happening, confusion, difficulty thinking clearly or responding appropriately to mental status questions, and being unable to describe events immediately before or after the trauma event.

Impairment, Disability, and Psychiatric Sequelae

TBI survivors, particularly those with moderate to severe injuries, experience a range of motor-sensory (Ponsford et al., 2014), cognitive (Draper & Ponsford, 2008), and behavioral impairments (Sabaz et al., 2014) that create significant challenges in areas of occupation, relationships, and independent living (Tyerman, 2012; McRae, Hallab, & Simpson, 2016; Agyemang, Marwitz, & Kreutzer, 2017). Psychiatric disorders among those with TBI are common, with depression being the most frequently diagnosed. The etiology of psychiatric symptoms is complicated. In many cases organic and psychosocial factors contribute. Among 559 consecutively hospitalized adults with complicated mild to severe TBI, Bombardier et al. (2010) found that, during the first year post-injury, 53.1% met criteria for MDD. This is about eight times greater than would be expected in the general population. Research has found that these high rates continue long after injury.

Progressive Conditions

AMYOTROPHIC LATERAL SCLEROSIS/LOU GEHRIG'S
DISEASE/MOTOR NEURON DISEASE

Description and Epidemiology

ALS is a condition that involves degeneration of lower and upper motor neurons. As nerve cells stop working, the individual with the condition loses the ability to engage muscles. The term has also been used more generally to refer to motor neuron syndromes (e.g., progressive muscular atrophy [PMA]; Clark, Pritchard, & Sunak, 2005). Although first formally identified in 1874, the etiology of the disease remains unknown (Clark et al., 2005). Whereas approximately 5–10% of diagnoses appear in families with a history of the condition ("familial ALS"), most often it seems to occur "at random." Study has focused on genetic and environmental factors. Men appear to be more at risk than women (1.4:1.0) (Clark et al., 2005) There are approximately 12,000–15,000 individuals in the United States living with the disease, with around 5,000 individuals receiving a new diagnosis each year (CDC, 2016c). Geographic (e.g., Island of Guam) and subpopulation (e.g., US Gulf War Veterans) disease clusters have been identified (Clark et al., 2005).

Survival/Life Expectancy Post-Diagnosis/Mortality

Age of onset is generally between 55 and 75, with average life expectancy post-diagnosis being 2–5 years (CDC, 2016c). Among those with "familial ALS," post-diagnosis life expectancy is shorter at 2 years (CDC, 2016c).

Impairment, Disability, and Psychiatric Sequelae

ALS-related paralysis results secondarily to the individual's inability to engage his muscles. Persons with the condition experience progressive weakness, with the eventual inability to control their breath. Bronchopneumonia and pneumonia have been documented as the most frequent causes of death (Corcia et al., 2008). Although initially ALS was defined as solely a disorder of upper and lower motor neuron dysfunction, more recently it has been recognized that cognitive impairment is also common. It is estimated that 50% of those with ALS have some level of cognitive impairment (Lomen-Hoerth et al., 2003). Depression is also relatively common, though reported rates vary (e.g., 37% were mild–moderately depressed, 13% were moderately–severely depressed, and 6% were severely depressed; MDD, 16.2–25%)

(Wicks et al., 2007). Given the lack of understanding about the triggers of ALS, treatments largely focus on the management of symptoms arising from the disease rather than the disease process itself. Nonetheless, recent advances regarding the identification of genetic factors underlying at least some forms of ALS are providing hope for the development of novel disease-modifying treatments (Riva, Agosta, Lunetta, Filippi, & Quattrini, 2016).

EPILEPSY

Description and Epidemiology

Epilepsy is a set of neurological conditions characterized by seizures. Approximately 4.3 million individuals in the United States (CDC, 2016f) and 50 million individuals worldwide are affected by epilepsy, with 90% of cases identified in developing regions (WHO, 2016a). To be diagnosed with epilepsy, one must experience two or more unprovoked seizures. Among those with epilepsy, treatment is effective approximately 70% of the time; however, 75% of individuals in developing counties do not received necessary medications (WHO, 2016a).

Although the defining symptom of epilepsy is spontaneous epileptic seizures, an abundance of evidence suggests that epilepsy is a "complex set of brain disorders" associated with a spectrum of cognitive, behavioral, and psychiatric symptoms (Berg, 2011, p. 10). Among those with childhood onset, approximately a quarter of individuals have seizures that occur in association with identifiable structural brain lesions likely secondary to prenatal and perinatal events (e.g., strokes, developmental malformations) (Berg, 2011). Onset among adults is most often associated with a trauma to the brain, stroke, or tumor.

Survival/Life Expectancy Post-Diagnosis/Mortality

Compared to members of the general population, risk of premature death among those with epilepsy is up to three times higher, with the highest rates being found in low- and middle-income countries and in rural areas (WHO, 2016a). Certainly, if present, malignant underlying causes (e.g., brain tumor) can contribute to decreased survival times. Periods of prolonged seizures or multiple seizures over a brief period of time (status epilepticus) can also cause death. Sudden unexplained death in epilepsy (SUDEP) is also a cause of early mortality among those with epilepsy, with 1.16 cases of SUDEP for every 1,000 people with epilepsy (Thurman, Hesdorffer, & French, 2014). Although the mechanisms of death remain unknown, possible factors include pauses in breathing or dangerous heart rhythms (CDC, 2016f). That being said, "most individuals with epilepsy live a full life span" (Sperling, 2001).

Impairment, Disability, and Psychiatric Sequelae

Although individuals with early and late onset of this disorder appear to be at risk for poor psychosocial and cognitive outcomes, those with childhood onset seem to face even more significant disability (Berg, 2011). In particular, those with very early onset (e.g., <2 years of age) and frequent uncontrolled seizures seem to face the greatest challenges (Berg, 2011). Among adults, Taylor and colleagues (2010) compared the cognitive profile of newly diagnosed patients with epilepsy with healthy volunteer, and their findings supported that cognitive impairment may be associated with epileptogenesis the longitudinal and often gradual process that results in the development of epilepsy (McNamara, Huang, & Leonard, 2006). Most significant deficits were found in the areas of memory and psychomotor speed. Patients with epilepsy also reported greater mood disturbance. Emerging evidence suggests that, particularly among those with mesial temporal lobe epilepsy, deficits may be progressive (Berg, 2011). Side effects of antiepileptic medications also seem to impact cognitive functioning (Taylor et al., 2010).

Using a large Canadian national population health survey, Tellez-Zenteno, Patten, Jette, Williams, and Wiebe (2007) assessed the population-based prevalence of psychiatric conditions associated with epilepsy. Findings suggested that individuals with epilepsy were more likely than individuals without epilepsy to report lifetime anxiety disorders, with an odds ratio of 2.4 (95% CI, 1.5–3.8). After adjusting for covariates, lifetime history of depression was also significantly greater than for the general population.

HUNTINGTON DISEASE

Description and Epidemiology

HD is an autosomal dominant movement disorder. The HD gene has been isolated on chromosome 4, and, as such, direct mutation analysis makes it possible to detect those at risk (Baliko, Csala, & Czopf, 2004). Although as the disease progresses all areas of the brain are vulnerable to deterioration, the striatum is the primary structure affected by HD (Wetzel, Gehl, Dellefave-Castillo, Schiffman, & Shannon, 2011). The prevalence rate of HD is reported at 7–10 per 100,000 (Harper, 1996). Disease onset typically occurs between the ages of 35 and 44.

Survival/Life Expectancy Post-Diagnosis/Mortality

Individuals with HD experience a significantly shortened life span, with an average life expectancy of 20 years post-diagnosis (Paulsen, Hoth, Nehl, & Steirman, 2005).

Impairment, Disability, and Psychiatric Sequelae

In discussing ethical challenges associated with presymptomatic testing, Bird (1999) notes that HD is a degenerative brain disorder that occurs in the prime of life and involves a socially embarrassing and disabling movement disorder and serious cognitive and behavioral changes. At present there is no cure or even effective treatment. Moreover, "there is a 50% risk of the same disorder" in offspring (Bird, 1999, p. 1289). Dewhurst and colleagues published an article in 1970 titled "Socio-Psychiatric Consequences of Huntington's Disease." Families of 102 patients were followed for 16 years. This included 20 pedigrees involving 50 individuals with HD. The researchers identified a "high incidence of psychiatric, sexual, and social features of illness" which antedated institutionalization (Dewhurst, Oliver, & McKnight, 1970, p. 258). Thirty-eight percent of the marriages ended. The negative impact on children and families of those with the disease was also highlighted.

Work by Cummings (1995) suggests that psychiatric symptoms occur in 35–75% of individuals. Personality changes, affective disorders, and psychosis are common (Cummings, 1995). Evidence suggests that psychiatric symptoms often predate motor signs by as much as 10 years (Berrios et al., 2001; Campodonioco, Codori, & Brandt, 1996). Serious depression is common (9–44%) (Harper, 1996, pp. 85–93).

MULTIPLE SCLEROSIS

Description and Epidemiology

MS is a chronic condition characterized by "episodes of focal disorders of the optic nerves, spinal cord, and brain which may remit to a varying extent and recur over a period of many years" (Ropper & Brown, 2005b, p. 771). It affects approximately 400,000 individuals in the United States and 2.5 million individuals worldwide (National Multiple Sclerosis Society, n.d.). Diagnosis generally occurs between the ages of 20 and 50 (National Multiple Sclerosis Society, 2015). Although the etiology of MS is not well understood, data suggest that a combination of genetic susceptibility and some environmental factors likely "evoke" the disease (Ropper & Brown, 2005b, p. 775).

Survival/Life Expectancy Post-Diagnosis/Mortality

Research suggests that those with MS have a life expectancy of 7 years less than those without the condition (National Multiple Sclerosis Society, 2015).

Impairment, Disability, and Psychiatric Sequelae

Impairments associated with sensory and motor loss, fatigue, blindness, poor balance, pain, cognitive functioning, and depression are frequent (Turner, Williams, Bowen, Kivlahan, & Haselkorn, 2006). Worldwide, studies suggest that 12–25% of MS patients examined either at or post-diagnosis have been admitted to a psychiatric inpatient unit or received psychiatric outpatient treatment (Stenager & Jensen, 1988).

Depression is the most common psychiatric disorder among those with MS (Wallin, Wilken, Turner, Williams, & Kane, 2006), with a reported lifetime prevalence as high as 50% and an annual prevalence of 20% or higher (Siegert & Abernethy, 2005). For example, Sadovnick et al. (1996) found that by age 59 the lifetime rate of depression among those with MS was 50.3%. The etiology of depression among those with this condition is multifactorial and complex. Organic and psychosocial factors contribute. Moreover, findings regarding the association between depression and degree of physical disability have been mixed (Feinstein, 2011). This is likely associated with the diversity of the disease and complicated relationships between physical impairment and psychosocial functioning. Nevertheless, existing research supports links between depression and structural brain changes, immune dysfunction (Wallin et al., 2006), and psychosocial factors (i.e., uncertainty, inadequate coping strategies, helplessness, loss of recreational opportunities, poor-quality relationship, high levels of stress and fatigue, and cognitive impairment). Lynch, Kroencke, and Denney (2001) identified four independent risk factors of depression among those with MS including (1) emotion based-coping, (2) uncertainty, (3) loss of hope, and (4) degree of physical disability.

PARKINSON'S DISEASE

Description and Epidemiology

PD is a motor system disorder that is the result of the loss of dopamine-producing brain cells. Most individuals are diagnosed with the condition at age 60 or older (NINDS, 2015). That being said, approximately 5–10% of those with PD are diagnosed before the age of 50. Though data suggests that 500,000 individuals in the United States are living with PD, some experts believe that when one includes mis- or undiagnosed individuals, the number is much higher (e.g., 1 million) (NINDS, 2015). The etiology of the disease remains unknown. Research implicates genetic and environmental factors.

Survival/Life Expectancy Post-Diagnosis/Mortality

Work by Ishihara, Cheesbrough, Brayne, and Schrad (2007) suggests that for patients with PD living in the United Kingdom, life expectancy is decreased when compared to that of the general population. Age at onset plays a significant role. Specifically, the researchers found that in those with "onset between 25 and 40 years, estimated life expectancy was reduced from a mean of 49 to 38 years; in those with onset between 40 and 65 years, life expectancy was reduced from a mean of 31 to 21 years; and in those with an onset at or above 65 years, average life expectancy was reduced from a mean of 9 to 5 years" (p. 1305).

Impairment, Disability, and Psychiatric Sequelae

Symptoms include tremor, trembling in hands, arms, legs, jaw, and face; rigidity or stiffness of the limbs and trunk; bradykinesia (slowness of movement); postural instability; or impaired balance and coordination (NINDS, 2015). Advancing PD is associated with freezing (brief inability to start or continue rhythmic, repeated movements), falling, and/or dementia (Olanow, Stern, & Sethi, 2009). Despite the fact that there is no cure, there are effective treatment options (symptom control) for those with PD (e.g., dopamine replacement strategies) including deep brain stimulation (DBS) for those with more refractory symptoms (Olanow et al., 2009). Depression and challenges with sleep are also frequently noted. A systematic review found that the prevalence of psychological distress was widespread among people with PD (MDD, 17%; minor depression, 22%; dysthymia, 13%; Reijnders, Ehrt, Weber, Aarsland, & Leentjens, 2008).

Conclusion

A summary of information regarding the eight neurological conditions addressed in this book was provided in this chapter. To date, discussion regarding the similarities and differences among these different conditions that modulate the risk for suicidal thoughts and behaviors has been limited. The eight conditions incorporate a complex mosaic of disease- and injury-related factors that can potentially contribute to suicide risk (see Table 2.3 for some key domains). In terms of differences, the neurological conditions have widely varying ages of onset. The likelihood of a suicidal reaction to the onset of a neurological condition will be influenced by the background age-related prevalence rate and risk factors for suicidal thoughts and behaviors for the general population. There is also a broad spectrum of life expectancy associated

TABLE 2.3

Similarities and differences across conditions

	Nonprogressive conditions			Progressive conditions				
	CVA	SCI	TBI	ALS	Epilepsy	HD	MS	PD
Age of Onset								
Early in Life		X	X		X	X	X	
Later in Life	X		X	X	X			X
Life Expectancy Post-Onset								
Markedly Limited	X			X	X	X		
Etiology of condition								
Disease	X	X		X	X	X	X	X
Injury		X	X		X			
Functional Impairment Post-Onset Predominantly								
Physical	X	X	X	X		X	X	X
Cognitive	X		X		X	X	X	X
Psychiatric Symptoms Post-Onset	X	X	X	X	X	X	X	X
Treatments target								
Manage symptoms	X	X	X	X	X	X	X	X
Cure condition								
Uncertainly of diagnosis/onset					X	X	X	
Treatment for condition increases suicide risk					X			X

See Strauss et al. (2006).

CVA, cerebrovascular accident; SCI, spinal cord injury; TBI, traumatic brain injury; ALS, amyotrophic lateral sclerosis; HD, Huntington's disease; MS, multiple sclerosis; PD, Parkinson's disease.

with these conditions, and there may be a sharper impact associated with those conditions that significantly shorten life expectancy. Furthermore, differences in etiology also play a role, as people with a TBI or SCI may have sustained their condition due to risky behavior (e.g., a suicide attempt), and this can have ongoing consequences post-injury. In contrast, some neurological conditions have a period of uncertainty associated with an extended prodromal period. Subsequently, a confirmed diagnosis can act as the trigger for an acute suicidal crisis. Finally, treatments (neurosurgery, pharmacotherapy) for some neurological conditions may actually exacerbate suicide risk.

Alongside such differences, significant heterogeneity exists among the conditions. Most cause a range of both cognitive, physical, and behavioral impairment with associated disabilities. Increased levels of psychiatric symptoms, particularly depression, are universal across the conditions. Finally, the treatment across conditions generally targets symptom management, with few avenues for a cure developed to date. In subsequent chapters, we will explore both the commonalties and differences across the eight types of neurodisability. This investigation has the potential to improve our understanding of key factors associated with increased suicide risk, improve evidence-informed clinical decision-making, and lay a foundation for the design and implementation of novel research methods.

Implications for Clinicians

1. Though underlying mechanisms and sequelae associated with neurodisabilities vary, all eight conditions highlighted are associated with increased psychiatric sequelae, and all but one condition (PD) have been linked to an increased risk for death by suicide.
2. Increased understanding regarding cognitive, physical, and behavioral impairments, as well as associated disabilities, will assist providers in identifying potential risk factors and warning signs for suicide.

References

Agyemang, A., Marwitz, J., & Kreutzer, J. (2017). Marital satisfaction, stability, and conflict among treatment seeking couples after traumatic brain injury. *Archives of Physical Medicine and Rehabilitation, 98*(10), e81.

Anderson, C. J., Vogel, L. C., Chlan, K. M., Betz, R. R., & McDonald, C. M. (2007). Depression in adults who sustained spinal cord injuries as children or adolescents. *Journal of Spinal Cord Medicine, 30*(Suppl 1), S76–S82.

Baliko, L., Csala, B., & Czopf, J. (2004). Suicide in Hungarian Huntington's disease patients. *Neuroepidemiology, 23*(5), 258–260. doi:10.1159/000079953

Berg, A. T. (2011). Epilepsy, cognition, and behavior: The clinical picture. *Epilepsia, 52*(Suppl 1), S76–82. doi:10.1111/j.1528-1167.2010.02905.x

Berrios, G. E., Wagle, A. C., Marková, I. S., Wagle, S. A., Ho, L. W., Rubinsztein, D. C., . . . Hodges, J. R. (2001). Psychiatric symptoms and CAG repeats in a neurologically asymptomatic

Huntington's disease gene carriers. *Psychiatry Research, 102*(3), 217–225. doi:10.1016/S0165-1781(01)00257-8

Bird, T. D. (1999). Outrageous fortune: The risk of suicide in genetic testing for Huntington disease. *American Journal of Human Genetics, 64*(5), 1289–1292.

Bombardier, C. H., Fann, J. R., Temkin, N. R., Esselman, P. C., Barber, J., & Dikmen, S. S. (2010). Rates of major depressive disorder and clinical outcomes following traumatic brain injury. *JAMA, 303*(19), 1938–1945. doi:10.1001/jama.2010.599

Bombardier, C. H., Richards, J. S., Krause, J. S., Tulsky, D., & Tate, D. G. (2004). Symptoms of major depression in people with spinal cord injury: Implications for screening. *Archives of Physical Medicine and Rehabilitation, 85*(11), 1749–1756. doi:10.1016/j.apmr.2004.07.348

Boysen, G., Marott, J. L., Gronbaek, M., Hassanpour, H., & Truelsen, T. (2009). Long-term survival after stroke: 30 years of follow-up in a cohort, the Copenhagen City Heart Study. *Neuroepidemiology, 33*(3), 254–260. doi:10.1159/000229780

Campodonico, J. R., Codori, A. M., & Brandt, J. (1996). Neuropsychological stability over two years in asymptomatic carriers of the Huntington's disease mutation. *Journal of Neurology, Neurosurgery, and Psychiatry, 61*(6), 621–624. doi:10.1136/jnnp.61.6.621

Centers for Disease Control and Prevention (CDC). (n.d.). Getting the stat on traumatic brain injury in the United States. Retrieved from https://www.cdc.gov/traumaticbraininjury/pdf/blue_book.pdf

Centers for Disease Control and Prevention (CDC). (2016a). Epilepsy fast facts. Retrieved from http://www.cdc.gov/epilepsy/basics/fast_facts.htm

Centers for Disease Control and Prevention (CDC). (2016b). Injury prevention & control: Traumatic brain injury and concussion. Retrieved from https://www.cdc.gov/traumaticbraininjury/get_the_facts.html

Centers for Disease Control and Prevention (CDC). (2016c). National Amyotrophic Lateral Sclerosis (ALS) registry. Retrieved from http://wwwn.cdc.gov/ALS/WhatisALS.aspx

Centers for Disease Control and Prevention. (2016d). Report to Congress: Traumatic brain injury in the United States. Retrieved from http://www.cdc.gov/traumaticbraininjury/pubs/tbi_report_to_congress.html

Centers for Disease Control and Prevention. (2016e). Stroke. Retrieved from http://www.cdc.gov/stroke/

Centers for Disease Control and Prevention. (2016f). Sudden unexpected death in epilepsy. http://www.cdc.gov/epilepsy/basics/sudep/

Chan, R. C. (2000). Stress and coping in spouses of persons with spinal cord injuries. *Clinical Rehabilitation, 14*, 137–144.

Clark, J., Pritchard, C., & Sunak, S. (2005). Amyotrophic lateral sclerosis: A report on the state of research into the cause, cure, and prevention of ALS. Retrieved from http://www.researchals.org/uploaded_files/mdph_alsreport_211aDS.pdf

Corcia, P., Pradat, P., Salachas, F., Bruneteau, G., le Forestier, N., Seilhean, D., . . . Meininger, V. (2008). Causes of death in a post-mortem series of ALS patients. *Amyotrophic Lateral Sclerosis, 9*(1), 59–62. doi:10.1080/17482960701656940

Cummings, J. L. (1995). Behavioral and psychiatric symptoms associated with Huntington's disease. *Advances in Neurology, 65*, 179–186.

Department of Veterans Affairs & Department of Defense, Management of Concussion-mild Traumatic Brain Injury (mTBI). (2016). Clinical practice guideline: Management of concussion/mild traumatic brain injury. Retrieved from https://www.healthquality.va.gov/guidelines/rehab/mtbi/

Dewhurst, K., Oliver, J. E., & McKnight, A. L. (1970). Socio-psychiatric consequences of Huntington's disease. *British Journal of Psychiatry, 116*(532), 255–258. doi:10.1192/bjp.116.532.255

Draper, K., & Ponsford, J. (2008). Cognitive functioning ten years following traumatic brain injury and rehabilitation. *Neuropsychology, 22*(5), 618.

Dryden, D. M., Saunders, L. D., Rowe, B. H., May, L. A, Yiannakoulias, N., Svenson, L. W., . . . Voaklander, D. C. (2005). Depression following traumatic spinal cord injury. *Neuroepidemiology, 25*, 55–61.

Feintsein, A. (2011). Multiple sclerosis and depression. *Multiple Sclerosis, 17*(11), 1276–1281. doi:10.1177/1352458511417835

Gill, M. (1999). Psychosocial implications of spinal cord injury. *Critical Care Nursing Quarterly, 22*, 1–7.

Go, A. S., Mozaffarian, D., Roger, V. L., Benjamin, E. J., Berry, J. D. Borden, W. B., . . . Turner, M. B. (2013). Heart Disease and Stroke Statistics—2013 Update: A report from the American Heart Association. Centers for Disease Control and Prevention, National Center for Health Statistics. Compressed Mortality File 1999–2009. Retrieved from https://www.ncbi.nlm.nih.gov/pmc/articles/PMC5408511/pdf/nihms846234.pdf

Göthe, F., Enache, D., Wahlund, L. O., Winblad, B., Crisby, M., Lökk, J., & Aarsland, D. (2012). Cerebrovascular diseases and depression: Epidemiology, mechanisms, and treatment. *Panminerva Medica, 54*(3), 161–170.

Hankey, G. J. (2003). Long-term outcome after ischaemic stroke/transient ischaemic attack. *Cerebrovascular Disease, 16*(Suppl 1), 14–19. doi:10.1159/000069936

Harper, P. S. (Ed.). (1996). *Huntington's disease* (2nd ed.). London: WB Saunders.

Harrison-Felix, C. L., Whiteneck, G. G., Jha, A., DeVivo, M J., Hammond, F. M., & Hart, D. M. (2009). Mortality over four decades after traumatic brain injury rehabilitation: A retrospective cohort study. *Archives of Physical Medicine and Rehabilitation, 90*(9), 1506–1513. doi:10.1016/j.apmr.2009.03.015

Ishihara, L. S., Cheesbrough, A., Brayne, C., & Schrad, A. (2007). Estimated life expectancy of Parkinson's patients compared with the UK population. *Journal of Neurology, Neurosurgery & Psychiatry, 78*, 1304–1309. doi:10.1136/jnnp.2006.100107

Kennedy, P., Evans, M., & Sandhu, N. (2009). Psychological adjustment to spinal cord injury: The contribution of coping, hope and cognitive appraisals. *Psychology, Health and Medicine, 14*, 17–33.

Kennedy, P., & Rogers, B. A. (2000). Anxiety and depression after spinal cord injury: A longitudinal analysis. *Archives of Physical Medicine & Rehabilitation, 81*, 932–937.

Lees, R., Fearon, P., Harrison, J. K., Broomfield, N. M., & Quinn, T. J. (2012). Cognitive and mood assessment in stroke research: Focused review of contemporary studies. *Stroke, 43*(6), 1678–1680. doi:10.1161/STROKEAHA.112.653303

Lincoln, N. B., Brinkmann, N., Cunningham, S., Dejaeger, E., De Weerdt, W., Jenni, W., . . . De Wit, L. (2013). Anxiety and depression after a stroke: A 5 year follow-up. *Disability and Rehabilitation, 35*(2), 140–145. doi:10.3109/09638288.2012.691939

Lomen-Hoerth, C., Murphy, J., Langmore, S., Kramer, J. H., Olney, R. K., & Miller, B. (2003). Are amyotrophic lateral sclerosis patients cognitively normal? *Neurology, 60*(7), 1094–1097. doi:10.1212/01.WNL.0000055861.95202.8D

Lynch, S. G., Kroencke, D. C., & Denney, D. R. (2001). The relationship between disability and depression in multiple sclerosis: The role of uncertainty, coping, and hope. *Multiple Sclerosis, 7*(6), 411–416. doi:10.1177/135245850100700611

McNamara, J. O., Huang, Y. Z., & Leonard, A. S. (2006). Molecular signaling mechanisms underlying epileptogenesis. *Science STKE, 6*(356), re 12. doi:10.1126/stke.3562006re12

McRae, P., Hallab, L., & Simpson, G. K. (2016). Navigating employment pathways and support following acquired brain injury: Client perspectives. *Australian Journal of Rehabilitation Counseling, 22*, 76–92.

Mozzafarian, D., Benjamin, E. J., Go, A. S., Arnett, D. K., Blaha, M. J., Cushman, M., . . . American Heart Association Statistics Committee and Stroke Statistics Subcommittee (2015). Heart disease and stroke statistics—2015 update: A report from the American Heart Association. *Circulation,* e29–322.

National Institute of Neurological Disorders and Stroke (NINDS). (2015). Parkinson' disease: Challenges, progress, and promise. Retrieved from https://www.ninds.nih.gov/Disorders/Patient-Caregiver-Education/Preventing-Stroke

National Institute of Neurological Disorders and Stroke (NINDS). (2016a). Brain basics: Preventing stroke. Retrieved from http://www.ninds.nih.gov/disorders/stroke/preventing_stroke.htm

National Institute of Neurological Disorders and Stroke (NINDS). (2016b). NINDS Parkinson's disease information page. Retrieved from http://www.ninds.nih.gov/disorders/parkinsons_disease/parkinsons_disease.htm

National Multiple Sclerosis Society. (n.d.) Research fact sheet. Retrieved from http://main.nationalmssociety.org/docs/HOM/ResearchFactSheet.pdf

National Multiple Sclerosis Society. (2015). Multiple sclerosis: Just the facts. Retrieved from http://www.nationalmssociety.org/NationalMSSociety/media/MSNationalFiles/Brochures/Brochure-Just-the-Facts.pdf

National Spinal Cord Injury Statistical Center. (2016). Spinal cord injury facts and figures at a glance. Retrieved from https://www.nscisc.uab.edu/Public/Facts%202016.pdf

Olanow, C. W., Stern, M. B., & Sethi, K. (2009). The scientific and clinical basis for the treatment of Parkinson disease (2009). *Neurology, 72*(21 Suppl 4), S1–S136. doi:10.1212/WNL.0b013e3181a1d44c

Paulsen, J. S., Hoth, K. F., Nehl, C., & Stierman, L. (2005). Critical periods of suicide risk in Huntington's disease. *American Journal of Psychiatry, 162*(4), 725–731. doi:10.1176/appi.ajp.162.4.725

Ponsford, J. L., Downing, M. G., Olver, J., Ponsford, M., Acher, R., Carty, M., & Spitz, G. (2014). Longitudinal follow-up of patients with traumatic brain injury: Outcome at two, five, and ten years post-injury. *Journal of Neurotrauma, 31*(1), 64–77. doi:10.1089/neu.2013.2997

Reijnders, J. S., Ehrt, U., Weber, W. E., Aarsland, D., & Leentjens, A. F. (2008). A systematic review of prevalence studies of depression in Parkinson's disease. *Movement Disorders, 23*(2), 183–189.

Riva, N., Agosta, F., Lunetta, C., Filippi, M., & Quattrini, A. (2016). Recent advances in amyotrophic lateral sclerosis. *Journal of Neurology, 263*, 1241–1254. http://doi.org/10.1007/s00415-016-8091-6

Roger, V. L., Go, A. S., Lloyd-Jones, D. M., Benjamin, E. J., Berry, J. D., Borden, W. B., . . . Turner, M. B. (2012). Heart disease and stroke statistics-2012 update: A report from the American Heart Association. *Circulation, 125*, e2–e220. doi:10.1161/CIR.0b013e31823ac046

Ropper, A. H., & Brown, R. H. (Eds.). (2005a). Cerebral vascular disease. In A. Ropper & R. Brown (Eds.), *Adams and Victor's principles of neurology* (8th ed., pp. 660–746). New York: McGraw Hill.

Ropper, A. H., & Brown, R. H. (Eds.). (2005b). Multiple sclerosis and allied demyelinative diseases. In A. Ropper & R. Brown (Eds.), *Adams and Victor's principles of neurology* (8th ed., pp. 771–798). New York: McGraw Hill.

Ropper, A. H., & Brown, R. H. (Eds.). (2005c). Diseases of the spinal cord. In A. Ropper & R. Brown (Eds.), *Adams and Victor's principles of neurology* (8th ed., pp. 1049–1091). New York: McGraw Hill.

Sabaz, M., Simpson, G. K., Walker, A. J., Rogers, J. M., Gillis, I., & Strettles, B. (2014). Prevalence, comorbidities, and correlates of challenging behavior among community-dwelling adults with severe traumatic brain injury: A multicenter study. *Journal of Head Trauma Rehabilitation, 29*(2), E19–E30.

Sadovnick, A. D., Remick, R. A., Allen, J., Swartz, E., Yee, I. M., Eisen, K., . . . Paty, D. W. (1996). Depression and multiple sclerosis. *Neurology, 46*(3), 628–632. doi:10.1212/WNL.46.3.628

Siegert, R. J., & Abernethy, D. A. (2005). Depression in multiple sclerosis: A review. *Journal of Neurology, Neurosurgery, and Psychiatry, 76*(4), 469–475. doi:10.1136/jnnp.2004.054635

Sperling, M. R. (2001). Sudden death in epilepsy. *Epilepsy Current, 1*(1): 21–23, doi:10.1046/j.1535-7597.2001.00012.x

Stenager, E., & Jensen, K. (1988). Multiple sclerosis: Correlation of psychiatric admissions to onset of initial symptoms. *Acta Neurologica Scandinavica, 77*(5), 414–417. doi:10.1111/j.1600-0404.1988.tb05928.x

Strauss, D. J., Devivo, M. J., Paculdo, D. R., & Shavelle, R. M. (2006). Trends in life expectancy after spinal cord injury. *Archives of Physical Medicine and Rehabilitation, 87*(8), 1079–1085.

Taylor, J., Kolamunnage-Dona, R., Marson, A. G., Smith, P. E., Aldenkamp, A. P., & Baker, G. A. (2010). Patients with epilepsy: Cognitively compromised before the start of antiepileptic drug treatment? *Epilepsia, 51*(1), 48–56. doi:10.1159/j.1528-1167.2009.02195.x

Terrio, H, Brenner, L. A., Ivins, B., Cho, J. M., Helmick, K., Schwab, K, . . . Warden, D. (2009). Traumatic brain injury screening: Preliminary findings regarding prevalence and sequelae in a US Army Brigade Combat Team. *Journal of Head Trauma Rehabilitation, 24*(1), 14–23.

Tellez-Zenteno, J. F., Patten, S. B., Jette, N., Williams, J., & Wiebe, S. (2007). Psychiatric comorbidity in epilepsy: A population-based analysis. *Epilepsia, 48*(12), 2336–2344. doi:10.1111/j.1528-1167.2007.01222.x

Thurman, D. J., Branche, C. M., & Sniezke, J. E. (1998). The epidemiology of sports-related traumatic brain injuries in the United States: Recent developments. *Journal of Head Trauma and Rehabilitation, 13*(2), 1–8.

Thurman, D. J., Hesdorffer, D. C., & French, J. A. (2014). Sudden unexpected death in epilepsy: Assessing the public health burden. *Epilepsia, 55*(10), 1479–1485.

Turner, A. P., Williams, R. M., Bowen, J. D., Kivlahan, D. R., & Haselkorn, J. K. (2006). Suicidal ideation in multiple sclerosis. *Archives of Physical Medicine and Rehabilitation, 87*(8), 1073–1078.

Tyerman, A. (2012). Vocational rehabilitation after traumatic brain injury: Models and services. *NeuroRehabilitation, 31*, 51–62.

Ventura, T., Harrison-Felix, C., Carlson, N., Diguiseppi, C., Gabella, B., Brown, A., ... Whiteneck, G. (2010). Mortality after discharge from acute care hospitalization with traumatic brain injury: A population-based study. *Archives of Physical Medicine and Rehabilitation, 91*(1), 20–29. doi:10.1016/j.apmr.2009.08.151

Wallin, M. T., Wilken, J. A., Turner, A. P., Williams, R. M., & Kane, R. (2006). Depression and multiple sclerosis: Review of a lethal combination. *Journal of Rehabilitation Research and Development, 43*(1), 45–62. doi:10.1682/JRRD.2004.09.0117

Wetzel, H. H., Gehl, C. R., Dellefave-Castillo, L., Schiffman, J. F., & Shannon, K. M. (2011). Suicidal ideation in Huntington disease: The role of comorbidity. *Psychiatry Research, 188*(3), 372–376. doi:10.1016/j.psychres.2011.05.006

Wicks, P., Abrahams, S., Masi, D., Hejda-Forde S., Leigh, P. N., & Goldstein, L. H. (2007). Prevalence of depression in a 12-month consecutive sample of patients with ALS. *European Journal of Neurology, 14*(9), 993–1001. doi:10.1111/j.1468-1331.2007.01843.x

World Health Organization (WHO). (2011). World report on disability. Retrieved from http://whqlibdoc.who.int/publications/2011/9789240685215_eng.pdf

World Health Organization (WHO). (2016a). Epilepsy: Fact sheet. Retrieved from http://www.who.int/mediacentre/factsheets/fs999/en/index.html

World Health Organization (WHO). (2016b). *World Health Statistics 2016: Monitoring health for the SDGs*. Geneva: Author.

3   Understanding Suicide

Introduction

In this chapter information will be provided to increase understanding regarding suicidal thoughts and behaviors, as well as clinical concepts and terms associated with self-directed violence (SDV). To provide a broad context from which information regarding those with neurodisability can be examined, data presented will pertain to the general population. Information to be discussed includes epidemiology of suicide in the general population, SDV nomenclature, key clinical concepts (suicidal intent, ambivalence, lethality, possibility of interruption/rescue), risk/protective factors and warning signs, and the newly released *Diagnostic and Statistical Manual of Mental Disorders* (DSM-5) condition for which further research is required, Suicide Behavior Disorder (American Psychiatric Association, 2013).

Epidemiology and Clinical Features of Suicidal Thoughts and Behaviors in the General Population

Worldwide, almost 800,000 million people per year die by suicide (World Health Organization [WHO], Suicide Prevention, 2013). Over the past 45 years, suicide rates have increased by 60%. In the United States, suicide is the tenth leading cause of death. According to 2016 data from the Centers for Disease Control (CDC), there were 45,000 suicides in the United States (NCHS Fact Sheets, 2015). That is, 1 suicide every 12 minutes. Moreover, some cohorts, such as US military veterans, are at increased risk. Accounting for age and gender, in 2016 the suicide rate was 1.5 times greater for Veterans than for non-Veterans. Moreover, suicide rates among younger Veterans (18–34) continue to increase. When compared to other age groups, Veterans 18–34 had the highest rate (45/100,000; 2016 data). Nonetheless, Veterans who sought Veterans Health Administration (VHA) care had a lower increase in rate than those who did not.

Specific estimates regarding worldwide suicide attempts per year are hard to identify. This in part is related to the heterogeneous nature of suicidal behavior and the reality that many do not seek care after making an attempt. Maris, Berman, and Silverman (2000) suggested that a ratio of 8 suicide attempts to every suicide is conservative. Two common ways of reporting rates of suicide attempts are the number of people (1) who have made an attempt within the previous year and (2) with a lifetime history of attempts. According to the CDC, in 2016, 1.3 million Americans attempted suicide. Moreover, lifetime estimated rates of suicide attempts vary by ethnic group (Oquendo, Lizardi, Greenwald, Weissman, & Mann, 2004). Oquendo and colleagues (2004) combined data from multiple surveys and found that percentages of cohorts with a lifetime history of suicide attempt varied from 1.94 (Cuban) to 9.05 (Puerto Rican). Percentages among whites and blacks were 3.26 and 2.69, respectively.

Suicide attempts are one of the strongest predictors of suicide (Mann, Waternaux, Haas, & Malone, 1999). However, this finding needs to be tempered by the fact that up to 70% of people who die by suicide do so on their first attempt (Mann et al., 1999). Furthermore, Hawton (2007) observed that the vast majority of individuals who attempt suicide (even those surviving very serious attempts) neither go on to die by suicide nor make a subsequent attempt using another method.

Although, suicide ideation (SI; SI and suicidal thoughts will be used interchangeably) is an almost universal precondition for action, great challenges exist in terms of estimating the percentage of the population with a history of thinking about ending their own lives. Linehan and Laffaw (1982) suggested that 31% of the clinical population and 24% of the general population have considered suicide at some time in their lives. Thoughts can be conceptualized as lying along a continuum, from SI with no intent and fleeting ("Thoughts about ending my life pop into my head but I don't want to kill myself") to active and chronic ("Each and every day I think about the steps I will take to kill my-self"). According to the CDC, in 2016, 9.8 million American adults thought about suicide. Based on these numbers, it is clear that many individuals think about suicide but do not engage in suicidal behavior. That being said, a 13-year follow-up study by Kuo, Gallo, and Tien (2001) found that people who reported SI at baseline were more likely to report having attempted suicide at follow-up (RR = 6.09; 95% CI, 2.58–14.36).

In terms of factors associated with SI among an international general population cohort, Casey et al. (2006) found that being married and negative life events lowered and increased, respectively, the risk. The researchers also explored risk factors among those with "serious ideation" and found that whereas concern shown by others decreased risk, severity of depression increased risk.

Suicide Nomenclature

Clinicians, researchers and policymakers have been challenged by the lack of universally agreed upon definitions for suicide and associated terms. Seminal work in this area was published by O'Carroll et al. (1996) in the article "Beyond the Tower of Babel: A Nomenclature for Suicidology." The authors correctly noted that it was "past time to take concrete (if incremental) steps to rectify this state of affairs" and suggested that the field adopt a set of commonly understood, logically defined terms that could be used as a type of "shorthand" to facilitate communication regarding "more subtle phenomena" (p. 238). O'Carroll and colleagues, along with others, have also highlighted that common definitions are critical for implementation of evidence-based suicide risk assessment and treatment, sound research methodology, and accurate epidemiological analysis (O'Carroll et al., 1996; Institute of Medicine, 2002). Moreover, the lack of uniform definitions has led to confusion and misunderstanding, such as what constitutes a suicide attempt, how one distinguishes between nonsuicidal and suicidal thoughts and behaviors, and the meaning and use of related concepts. Terms originally proposed by O'Carroll et al. (1996) were conceptualized as falling under the heading of "self-injurious thoughts and behaviors" and included risk-taking thoughts and behaviors and suicide-related thoughts and behaviors.

Work in this area was further by Silverman who, in his 2006 paper, "The Language of Suicidology," provided the following frequently referenced historical definitions for suicide and suicide attempts. For example, Durkheim defined suicide as "All cases of death resulting directly from a positive or negative action of the victim himself, which he knows will produce the result" (p. 522). Silverman (2006) also highlighted the importance of removing stigmatizing terminology (e.g., failed completion, suicide victim).

In an attempt to address these and other remaining issues, individuals at the Centers for Disease Control in collaboration with clinical researchers at the Rocky Mountain Mental Illness Research Education and Clinical Center (MIRECC) finalized terms to be included in the Self-Directed Violence Classification System (SDVCS). The SDVCS is a taxonomy of terms and corresponding definitions for thoughts and behaviors related to both suicidal and nonsuicidal SDV (Brenner et al., 2011). Terms and definitions included in the SDVCS were informed by the work of experts in the field of suicidology (Posner, Oquendo, Gould, Stanley, & Davies, 2007; Silverman, Berman, Sanddal, O'Carroll, & Joiner, 2007a; Silverman, Berman, Sanddal, O'Carroll, & Joiner, 2007b) and have benefited from previously proposed nomenclatures (Beck et al., 1973; O'Carroll et al., 1996). Moreover, in 2010 and 2011, the nomenclature was formally adopted by the US Department of Veterans Affairs and the US Department of Defense (William Schoenhand, written communication, April 2010; Jo Ann Rooney, written communication, October 2011). The adoption of the SDVCS within these departments is a critical step in the process of implementing a common nomenclature within large healthcare systems.

The 22 terms included in the SDVCS are mutually exclusive, culture and theory neutral, and encompass the broad spectrum of suicidal and nonsuicidal thoughts and behaviors (Brenner et al., 2011). More specifically, the SDVCS consists of two types of terms (i.e., thoughts and behaviors), which are broken down into six subtypes, two of which are related to SDV thoughts. These terms are nonsuicidal SDV ideation and suicidal ideation. The four additional subtypes are related to SDV: preparatory, nonsuicidal SDV, undetermined SDV, and suicidal SDV. Modifiers associated with suicidal intent (definitions provided in Table 3.1), injury and/or interruption by self or other are also used to further describe specific thoughts or behaviors (Brenner et al., 2011). For more information regarding terms and key definitions see Table 3.1. Additional tools have been developed to facilitate use of the SDVCS, including the Clinical Tool, an Online-Decision Tree, and a Smartphone Web Browser, all of which are available on the Rocky Mountain Website (https://www.mirecc.va.gov/visn19/education/nomenclature.asp). The SDVCS Clinical Tool is also presented in Figure 3.1.

TABLE 3.1

Key terms with definitions[a]

Key term	Definition
Risk factors	Population-based information regarding potential sources of increased risk. Ultimately, epidemiologically based risk factors do not allow for prediction of who will die by suicide.
Self-directed violence[a]	Behavior that is self-directed and deliberately results in injury or the potential for injury to oneself.
Suicide attempt [a]	A nonfatal self-inflicted potentially injurious behavior with any intent to die as a result of the behavior.
Suicidal ideation [a]	Thoughts of engaging in suicide-related behavior.
Suicidal intent [a]	There is past or present evidence (implicit or explicit) that an individual wishes to die, means to kill him- or herself, and understands the probable consequences of his or her actions or potential actions. Suicidal intent can be determined retrospectively and in the absence of suicidal behavior.
Suicide [a]	Death caused by self-inflicted injurious behavior with any intent to die as a result of the behavior.
Warning signs	Precipitating emotions, thoughts, or behaviors to suicidal behavior. Warning signs are proximal to the suicidal behavior and imply imminent risk (Rudd et al., 2006).

[a] SDVCS definition.

Additional Key Clinical Concepts

Four interrelated clinical concepts are also important in understanding suicidal thoughts and behaviors. These are SI, ambivalence, lethality of the means, and the possibility of interruption by others. An appreciation of these concepts is important in any assessment and management of suicidal thoughts and behaviors.

SUICIDAL INTENT

The SDVCS definition of intent is provided in Table 3.1. Because "intent" is an internal state, it can be difficult to assess. Internationally, the official determination of

Self-Directed Violence (SDV) Classification System
Clinical Tool

BEGIN WITH THESE 3 QUESTIONS:

1. Is there any indication that the person engaged in self–directed violent <u>behavior</u> that was lethal, preparatory, or potentially harmful? (Refer to Key Terms on reverse side)
   If NO, proceed to Question 2
   If YES, proceed to Question 3

2. Is there any indication that the person had self-directed violence related <u>thoughts?</u>
   If NO to Questions 1 and 2, there is insufficient evidence to suggest self-directed violence → NO SDV TERM
   If YES, proceed to Decision Tree A

3. Did the behavior involve any <u>injury</u> or did it result in death?
   If NO, proceed to Decision Tree B
   If YES, proceed to Decision Tree C

DECISION TREE A: THOUGHTS

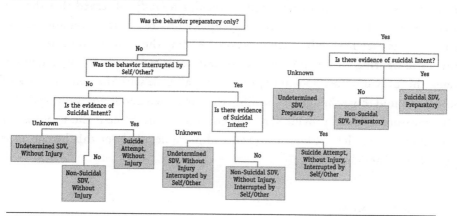

DECISION TREE B: BEHAVIORS, WITHOUT INJURY

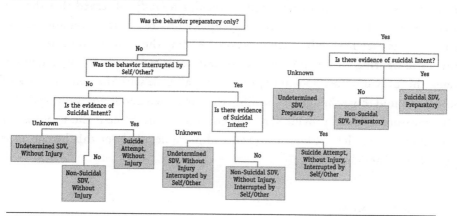

DECISION TREE C: BEHAVIORS, WITHOUT INJURY

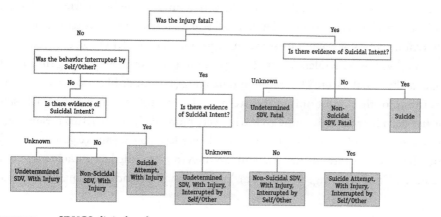

FIGURE 3.1 SDVCS clinical tool.

a suicide is typically made through coronial or medico-legal processes (Värnik et al., 2010). In coronial systems, establishing the presence of SI "beyond reasonable doubt" is a precondition for a finding of suicide (Linsley, Schapira, & Kelly, 2001), whereas, in medico-legal systems, the presence of intent has only to be established "on the balance of probabilities" (Värnik et al., 2010).

Standardized measures, such as the Beck Scale for Suicide Ideation (BSS), have items to measure SI (Beck & Steer, 1993). For example, the BSS has two items: one asks about lifetime history of suicide attempts and the second asks about the level of intent to die of the most recent attempt. The options for rating the strength of intent are mild, moderate, and severe. The level of intent that a person has to die is rarely stable and, as such, changes over time. More information about the significance of suicide intent is provided later in the chapter.

AMBIVALENCE

Ambivalence is associated with intent. Shneidman (1985) observed that the key characteristic of the state of mind of people who are suicidal is ambivalence; namely, that they have mixed feelings about ending their life, with some part of them still wanting to live. The presence of ambivalence is clinically important because this provides the opportunity to form an alliance with the person at risk of suicide around those thoughts or feelings the person has about not wanting to die. One measure that can provide some insight into ambivalence is the Reasons for Living Inventory (RLI; Linehan, 1985), and more detail about this Inventory is provided in later chapters.

LETHALITY OF MEANS

Maris et al. (2000) define *lethality* as "the probability or medical certainly that an action, method, or condition will in fact kill you . . . lead to a fatal outcome," (p. 32). Different methods of suicide are sometimes grouped into violent (e.g., gun, hanging, drowning) versus nonviolent means (e.g., poisoning). Research regarding the means supports the lethal nature of firearms and hanging (Elnour & Harrison, 2008). One hypothesis for the almost universal pattern of higher rates of male versus female suicide has been that males in some countries were more likely to use lethal means (e.g., gun, hanging) while females typically used lower lethality means (e.g., poisoning) which have higher rates of survival and are therefore recorded as a suicide attempt (Denning, Conwell, King, & Cox, 2000). Although this trend still remains, over the past several years, the rate of suicide by firearm among females has been increasing (Hoyert, Heron, Murphy, & Kung, 2003; Xu, Murphy, Kochanek, & Bastian, 2013). According to the National Center for Health Statistics' National Vital Statistics Reports on yearly Final Death data, 2,080 and 2,934 females died by suicide with firearms in 2003 and 2013, respectively. That is, between 2003 and 2013, there was a more than 41% increase in the number of females who used firearms as lethal means of suicide (Hoyert et al., 2003; Xu et al., 2013).

Approaches have been developed to measure the lethality of suicide attempts, including the Lethality of Suicide Attempts Rating Scale (LSARS; Smith, Conroy, & Ehler, 1984) and the Lifetime Suicide Attempt Self Injury Interview (L-SASI; Linehan & Comtois, 1996). The LSARS is a reliable and valid 9-point scale that can be used to characterize behavior. Categories range from death being an impossible outcome of the suicide-related behavior to death being almost certain regardless of intervention. In the LSARS, information on potentially lethal doses for adult medications (prescription and nonprescription) is provided. This table was updated in 2003 by Berman, Shepherd, and Silverman (Lethality of Suicide Attempt Rating Scale-updated; the LSARS-II). Further information regarding this measure will be provided in Chapter 6. The L-SASI is a brief structured interview regarding lifetime history of SDV that allows for behaviors to be categorized into suicidal and nonsuicidal acts and scored in terms of lethality. Psychometric properties have been established including good interrater reliability and adequate validity (Linehan, Comtois, Brown, Heard, & Wagner, 2006).

It is a mistake to infer seriousness of intent from the lethality of the means (Denning et al., 2000). For example, just because a person took an overdose and survived should not automatically lead to the inference that "they weren't really serious." In a study of suicide attempts after traumatic brain injury (TBI; Simpson & Tate, 2005), no correlation was found between levels of intent to die (as measured by the BSS) and the lethality of the means (LSARS). Beck, Beck, and Kovacs (1975) have argued that the lack of association could be due to the mediating effect of the preconceptions that the person had about the potential lethality of their chosen means. For example, a client who tries to insert an air bubble in his veins by means of a syringe and just ends up with a small swelling on his arm may have been sure that his chosen means was going to be fatal. The corollary of this focus on means is the importance of restricting people's access to lethal means of killing themselves as one aspect of suicide prevention. This issue is addressed in a number of the later chapters.

Methods of choice vary between different countries and among different races within countries. For example, among men and women in India and Japan who died by suicide, hanging was the most favored methods (Kanchan, Menon, & Menezes, 2009; Ojima, Nakamura, & Detels, 2004). Among those who died by suicide in the United States, firearms were the most common means. That being said, among Asians in the United States, hanging was more frequent than in other cohorts (Kanchan et al., 2009; Ojima et al., 2004). The cross-cultural differences in suicidal thoughts and behavior in the context of neurodisability is the subject of Chapter 11.

POSSIBILITY OF INTERRUPTION OR RESCUE

An additional clinical concept that needs to be considered and which is related to the issues of intent/ambivalence and the lethality of means is the possibility of interruption by other or rescue. In the earlier section on intent, the important issue of ambivalence was mentioned. One way that this ambivalence may be observed is in the extent to which a person attempting suicide leaves open the possibility of being found by another. This is reflected in the SDCVC taxonomy by the inclusion of the SDCVC modifier "interrupted by self or other." Weisman and Worden (1972) developed an assessment scale called the Risk-Rescue Rating Scale which quantified the extent to which people left the door open for rescue when making suicide attempts. Clinically, if someone takes an overdose in their bedroom while there are other people in the house, there is a high likelihood that the person will be discovered in time. In contrast, if someone takes a firearm and drives out into a remote area of country and then pulls the trigger, there is a very low chance that they will be discovered.

Risk and Protective Factors and Warning Signs for Suicide in the General Population

Although suicide has a low base rate, the number of deaths by suicide is not uniform across the population. People with certain characteristics or risk factors are at higher levels of risk, and this helps to provide a focus for the resources dedicated to suicide prevention. Some risk factors are permanent and nonmodifiable (e.g., male gender), while others can be modified (e.g., depression). Maris et al. (2000) provide a summary of this work, which consists of 62 empirically identified risk factors for suicide in addition to 17 protective factors (see Table 3.2). Whereas risk factors provide population-based information regarding potential sources of

TABLE 3.2

Risk and protective factors

Risk factors	Protective factors
Psychological factors	**Positive personal traits**
Suicide of someone close[a]	Help-seeking[a]
Suicide bereavement[a,d]	Impulse control[a]
Loss of loved one (grief)[a]	Strong problem-solving skills[a,c,d]
Loss of relationship (i.e., divorce, separation)[a]	Good coping strategies[a,c,d]
Loss of status, respect, or rank; failure[a,b]	Sense of identity[a,b]
Prior suicide attempt[b,c,d,e]	Good self-esteem[a]
Impulsivity[c,e]	Use of leisure time[a]
Social factors	Identifying future goals[a]
Stressful life events (acute) (e.g., being fired, breakups, arrested)[a,c]	Religious or cultural beliefs about meaning or value of life[a-c]
Chronic financial problems (e.g., unemployment, homelessness, debt)[a-c]	Resilience[a,d]
Chronic legal problems (e.g., DUI, incarceration)[a]	**Social support system**
Poor interpersonal relationships[a]	Strong interpersonal relationships[a-d]
Geographic isolation from support/living alone[a-c,e]	Employment[a]
Barriers to accessing mental health care[a]	Married[a]
Change in intensity of mental health care[a, b]	Responsibilities to others[a]
Mental health conditions[d]	Sense of belonging[a,b]
History of depressive/dipolar disorder[a,c,e]	Safe and stable environment[a,d]
Current Major Depressive Disorder[a,c,e]	**Access to healthcare**[a,d]
Current comorbid anxiety or substance abuse disorder with a major medical diagnosis[b]	Restriction on lethal means of suicide[d]
Personality disorder[a,c,e]	Positive therapeutic relationship[c]
Schziophreania[a,b,c,e]	**Other**
Anxiety disorders[a,b,c]	Pregnancy[c]
Substance abuse disordesr[a,c,e]	
Eating disorder[a,c]	
Sleep disturbance[a]	
Medical conditions[d]	
Traumatic brain injury[a,c]	
Terminal disease[a,c]	
HIV/AIDS[a,c]	
Worsening chronic illness or chronic pain[a]	
New diagnosis of major illness[a]	

(continued)

TABLE 3.2 CONTINUED

Risk factors	Protective factors
Groups at higher risk and non-modifiable risk factors and groups at higher risk	
Age (young & elderly) [a-d]	
Gender (male) [a-d]	
Race (white) [a,b]	
Child maltreatment [a-c,e]	
Sexual trauma [a]	
Lower education level	
Sexual orientation (LGBT) [a,d,e]	
Marital status (divorced, separated, widowed) [a,c]	

[a] VA/DoD Clinical Practice Guideline.
[b] Wasserman and Wasserman (2009).
[c] Rudd (2012).
[d] US Department of Health and Human Services (HHS) (2012).
[e] Maris, Berman, and Silverman (2000).

increased risk, they have limited utility in predicting individual behaviors. That is, an individual could possess multiple risk factors for suicidal behavior and never engage in such actions, or, conversely, one could possess no risk factors and engage in lethal SDV.

Further support for this is provided by Crocker, Clare, and Evans (2006) who conducted qualitative interviews with elderly adults who had recently made a suicide attempt to capture their subjective experience regarding factors that had contributed towards their engagement in SDV. Three themes emerged: (1) "struggle (experiencing life as a struggle before and after the attempt, and in relation to growing older)," (2) "control (trying to maintain control over life before the attempt, and following it either failing or succeeding to regain control)," and (3) "visibility (feeling invisible or disconnected from others and trying to fight against this before the attempt and either becoming more or less connected afterwards)" (p. 638). Moreover, factors often identified in the literature were generally "absent" or "construed" by interviewees as not being relevant to their attempt.

Among risk factors that have been identified, several have been shown to predict future behavior. Data suggest that one of the most salient is past suicidal behavior (Harris & Barraclough, 1997). Evidence also exists for the relationship between hopelessness and SDV (Beck, Brown, Berchick, Stewart, & Steer, 1990; Beck, Brown, &

Steer, 1989). Suominen, Isometsa, Ostamo, and Lonnqvst (2004) explored risk factors for suicide among 224 Finish individuals referred for services after a suicide attempt. At 12-year follow-up a high level of SI was identified as a significant predictor of both subsequent death and suicide following a suicide attempt. In fact, a high SI score at the index attempt seemed to be a more robust predictor of death by suicide than previous attempts or hopelessness. Also notable was that a fifth of the cohort died during the 12-year follow-up period (all cause), with 8% dying by suicide.

Often discussed within the theoretical literature are protective factors, which are defined within the US National Strategy for Suicide Prevention (2012) "as conditions that promote strength . . . and ensure that vulnerable individuals are supported and connected with others during difficult times, thereby making suicidal behaviors less likely" (p. 13). Frequently, protective factors are misconceptualized as the opposite of risk factors (US Department of Health and Human Services [HHS], 2012). This in part may be related to the lack of research regarding societal, community, relationship, and individual factors believed to promote resilience in response to stress. Examples of protective factors vary and range from reasons for living to access to mental health care. Again, caution is warranted regarding extrapolating findings regarding population-derived protective factors when conceptualizing an individual's overall risk for suicide. For example, using a nationally representative sample, Israeli researchers found level of religiosity to be inversely associated with self-injurious thoughts or behaviors among adolescents (Amit et al., 2014). That being said, for any individual patient, a high level of religiosity should not be confused with no risk for suicide.

More recent efforts encourage a focus on warning signs—person-specific thoughts, feelings, and/or behaviors that precipitate suicidal thoughts and behaviors. Whereas suicide risk factors are often distal in nature, warning signs are proximal to the suicidal behavior and imply imminent risk (Rudd et al., 2006). Identification of warning signs requires sitting down with the at-risk individual to identify poignant thoughts, feelings, and behaviors. The potential contribution of this approach to suicide prevention after neurodisability will be discussed in later chapters.

DSM-V: Suicide Behavior Disorder

In the fifth edition of the DSM (American Psychiatric Association, 2013), section III, Emerging Measures and Models, proposed criteria are presented for conditions "on which future research is encouraged." One of the conditions described is Suicide Behavior Disorder. Diagnostic criteria are presented in Table 3.3. Proposed specifiers

TABLE 3.3

Suicidal Behavior Disorder (DSM-V)

Proposed criteria

A. Within the last 24 months, the individual has made a suicide attempt.

   Note: A suicide attempt is a self-initiated sequence of behaviors by an individual who, at the time of initiation, expected that the set of actions would lead to his or her own death. The "time of initiation" is the time when a behavior took place that involved applying the method.)

B. The act does not meet criteria for nonsuicidal self-injury—that is, it does not involve self-injury directed to the surface of the body undertaken to induce relief from a negative feeling/cognitive state or to achieve a positive mood state.

C. The diagnosis is not applied to suicidal ideation or to preparatory acts.

D. The act was not initiated during a state of delirium or confusion.

E. The act was not undertaken solely for a political or religious objective.

Specify if:

- **Current:** Not more than 12 months since the last attempt.
- **In early remission:** 12–24 months since the last attempt.

pertain to violence of the method, medical consequences of the behavior, and degree of planning versus impulsiveness of the event. As noted earlier, further research regarding this proposed condition among those with neurodisability is warranted.

Conclusion

Worldwide, suicide is a significant public health concern. Although research has increased knowledge regarding risk and protective factors, rates of death by suicide are not significantly declining. Nevertheless, gains continue to be made that are expected to facilitate suicide prevention efforts. These include adoption of a standard nomenclature within several large departments of the US government and increased understanding regarding the importance of warning signs and comprehensive assessment of intent. Moreover, implications associated with the proposed DSM-V condition of Suicide Behavior Disorder remain to be seen.

Implications for Clinicians

1. Suicide is a leading cause of death, particularly among younger cohorts; compared to members of the general population, specific groups (e.g., US military veterans) are at increased risk for death by suicide.

2. Clinicians, researchers, and policymakers have long struggled to identify a common nomenclature of suicide-related terms. The SDVCS is a taxonomy of terms and corresponding definitions for thoughts and behaviors related to both suicidal and nonsuicidal SDV that can help to guide clinical and research practice, as well as policy decision-making (https://www.mirecc.va.gov/visn19/education/nomenclature.asp).

3. Whereas risk factors, which are based on epidemiological data, may help to identify potential indicators of risk, risk factor data alone should not be relied on to gauge an individual's level of risk.

4. Warning signs—person-specific thoughts, feelings, or behaviors—can be used to help evaluate an individual's level of risk.

5. The clinical concepts of SI, ambivalence, lethality of means, and leaving open the possibility of rescue are important in the ongoing assessment and treatment of people with suicidal thoughts and behaviors after neurodisability.

References

American Psychiatric Association. (2013). *Diagnostic and statistical manual of mental disorders, fifth edition*. Arlington, VA, American Psychiatric Association.

Amit, B. H., Krivoy, A., Mansbach-Kleinfeld, I., Zalsman, G., Ponizovsky, A. M., Hoshen, M., . . . Shoval, G. (2014). Religiosity is a protective factor against self-injurious thoughts and behaviors in Jewish adolescents: Findings from a nationally representative survey. *European Psychiatry, 29(8)*, 509–513.

Beck, A. T., Beck, R., & Kovacs, M. (1975). Classification of suicidal behaviours: I: Quantifying intent and medical lethality. *American Journal of Psychiatry, 132*, 285–287.

Beck, A. T., Brown, G., Berchick, R. J., Stewart, B. L., & Steer, R. A. (1990). Relationship between hopelessness and ultimate suicide: A replication with psychiatric outpatients. *American Journal of Psychiatry, 147(2)*, 190–195.

Beck, A. T., Brown, G., & Steer, R. A. (1989). Prediction of eventual suicide in psychiatric inpatients by clinical ratings of hopelessness. *Journal of Consulting and Clinical Psychology, 57(2)*, 309–310. doi:10.1037//0022-006X.57.2.309

Beck, A. T., Davis, J. H., Frederick, C. J., Perlin, S., Pokorny, A. D., Schulman, R. E., . .Wittlin, B. J. (1973). Classification and nomenclature. In Resnick, H. L. P., Hathore, B. C. (Eds.), *Suicide prevention in the seventies* (pp. 7–12). Washington, DC: US Government Printing Office.

Beck, A. T., & Steer, R. A. (1993). *Beck Scale for Suicidal Ideation*. San Antonio, TX: Psychological Corporation; 1993.

Berman, A. L., Shepherd, G., & Silverman, M. M. (2003). The LSARS-II: Lethality of Suicide Attempt Rating Scale-updated. *Suicide and Life- Threatening Behavior, 33*, 261–276.

Brenner, L. A., Breshears, R. E., Betthauser, L. M., Bellon, K. K., Holman, E., Harwood, E., . . Nagamoto, H. T. (2011). Implementation of a suicide nomenclature within two VA healthcare settings. *Journal of Clinical Psychology in Medical Settings, 18(2)*, 116–128.

Casey, P. R., Dunn, G., Kelly, B. D., Birkbeck, G., Dalgard, O. S., Lehtinen, V., . . Dowrick, C. (2006). Factors associated with suicidal ideation in the general population: Five-centre analysis from the ODIN study. *The British Journal of Psychiatry,189*, 410–415. doi:10.1192/bjp.bp.105.017368

Centers for Disease Control and Prevention, National Center for Injury Prevention and Control. Web-based Injury Statistics Query and Reporting System (WISQARS) [online]. (2015). Retrieved from http://www.cdc.gov/injury/wisqars/index.html

Crocker, L., Clare, L., & Evans, K. (2006). Giving up or finding a solution? The experience of attempted suicide in later life. *Aging and Mental Health,10*(6), 638–647. doi:10.1080/13607860600640905

Denning, D. G., Conwell, Y., King, D., & Cox, C. (2000). Method choice, intent and gender in completed suicide. *Suicide and Life Threatening Behavior, 30*(3), 282–288.

Department of Veterans Affairs (2016, July 15). VA Suicide Prevention Program: Facts About Veteran Suicide, July 2015. Retrieved from http://www.va.gov/opa/publications/factsheets/Suicide_Prevention_FactSheet_New_VA_Stats_070616_1400.pdf.

Elnour, A., & Harrison, J. (2008). Lethality of suicide methods. *Injury Prevention, 14*(1), 39–45.

Harris, E. C., & Barraclough, B. (1997). Suicide as an outcome for mental disorders: A meta-analysis. *British Journal of Psychiatry, 170*, 205–228. doi:10.1192/bjp.1703.205

Hawton, K. (2007). Restricting access to methods of suicide: Rationale and evaluation of this approach to suicide prevention. *Crisis, 28*(1), 4–9. doi:10.1027/0227-5910.28.S1.4

Hoyert, D. L., Heron, M. P., Murphy, S. L., & Kung, H. (2006). Deaths: Final data for 2003. *National Vital Statistics Reports, 54*(13). (DHHS Publication No. [PHS] 2006-1120). Hyattsville, MD: National Center for Health Statistics. Retrieved from http://www.cdc.gov/nchs/data/nvsr/nvsr54/nvsr54_13.pdf

Institute of Medicine; Board on Neuroscience and Behavioral Health; Committee on Pathophysiology and Prevention of Adolescent and Adult Suicide. (2002). In Goldsmith, S. K., Pellmar, T. C., Kleinman, A. M., Bunney, W. E. (Eds.), *Reducing suicide: A national imperative* (p. 375). Washington, DC: The National Academies Press. Retrieved from https://www.nap.edu/catalog/10398/reducing-suicide-a-national-imperative

Kanchan, T., Menon, A., & Menezes, R. G. (2009). Methods of choice in completed suicides: Gender differences and review of literature. *Journal of Forensic Sciences, 54*(4), 938–942. doi:10.1111/j.1556-4029.2009.01054.x

Kuo, W., Gallo, J. J., & Tien, A. Y. (2001). Incidence of suicide ideation and attempts in adults: The 13-year follow-up of a community sample in Baltimore, Maryland. *Psychological Medicine, 31*(7), 1181–1191.

Linehan, M. M. (1985). The reasons for living inventory. In Keller, P., & Ritt, L. (Eds.), *Innovations in clinical practice* (pp. 321–330). Sarasota, FL: Professional Resource Exchange.

Linehan, M. M., & Comtois, K. A. (1996). *Lifetime parasuicide history*. Seattle, WA: University of Washington, Department of Psychology.

Linehan, M. M., Comtois, K. A., Brown, M. Z., Heard, H. L., & Wagner, A. (2006). Suicide Attempt Self-Injury Interview (SASII): Development, reliability, and validity of a scale to assess suicide attempts and intentional self-injury. *Psychological Assessment, 18*, 303–312.

Linehan, M. M., & Laffaw, J. A. (1982). Suicidal behaviors among clients at an outpatient psychology clinic versus the general population. *Suicide and Life Threatening Behavior, 12*(4), 234–239.

Linsley, K. R., Schapira, K., & Kelly, T. P. (2001). Open verdict v. suicide: Importance to research. *British Journal of Psychiatry, 178,* 465–468.

Mann, J. J., Waternaux, C., Haas, G. L., & Malone, K. M. (1999). Towards a clinical model of suicidal behaviour in psychiatric patients. *American Journal of Psychiatry, 156,* 181–189.

Maris, R. W., Berman, A. L., & Silverman, M. M. (2000). *Comprehensive textbook of suicidology* (pp. 414–415; 536–561). New York: The Guilford Press.

O'Carroll, P. W., Berman, A. L., Maris, R. W., Moscicki, E. K., Tanney, B. L., & Silverman, M. M. (1996). Beyond the Tower of Babel: A nomenclature for suicidology. *Suicide and Life-Threatening Behavior, 26*(3), 237–252. doi:10.1111/j.1943-278X.1996.tb00609.x

Ojima, T., Nakamura, Y., & Detels, R. (2004). Comparative study about methods of suicide between Japan and the United States. *Journal of Epidemiology and General Health, 14*(6), 187–192.

Oquendo, M. A., Lizardi, D., Greenwald, S., Weissman, M. M., & Mann J. J. (2004). Rates of lifetime suicide attempt and rate of lifetime major depression in different ethnic groups in the United States. *Acta Psychitric Sandanavia, 110*(6), 446–451.

Posner, K., Oquendo, M. A., Gould, M., Stanley, B., & Davies, M. (2007). Columbia Classification Algorithm of Suicide Assessment (C-CASA): Classification of suicidal events in the FDA's pediatric suicidal risk analysis of antidepressants. *The American Journal of Psychiatry, 164*(7), 1035–1043. doi:10.1176/appi.ajp.164.7.1035

Reger, M. A., Smolenski, M. P. H., Skopp, N. A., Metzger-Abamukang, M. J., Kang, H. K., Bullman, T. A, . . . Gahm, G. A. (2015). Risk of suicide among US military service members following Operation Enduring Freedom or Operation Iraqi Freedom deployment and separation from the US military. *JAMA Psychiatry, 72*(6), 561–569. doi:10.1001/jamapsychiatry.2014.3195

Rudd, M. D. (2012). The clinical risk assessment interview. In R. I. Simon & R. E. Hales (Eds.), *The American Psychiatric Publishing textbook of suicide assessment and management* (pp. 57–73). Washington, D.C.: American Psychiatric Publishing.

Rudd, M. D., Berman, A. L., Joiner, T. E., Jr., Nock, M. K., Silverman, M. M., Mandrusiak, M., . . . Witte, T. (2006). Warning signs for suicide: Theory, research, and clinical applications. *Suicide and Life-Threatening Behavior, 36*(3), 255–262. doi:10.1521/suli.2006.36.3.255

Shneidman, E. S. (1985). *Definition of suicide.* New York: John Wiley and Sons.

Silverman, M. (2006). The language of suicidology. *Suicide and Life-Threatening Behavior, 36*(5), 519–532.

Silverman, M. M., Berman, A. L., Sanddal, N. D., O'Carroll, P. W., & Joiner, T. E. (2007a). Rebuilding the tower of Babel: A revised nomenclature for the study of suicide and suicidal behaviors. Part 1: Background, rationale, and methodology. *Suicide and Life-Threatening Behavior, 37*(3), 248–263. doi:10.1521/suli.2007.37.3.248

Silverman, M. M., Berman, A. L., Sanddal, N. D., O'Carroll, P. W., & Joiner, T. E. (2007b). Rebuilding the tower of Babel: A revised nomenclature for the study of suicide and suicidal behaviors. Part 2: Suicide-related ideations, communications, and behaviors. *Suicide and Life-Threatening Behavior, 37*(3), 264–277. doi:10.1521/suli.2007.37.3.264

Simpson, G. K., & Tate, R. L. (2005). Clinical features of suicide attempts after traumatic brain injury. *Journal of Nervous and Mental Disease, 19*, 680–685.

Smith, K., Conroy, R. W., & Ehler, B. D. (1984). Lethality of Suicide Attempt Rating Scale. *Suicide and Life-Threatening Behavior, 14*, 215–242.

Suominen, K., Isometsa, E., Ostamo, A., & Lonnqvist, J. (2004). Level of suicidal intent predicts overall mortality and suicide after attempted suicide: A 12-year follow-up study. *BMC Psychiatry, 4*, 11. doi: 10.1186/1471-244X-4-11

US Department of Health and Human Services (HHS) Office of the Surgeon General and National Action Alliance for Suicide Prevention. (2012). *2012 National Strategy for Suicide Prevention: Goals and Objectives for Action.* Washington, DC: HHS.

Värnik, P., Sisask, M., Värnik, A., Yur'yev, A., Kõlves, K., Leppik, L., . . . Wasserman, D. (2010). Massive increase in injury deaths of undetermined intent in ex-USSR Baltic and Slavic countries: hidden suicides? *Scandinavian Journal of Public Health, 38*(4), 395–403.

VISN 19 MIRECC SDV Classification Tool: Preliminary Questions—MIRECC Centers. (2011, June 27). MIRECC Centers Home. Retrieved from http://www.mirecc.va.gov/visn19/education/sdvtree/sdv_tree.asp

Wasserman, D., & Wasserman, C. (Eds.) (2009). *Suicidology and suicide prevention.* New York: Oxford University Press.

Weisman, A. D., & Worden, J. W. (1972). Risk-rescue rating in suicide assessment. *Archives of General Psychiatry, 26*, 553–560.

World Health Organization (WHO). (2013). *World Health Organization Suicide Prevention (SUPRE).* Retrieved from www.who.int/mental_health/prevention/suicide/suicideprevent/en/

Xu, J., Murphy, S. L., Kochanek, K. D., & Bastian, B. A. (2016). Deaths: Final data for 2013. *National Vital Statistics Report, 64*(2). (DHHS Publication No. 2016-1120). Hyattsville, MD: National Center for Health Statistics. Retrieved from http://www.cdc.gov/nchs/data/nvsr/nvsr64/nvsr64_02.pdf.

4   Theories of Suicide

Introduction

The purpose of this chapter is to outline a range of theories of suicide and their potential application to neurodisability. First, the sociological theories and insights provided by Durkheim, rational choice theory and a social ecological approach, will be briefly explored. This will be followed by canvassing psychological theories that have been applied to suicide including cognitive behavior theory, social learning theory, psychoanalytic approaches, and the construct of emotional dysregulation proposed in dialectical behavior therapy. Other theories that seek to account for the psychological mechanisms underpinning suicide, such as fluid vulnerability theory, overgeneralized memory, and the interpersonal-psychological theory of suicide, will also be covered. The few examples of the application of these theories to the understanding of suicidal behavior after neurodisability are highlighted throughout the chapter. The final section outlines a discussion on the application of a diathesis–stress framework to account for increased risk and eventual suicide after neurodisability.

Sociological and Social Ecological Theories of Suicide

Sociological approaches to suicide seek to understand broad patterns and contextual factors related to suicidal behavior observed both inter- and intranationally. Although suicide is ultimately an individual act, it is influenced by prevailing social, economic, and political circumstances. Such perspectives challenge us to think about which factors lead to increases or decreases in rates of suicidal behaviors at particular time points in history, and why discrepancies exist in rates among different countries, among different regions within countries, among different age groups and by sex.

DURKHEIM

Among sociologists, the enduring work of Emile Durkheim (1897/1992) has had the most profound influence on the field of suicidology. He proposed a quadripartite typology of suicide (egoistic, altruistic, anomic, fatalistic) arising from the extremes (excessive, deficient) of social integration and moral regulation within society, respectively. Social integration is self-explanatory. Moral regulation refers to the extent that laws, policies, and social norms influence individual behavior (Durkheim, 1893/1984). An outline of these four constructs and how they might apply to suicide in neurodisability can be found in Table 4.1.

RATIONAL CHOICE THEORY

Apart from the work of Durkheim, another body of theory identified with sociology and applied to diverse fields (e.g., economics, politics, organizational psychology, and terrorism studies) is rational choice theory (Satz & Ferejohn, 1994). This theory has also been applied to suicide. Werth and Holdwick (2000) define rational choice as "following a sound decision-making process, a person has decided, without being coerced by others, to end his or her life because of unbearable suffering associated with a terminal illness" (p. 513). As the term implies, a rational choice approach emphasizes the process of a person weighing the benefits versus the costs of self-inflicted death in the face of adverse circumstances that are unlikely to change in a meaningful way.

With regard to people with neurodisability, the issue of rational suicide has been raised (Wetzel, et al., 2011), most commonly in the context of physician-assisted suicide (Ganzini, Johnston, McFarland, Tolle, & Lee, 1998; Berkman,

TABLE 4.1

Durkheim's typology

Construct	Explanation	Possible application to neurodisability
Egoistic	Individual is poorly integrated into society (deficient integration). This link between social alienation/isolation and suicide risk still forms a central plank in contemporary theories of suicide and suicide research (Rudd, Trotter, & Williams, 2009).	Loss of social integration/social support breakdown of key relationships, loss of employment, and increased social isolation commonly reported (e.g., Jones et al., 2003; Wallin et al., 2006).
Altruistic	Overidentification (excessive integration) with a group, community, or society at the expense of personal identity and needs. Such suicides may be rationalized on the basis that the individual death serves a greater social good.	Desire among some people to end their life so that they do not continue to "be a burden" on family members or society (e.g., Brenner et al., 2009; Gaskill et al., 2011).
Anomie	The imbalance between the need for stability and a lack of regulation or rapidly changing regulation within society (deficient regulation). Anomie could result from "irregular" situations in economic (e.g., an economic crisis) or social realms (e.g., divorce).	The multiple significant and abrupt life changes that arise from traumatic brain injury (TBI; e.g., relationship changes, loss of job, diminished independence) can be likened to the preconditions associated with anomic suicide, including the common experience of uncertainty reported by many people with neurodisability, the rapidity of unexpected change to familiar life structures (e.g., such as valued social roles), and an associated existential crisis of meaning (Klonoff & Lage, 1995).

TABLE 4.1 CONTINUED

Construct	Explanation	Possible application to neurodisability
Fatalistic	Suicides arise when a person's right to freedom is circumscribed or taken away by social regulation (excessive regulation).	People with neurodisability often become highly dependent on others for care and/or supervision (Mackensie & Popkin, 1987; Pohjasvaara et al., 2001; Brenner et al., 2009). In addition, their opinions and preferences can be dismissed, ignored, or not considered by staff and/or family members in decision-making. Learned helplessness (Seligman, 1975) is a possible psychological mechanism through which such experiences of dependency and powerlessness might increase suicide risk after neurodisability (Moore & Stambrook, 1995).

Cavallo, Chesnut, & Holland, 1999). However, rational choice assumes that an individual has sufficient cognitive resources to undertake such an evaluative process. This condition could be met among people in the early stages of neurodegenerative conditions that ultimately result in impairments to cognition, but not as the course of the disease progresses (Almqvist, Bloch, Brinkman, Craufurd, & Hayden, 1999). Impairment of reasoning may also be compromised by co-occurring psychiatric symptoms, a commonly observed complication among progressive conditions. In contrast, sudden-onset conditions (e.g., traumatic brain injury [TBI], stroke) may cause severe cognitive impairments from the outset, limiting the capacity to engage in the process of reasoning associated with rational suicide. The topic of assisted suicide will be addressed in greater detail in Chapter 13.

SOCIAL ECOLOGY MODEL OF SUICIDE

Extending beyond sociological theory, the 2012 United States National Suicide Strategy (USDHHS, 2012) has proposed a social ecological model of suicide adapted from earlier work of Dahlberg and Krug (2002) (see Figure 4.1). The model recognizes the countervailing roles of risk and protective factors and posits that these factors influence the degree of suicide risk at four different levels: individual,

EXAMPLES OF RISK AND PROTECTIVE FACTORS IN A SOCIAL ECOLOGICAL MODEL

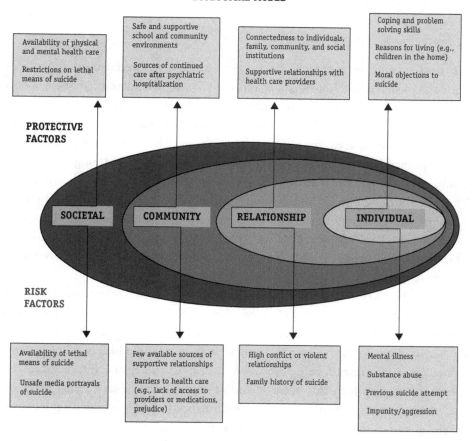

Adapted from: Dahlberg LL, Krug EG. Violence—a global public health problem. In: Krug E, Dahlberg LL, Mercy JA, Zwi AB, Lozano R, eds. World report on violence and health. Geneva, Switzerland: World Health Organization; 2002:1–56.

FIGURE 4.1 Social ecology model.
From USDHHS (2012).

relational, community, and societal. The model is expansive, integrating the understanding that suicide is not only closely linked to mental health and substance abuse problems but also shares risk/protective factors with forms of violence (self-directed, interpersonal) and other problems. The model suggests that approaches to suicide prevention can also generalize to the reduction or prevention of these other problems. Empirical support for these hypothesized relations were found in outcomes from US Air Force's suicide prevention program, which not only reduced suicidal behaviors but also family violence and homicide (Knox, Litts, Talcott, Feig, & Caine, 2003).

Psychological Theories

COGNITIVE BEHAVIOR THEORY

In Beck's cognitive approach (Beck, 1967), suicide was understood as a consequence of persistent hopelessness and depression. The genesis of these mood states derived from an individual's cognitive style. Predictable patterns of errors and distortions of thought processes gave rise to a cognitive triad of negative thoughts about oneself, the world, and the future. These cognitive processes are underpinned by cognitive schemas or generalized patterns of thought that then influence how particular situations, events, or challenges will be perceived. The negative outlook engendered by faulty cognitive processing influenced by such schemas can give rise to a sense of hopelessness which increases the likelihood of suicide (e.g., Beck, Brown, & Steer, 1989). Hopelessness is clinically important because it is a stronger predictor of suicide than depression (Beck, Brown, & Steer, 1989).

In further refinement on these original formulations, a construct of suicide schemas has been introduced (Wenzel, Brown, & Beck, 2008). Suicide schemas comprise beliefs directly related to the exacerbation of hopelessness and emergence of intent to die by suicide. These schemas reduce the likelihood of positive or adaptive information being processed in contrast to negative information. The mechanisms by which this occur include a suicide-relevant attentional bias (the selective processing of suicide-relevant information) and an over-general memory style, as originally suggested by Williams, Barnhoffer, & Crane (2006, see later discussion). Furthermore, the schemas form part of larger modes, which include broader interrelated cognitive, affective, motivational, physiological, and behavioral elements, activated simultaneously by salient internal and external events (Wenzel et al., 2008).

Significant levels of hopelessness have been reported among various neurodisability populations, including persons with amyotrophic lateral sclerosis (ALS), epilepsy, cerebrovascular accident (CVA), multiple sclerosis (MS), spinal cord injury (SCI), and TBI (Albert et al., 2005; Hackett, Hill, Hewison, Anderson, & House, 2010; Berman & Samuel 1993; Charlifue & Gerhart, 1991; Garden, Garrison, & Jain, 1990; Long & Miller, 1991; Lynch, Kroencke, & Denney, 2001; Pompili et al., 2007; Simpson & Tate, 2002). Hopelessness has been identified through qualitative interviews, in broader reports of depression symptom profiles (e.g., Jorge, Robinson, & Arndt, 1993), and through direct measurement by validated instruments (e.g., Pompili et al., 2007; Simpson & Tate, 2002). The strong correlation between hopelessness and suicide ideation (SI) reported in other clinical populations has also been found after TBI (Simpson & Tate, 2002).

SOCIAL LEARNING THEORY

Precepts from social learning theory have also been applied to suicide. A proportion of suicidal behavior is accounted for by imitative behavior (*copycat suicides*, also known as *contagion*). Clusters of suicide behavior can occur in spatial/temporal proximity (so-called *point clusters*) such as a high school (Brent et al., 1989) or a psychiatric hospital (Haw, 1994) or in temporal proximity alone (so-called *mass clusters*, known as the "Werther effect"), usually due to media reporting of suicides (e.g., celebrity suicide deaths). Social learning theory, which holds that most human behavior arises from observation and modeling of others, has been used to explain these clusters of behavior (Bandura, 1977).

Gould, Wallenstein, and Kleinman (1990) found that, in the United States, 2% of suicide deaths among those aged 15–19 years were accounted for by clustering, with the rate as high as 13% in some states. Joiner (1999) has suggested that point clusters may be better accounted for by *homophilly*, namely, that like-minded people with high suicide risk are attracted to one another than by social learning. However, a recent analysis has found support for the social learning hypothesis in point clusters independent of homophilly (Mesoudi, 2009). There is strong evidence that supports links between mass media reports of celebrity suicides and imitative suicide deaths (Stack, 2005); as a result, the United States and many other countries are establishing media codes of conduct in the reporting of suicide (US Department of Health and Human Services Office of the Surgeon General and National Action Alliance for Suicide Prevention, 2012; www.reportingonsuicide.com). To date, there is no evidence of clusters of suicidal behaviors among people with neurodisability, and, to the best of our knowledge, there are no case reports of individuals with neurodisability who have died by suicide as part of a mass cluster.

PSYCHOANALYTIC THEORY

Psychoanalytic theorists have developed a complex range of formulations and theories to account for suicide (Ronningstam, Weinberg, & Maltserger, 2009). This started with the work of Freud on melancholy and suicide (Freud, 1917), his later formulation of the death instinct (Menninger, 1938), and work by subsequent theorists on narcissism and suicide (e.g., Kernberg, 2001; Rosenfeld, 1971). An initial challenge for psychodynamic theorists was to address the paradox between the self-love of the ego and its participation in its self-destruction (Freud, 1957). Several putative dynamics of intrapsychic conflict have been advanced to account for suicide (Menninger, 1938).

One of these is Kohut's (1971) theory that self-destructive impulses are fueled not so much by suicidal impulses associated with depression, but rather are an expression of narcissistic rage. This concept has been applied to suicide after neurodisability. For example, it has been suggested that suicide after epilepsy was a form of aggression turned inward (Blumer, 2008). In relation to TBI, Klonoff and Lage (1995) have also drawn on the conception of narcissistic rage, which they characterize as the reaction of the self to its sense of helplessness and loss of integrity. The narcissistic rage can be directed outward at external causes perceived to be the cause of narcissistic insult or turned inward and expressed as self-destructive behavior, including suicide. Klonoff, Lage and Chiapello (1993) applied this construct of narcissistic rage to account for the catastrophic reaction often observed among people with a brain injury and first described by Goldstein (1963). Klonoff and Lage suggest that a growing awareness of the negative impacts of a TBI can lead to feelings of emptiness and worthlessness, with the result that "For some patients the suffering ego experiences narcissistic rage and may act to do away with the damaged self to wipe out the offending, disappointing reality of being damaged" (1995, p.18).

EMOTIONAL DYSREGULATION

Dialectical behavior therapy is a more behaviorally oriented variant of cognitive-behavior therapy, originally developed to treat people with borderline personality disorders, but now validated for the treatment of a number of different challenging clinical groups (Feigenbaum, 2007; Kliem, Kröger, & Kosfelder, 2010; Linehan, 1993). It has been particularly effective in the management of suicidal behaviors among such clients. There is strong empirical support for the efficacy of dialectical behavior therapy as a psychological treatment modality in reducing suicide risk (Mann et al., 2005).

Dialectical behavior therapy is underpinned by the contention that problems with emotional regulation lie at the core of psychopathology such as borderline personality disorder (Feigenbaum, 2007). Central to intervention is addressing skill deficits (e.g., problem-solving, emotional regulation, interpersonal effectiveness), a greater emphasis on behavioral change than on cognitive modification, and the crucial role of the therapeutic relationship as a vehicle for validation and creating a sense of hopefulness for change (Linehan, 1993). Linehan (1993) emphasized the importance of the continuous individual–environment interaction in influencing affect and behavior (environment–person system). Furthermore, individual variation in biology/physiology may result in some people being more vulnerable to negative stressors and sharp emotional shocks. Linehan (1993) also highlighted the impact of "invalidating environments," social contexts within which punitive and/or erratic reinforcement of suicidal behavior occurred.

Elements of dialectical behavior therapy have potential applicability to the understanding and treatment of suicide in neurodisability. As an underlying vulnerability, emotional dysregulation is a common consequence of various types of neurodisability (e.g., CVA, Huntington's disease [HD], TBI), arising from damage by disease or injury to the orbitofrontal region of the prefrontal cortex (Eslinger, 2008). A secondary cause of emotional dysregulation is also commonly observed, arising from the interactions among increased stressors, lowered stress thresholds, and reduced coping ability (Anson & Ponsford, 2006). Therapeutic elements highlighted in dialectical behavior therapy, such as the importance of behavioral approaches to managing emotional dyscontrol (such as irritability, lability), have also been documented in neurodisability (Alderman, 2003), although they have yet to be applied to suicide prevention.

Suicide-Specific Psychological Theories

FLUID VULNERABILITY THEORY

Rudd has proposed that suicidal states are fluid rather than static. Suicidal modes can be activated and deactivated, and each successive crisis increases the vulnerability (or priming) for future episodes. The various components of the suicidal mode (cognitive, affective, physiological, behavioral) become sensitized to subsequent triggering primarily through the suicidal belief system, the cognitive component of the suicidal mode. Rudd delineates a number of core cognitive beliefs commonly associated with the suicidal belief system (e.g., "I don't deserve to live; I can't fix this problem; I can't stand this pain"). Recent episodes provide a "cognitive scaffolding" for these core beliefs that increases vulnerability (a low threshold for future activation of the suicidal mode). This is underpinned by an interlinked susceptibility across cognitive (e.g., impaired problem-solving, attentional bias, over-general memory), biological (e.g., physiological and affective symptoms), and behavioral (e.g., limited skills in emotional self-regulation, interpersonal skills) domains of the suicidal mode (Rudd, Trotter, & Williams, 2009). Bryan and Clemens (2013) have suggested that the impairments from repeated TBIs can also increase the susceptibility for suicidal behaviors, particularly through increasing the impairments in neurological and neurocognitive function and the associated increase in risk of psychiatric symptoms.

In an observational study of TBI and suicide risk among a clinical sample of deployed military personnel, Bryan and Clemens (2013) found that repeated TBIs were associated with greater suicide risk after depression, TBI symptom severity, and posttraumatic stress disorder (PTSD) were controlled for. The authors suggest that the relationship between repeated TBIs and increasing SI could be explained by reference to the fluid vulnerability theory (Rudd, 2006).

OVER-GENERALIZED MEMORY

Williams and colleagues have posited that over-generalized autobiographical memory plays a key role in a causal pathway leading to suicidal behaviors (Williams et al., 2006). Over-general autobiographical memory results in greater limitations in capacity to range back over one's memories to identify reasons for living and accessing cognitions that support problem-solving and maintaining a sense of hope (Williams et al., 2006). Williams has found that this type of impairment is independent of depression, making a unique contribution to suicide risk. Applying this framework to an earlier formulation, the "cry of pain" model, Williams suggests that, in the face of situational stressors, an individual feels trapped but does not have the cognitive resources (i.e., problem-solving ability, capacity to maintain hope) to find a resolution to the stressor (Williams et al., 2006). As a result, hopelessness is likely to increase with an attendant elevation in suicide risk (Williams et al., 2006).

Disruptions to autobiographical memory have been demonstrated after neurodisability (e.g., Piolino et al., 2007). Impairments in problem-solving have also been widely documented (Kennedy & Coelho, 2005). However, investigation into the hypothesized linkages between such impairments and suicidality has received little research attention among neurodisability groups to date.

INTERPERSONAL-PSYCHOLOGICAL THEORY OF SUICIDE

Joiner's (2005) interpersonal-psychological theory of suicide has three interactive elements: burdensomeness (people at risk of suicide perceive themselves to be an unbearable burden on family, friends, and society), failed belongingness (the experience of thwarted efforts to establish and maintain social connection), and an acquired ability to engage in suicidal behavior stemming from an habituation to pain arising from exposure to multiple distressing life experiences. When these three elements co-exist and there is a desire to die, there is a high probability of imminent lethal suicidal behavior.

Brenner and Homaifar (2009) have sought to synthesize aspects of the International Classification of Functioning (WHO, 2001) with Joiner's work in a theory-driven approach to assessing suicide risk after TBI. The authors found evidence of both burdensomeness and failed belongingness in a qualitative study exploring triggers and protective factors for suicide among veterans with TBI (Brenner, Homaifar, Adler, Wolfman, & Kemp, 2009). Using this framework, clinicians can collect data on the impairments, limitations in activity, and restrictions in participation in accordance with the International Classification of Functioning model (Brenner et al., 2009). These data can be integrated with the assessment of the three elements of Joiner's model to formulate the risk of suicide among veterans with TBI.

Diathesis–Stress Model

The diathesis–stress model is the most common paradigm for understanding suicidal behavior in the field of suicidology. Roy and Sarchiapone (2009) define the diathesis as trait-related and independent of psychiatric diagnosis (i.e., a propensity to suicide), whereas the stressors are state-related and act as the trigger for suicidal behavior. Suicide risk factors may therefore be diathesis-related or stress-related. Mann and Arango (1992) proposed a range of biological, psychopathological, and psychosocial factors that could form a diathesis to suicide (see Table 4.2), a

TABLE 4.2

Diathesis–stress model - exemplars	
Diathesis	Stress
Low 5-HIAA in the cerebrospinal fluid	
Alcohol abuse	Acute substance intoxication
Substance abuse	Some type of crisis (financial, family, social)
	Contagion (Werther's effect; e.g., suicide of a celebrity)
Cluster B personality disorders	
Chronic physical illness	
Marital isolation	
Family history of suicide	
Low self-esteem	
Hopelessness	
Childhood history of physical or sexual abuse	

Adapted from Carballo, Akamnonu, and Oquendo (2008); Mann and Arango (1992); Mann (2003); Oquendo et al. (1997).

number of which have also been identified as risk factors for acquiring injury-related neurodisability (e.g., TBI, SCI).

In the limited discussion that has taken place exploring the application of this model to neurodisability, Oquendo and colleagues (2004) suggested that TBI-related frontal lobe impairments lead to disinhibition and/or impulsiveness which can act as a diathesis for suicide, while TBI-precipitated psychiatric illness can act as a stressor. In a discussion of the relative weight of underlying (distal) versus proximal risk factors for suicide after HD, Robins-Wahlin et al. (2000) suggested that psycho-social factors rather than genetic determinants act as the precipitant of suicide risk.

Conclusion

There has been limited application of sociological and psychological theories in the study of suicidal thoughts and behaviors after neurodisability. Despite this, many of the constructs across a range of theories would seem to have application in making sense of the patterns of suicidal thoughts and behaviors after neurodisability and the reasons that suicide risk is elevated. Theoretical constructs highlight the significance of hopelessness, poor problem-solving, the possibility of suicide frames, the impact of social dislocation as a consequence of neurodisability, and the weakening of social ties. The few areas where theory has been applied were highlighted, and the possibility for further development and testing of models such as the diathesis–stress paradigm or Joiners's interpersonal-psychological theory may well advance our understanding in the field.

Implications for Clinicians

1. Theory can provide useful insights to help us understand the clinical presentation of clients who are experiencing suicidal distress, even though there has been limited work done in applying such theories to neurodisability
2. Poor problem-solving; social isolation; the impact of acute emotional distress; the sense of feeling trapped, hopeless, and helpless; and perceiving suicide as a means of escape from what is experienced as unendurable pain appear in many of the theories.
3. Cognitive impairments in attention, memory, and executive function secondary to neurodisability may contribute to an increased level of suicide risk.
4. Theory provides a window into a number of the social and psychological processes that contribute to suicide risk.

5. Reducing the precipitating or aggravating factors and treating acute symptoms of distress seem to be important clinical considerations in formulating treatment responses to a suicidal crisis.

References

Albert, S. M., Rabkin, J. G., Del Bene, M. L., Tider, T., O'sullivan, I., Rowland, L. P., & Mitsumoto, H. (2005). Wish to die in end-stage ALS. *Neurology, 65*(1), 68–74.

Alderman, N. (2003). Contemporary approaches to the management of irritability and aggression following traumatic brain injury. *Neuropsychological Rehabilitation, 13*(1–2), 211–240.

Almqvist, E. W., Bloch, M., Brinkman, R., Craufurd, D., & Hayden, M. R. (1999). A worldwide assessment of the frequency of suicide, suicide attempts or psychiatric hospitalization after predictive testing for Huntington disease. *American Journal of Human Genetics, 64*(5), 1293–1304.

Anson, K., & Ponsford, J. (2006). Coping and emotional adjustment following traumatic brain injury. *Journal of Head Trauma Rehabilitation, 21*(3), 248–259.

Bandura, A. (1977). Self-efficacy: Toward a unifying theory of behavioral change. *Psychological Review, 84*(2), 191.

Beck, A. T. (1967). *Depression: Clinical, experimental and theoretical aspects.* New York: Harper and Row.

Beck, A. T., Brown, G., & Steer, R. A. (1989). Prediction of eventual suicide in psychiatric inpatients by clinical ratings of hopelessness. *Journal of Consulting and Clinical Psychology, 57*(2), 309–310.

Berkman, C. S., Cavallo, P. F., Chesnut, W. C., & Holland, N. J. (1999). Attitudes toward physician-assisted suicide among persons with multiple sclerosis. *Journal of Palliative Medicine, 2*(1), 51–63.

Berman, A. L., & Samuel, L. (1993). Suicide among people with multiple sclerosis. *Journal of NeuroRehabilitation, 7*(2), 53–62.

Blumer, D. (2008). Suicide: Incidence, psychopathology, pathogenesis, and prevention. In J. Engel & T. A. Pedley (Eds.), *Epilepsy: A comprehensive text book* (pp. 2196–2202). Philadelphia, PA: Lippincott Williams and Wilkins.

Brenner, L. A., & Homaifar, B. Y. (2009). Deployment-acquired TBI and suicidality: Risk and assessment. In L. Sher & A. Vilens (Eds.), *War and suicide* (pp. 17–43). New York: Nova Science.

Brenner, L. A., Homaifar, B. Y., Adler, L. E., Wolfman, J. H., & Kemp, J. (2009). Suicidality and veterans with a history of traumatic brain injury: Precipitating events, protective factors, and prevention strategies. *Rehabilitation Psychology, 54*(4), 390–397.

Brent, D. A., Kerr, M. M., Goldstein, C., Bozigar, J., Wartella, M., & Allan, M. J. (1989). An outbreak of suicide and suicidal behavior in a high school. *Journal of the American Academy of Child & Adolescent Psychiatry, 28*(6), 918–924.

Bryan, C. J., & Clemans, T. A. (2013). Repetitive traumatic brain injury, psychological symptoms, and suicide risk in a clinical sample of deployed military personnel. *JAMA Psychiatry, 70*(7), 686–691.

Carballo, J. J., Akamnonu, C. P., & Oquendo, M. A. (2008). Neurobiology of suicidal behavior. An integration of biological and clinical findings. *Archives of Suicide Research, 12*(2), 93–110.

Charlifue, S. W., & Gerhart, K. A. (1991). Behavioral and demographic predictors of suicide after traumatic spinal cord injury. *Archives of Physical Medicine and Rehabilitation, 72*(7), 488–492.

Dahlberg, L. L., & Krug, E. G. (2002). Violence—a global public health problem. In E. Krug, L. L. Dahlberg, J. A. Mercy, A. B. Zwi, & R. Lozano (Eds.), *World report on violence and health* (pp.1–56). Geneva, Switzerland: World Health Organization.

Durkheim, E. (1897/1992). *Suicide. A study in sociology.* London: Routledge.

Durkheim, E. (1893/1984). *The division of labour in society.* London: Macmillan.

Eslinger, P. J. (2008). The frontal lobes: Executive, emotional and neurological functions. In P. Mariën & J. Abutalebi (Eds.), *Neuropsyhcological research: A review* (pp. 379–407). New York: Psychology Press.

Feigenbaum, J. (2007). Dialectical behaviour therapy: An increasing evidence base. *Journal of Mental Health, 16*(1), 51–68.

Freud, S. (1957). Mourning and melancholia. In The Standard Edition of the Complete Psychological Works of Sigmund Freud, Volume XIV (1914–1916): On the History of the Psycho-Analytic Movement, Papers on Metapsychology and Other Works (pp. 237–258).

Ganzini, L., Johnston, W. S., McFarland, B. H., Tolle, S. W., & Lee, M. A. (1998). Attitudes of patients with amyotrophic lateral sclerosis and their care givers toward assisted suicide. *New England Journal of Medicine, 339*(14), 967–973.

Garden, F. H., Garrison, S. J., & Jain, A. (1990). Assessing suicide risk in stroke patients: Review of two cases. *Archives of Physical Medicine and Rehabilitation, 71*(12), 1003–1005.

Gaskill, A., Foley, F. W., Kolzet, J., & Picone, M. A. (2011). Suicidal thinking in multiple sclerosis. *Disability and Rehabilitation, 33*(17–18), 1528–1536.

Goldstein, K. (1963). The effect of brain damage on the personality. *Psychiatry, 15,* 245–260.

Gould, M. S., Wallenstein, S., & Kleinman, M. (1990). Time-space clustering of teenage suicide. *American Journal of Epidemiology, 131*(1), 71–78.

Hackett, M. L., Hill, K. M., Hewison, J., Anderson, C. S., & House, A. O.; Auckland Regional Community Stroke (ARCOS) Study; Stroke Outcomes Study (SOS2) Group. (2010). Stroke survivors who score below threshold on standard depression measures may still have negative cognitions of concern. *Stroke, 41*(3), 478–481.

Haw, C. M. (1994). A cluster of suicides at a London psychiatric unit. *Suicide and Life-Threatening Behavior, 24*(3), 256–266.

Joiner, T. E. Jr. (1999). The clustering and contagion of suicide. *Current Directions in Psychological Science, 8*(3), 89–92.

Joiner, T. E. (2005). *Why people die by suicide.* Cambridge, MA: Harvard University Press.

Jones, J. E., Hermann, B. P., Barry, J. J., Gilliam, F. G., Kanner, A. M., & Meador, K. J. (2003). Rates and risk factors for suicide, suicidal ideation and suicide attempts in chronic epilepsy. *Epilepsy and Behavior, 4,* 31–38.

Jorge, R. E., Robinson, R. G., & Arndt, S. (1993). Are there symptoms that are specific for depressed mood in patients with traumatic brain injury? *The Journal of Nervous and Mental Disease, 181*(2), 91–99.

Kennedy, M. R., & Coelho, C. (2005, November). Self-regulation after traumatic brain injury: A framework for intervention of memory and problem solving. *Seminars in Speech and Language, 26*(4), 242–255.

Kernberg, O. F. (2001). The suicidal risk in severe personality disorders: Differential diagnosis and treatment. *Journal of Personality Disorders, 15*(3), 195–208.

Kliem, S., Kröger, C., & Kosfelder, J. (2010). Dialectical behavior therapy for borderline personality disorder: A meta-analysis using mixed-effects modeling. *Journal of Consulting and Clinical Psychology, 78*, 936–951.

Klonoff, P. S., & Lage, G. A. (1995). Suicide in patients with traumatic brain injury: Risk and prevention. *Journal of Head Trauma Rehabilitation, 10*(6), 16–24.

Klonoff, P. S., Lage, G. A., & Chiapello, D. A. (1993). Varieties of the catastrophic reaction to brain injury: A self psychology perspective. *Bulletin of the Menninger Clinic, 57*(2), 227–241.

Knox, K. L., Litts, D. A., Talcott, G. W., Feig, J. C., & Caine, E. D. (2003). Risk of suicide and related adverse outcomes after exposure to a suicide prevention programme in the US Air Force: Cohort study. *British Medical Journal, 327*(7428), 1376.

Kohut, H.(1971). *The analysis of self.* New York: International Universities Press.

Linehan, M. M. (1993). *Cognitive-behavioural treatment of borderline personality disorder.* New York: Guilford.

Long, D. D., & Miller, B. J. (1991). Suicidal tendency and multiple sclerosis. *Health & Social Work, 16*(2), 104–109.

Lynch, S. G., Kroencke, D. C., & Denney, D. R. (2001). The relationship between disability and depression in multiple sclerosis: The role of uncertainty, coping, and hope. *Multiple Sclerosis, 7*(6), 411–416.

MacKenzie, T. B., & Popkin, M. K. (1987). Suicide in the medical patient. *International Journal of Psychiatric Medicine, 17*, 3–22.

Mann, J. J. (2003). Neurobiology of suicidal behaviour. *Nature Reviews. Neuroscience, 4*, 819–828.

Mann, J. J., & Arango, V. (1992). Integration of neurobiology and psychopathology in a unified model of suicidal behavior. *Journal of Clinical Psychopharmacology, 12*(2), 2S–7S.

Mann, J. J., Apter, A., Bertolote, J., Beautrais, A., Currier, D., Haas, A., . . . Mehlum, L. (2005). Suicide prevention strategies: A systematic review. *JAMA, 294*(16), 2064–2074.

Menninger, K. (1938). *Man against himself.* New York: Harcourt Brace.

Mesoudi A (2009). The cultural dynamics of copycat suicide. *PLoS ONE, 4*(9), e7252. doi:10.1371/journal.pone.0007252

Moore, A. D., & Stambrook, M. (1995). Cognitive moderators of outcome following traumatic brain injury: A conceptual model and implications for rehabilitation. *Brain Injury, 9*(2), 109–130.

Oquendo, M. A., Friedman, J. H., Grunebaum, M. F., Burke, A., Silver, J. M., & Mann, J. J. (2004). Suicidal behavior and mild traumatic brain injury in major depression. *The Journal of Nervous and Mental Disease, 192*(6), 430–434.

Oquendo, M. A., Malone, K. M., & Mann, J. J. (1997). Suicide: Risk factors and prevention in refractory major depression. *Depression and anxiety, 5*(4), 202–211.

Piolino, P., Desgranges, B., Manning, L., North, P., Jokic, C., & Eustache, F. (2007). Autobiographical memory, the sense of recollection and executive functions after severe traumatic brain injury. *Cortex, 43*(2), 176–195

Pohjasvaara, T., Vataja, R., Leppävuori, A., Kaste, M., & Erkinjuntti, T. (2001). Suicidal ideas in stroke patients 3 and 15 months after stroke. *Cerebrovascular Diseases, 12*(1), 21–26.

Pompili, M., Vanacore, N., Macone, S., Amore, M., Perticoni, G., Tonna, M., & della Misericordia, O. S. M. (2007). Depression, hopelessness and suicide risk among patients suffering from epilepsy. *Ann Ist Super Sanita, 43*(4), 425–429.

Robins Wahlin, T. B., Bäckman, L., Lundin, A., Haegermark, A., Winblad, B., & Anvret, M. (2000). High suicidal ideation in persons testing for Huntington's disease. *Acta Neurologica Scandinavica, 102*(3), 150–161.

Ronningstam, E., Weinberg, I., & Maltsberger, J. T. (2009). Psychoanalytic theories of suicide: Historical overview and empirical evidence. In D. Wasserman & C. Wasserman (Eds.), *Oxford textbook of suicidology and suicide prevention: A global perspective* (pp. 149–158), New York: Oxford University Press.

Rosenfeld, H. (1971). A clinical approach to the psychoanalytic theory of the life and death instincts: An investigation into the aggressive aspects of narcissism. *Journal of Psycho-Analysis, 52*, 169–178.

Roy, A., & Sarchiapone, M. (2009). Interaction of hereditary and environmental factors in the psychiatric disorders associated with suicidal behaviour. In D. Wasserman & C. Wasserman (Eds.), *Oxford textbook of suicidology and suicide prevention: A global perspective* (pp. 183–187), New York: Oxford University Press.

Rudd, M. D. (2006). Fluid vulnerability theory: A cognitive approach to understanding the process of acute and chronic suicide risk. In T. E. Ellis (Ed.), *Cognition and suicide: Theory, research and therapy* (pp. 355–368). Washington, DC: American Psychological Association.

Rudd, M. D., Trotter, D. R. M., & Williams, B. (2009). Psychological theories of suicidal behaviour. In D. Wasserman & C. Wasserman (Eds.), *Oxford textbook of suicidology and suicide prevention: A global perspective* (pp. 159–164). New York: Oxford University Press.

Satz, D., & Ferejohn, J. (1994). Rational choice and social theory. *The Journal of philosophy, 91*(2), 71–87.

Seligman, M. E. P. (1975). *Helplessness: On depression, development and death.* New York: WH Freeman/Times Books/Henry Bolt.

Simpson, G. K., & Tate, R. L. (2002). Suicidality after traumatic brain injury: Demographic, injury and clinical correlates. *Psychological Medicine, 32*(4), 687–697.

Stack, S. (2005). Suicide in the media: A quantitative review of studies based on nonfictional stories. *Suicide and Life-Threatening Behavior, 35*(2), 121–133.

US Department of Health and Human Services (USDHHS), Office of the Surgeon General, & National Action Alliance for Suicide Prevention. (2012). *2012 National strategy for suicide prevention: Goals and objectives for action.* Washington, DC: HHS.

Wallin, M. T., Wilken, J. A., Turner, A. P., & Williams, R. M. (2006). Depression and multiple sclerosis: Review of a lethal combination. *Journal of Rehabilitation Research and Development, 43*(1), 45–62.

Wenzel, A., Brown, G. K., & Beck, A. T. (2008). *Cognitive therapy for suicidal patients: Scientific and clinical applications.* Washington, DC: American Psychological Society.

Werth, J. L. Jr., & Holdwick, D. J. Jr. (2000). A primer on rational suicide and other forms of hastened death. *The Counseling Psychologist, 28*(4), 511–539.

Wetzel, H. H., Gehl, C. R., Dellefave–Castillo, L., Schiffman, J. F., Shannon, K. M., Paulsen, J. S., & Huntington Study Group. (2011). Suicidal ideation in Huntington disease: The role of comorbidity. *Psychiatry Research, 188*(3), 372–376.

Williams, J. M. G., Barnhoffer, T., & Crane, C. (2006). The role of overgeneral memory in suicide. In T. E. Ellis (Ed.), *Cognition and suicide: Theory, research and therapy* (pp. 173–192). Washington, DC: American Psychological Association.

World Health Organisation. (2001). *International classification of functioning, disability and health*. Geneva, Switzerland: World Health Organisation.

5 Neuroanatomy, Neurobiology, and Neuropsychology of Suicide

Introduction

Although the study of both neurodisability and suicide logically leads us to that host of thought and feelings, the brain, limited research has been conducted regarding the neuroanatomy, neurobiology, and/or neuropsychology of suicidal thoughts or behaviors among those with these conditions (see Table 5.1 for key definitions). This is despite the fact that neurodisability may predispose individuals to suicidal thoughts and/or behaviors, while at the same time decreasing their ability to cope with life stressors.

More work exists in each of these areas (neuroanatomy, neurobiology, and neuropsychology) regarding suicide, particularly among those with mental health conditions. Such efforts are focused on brain-based diatheses, independent of psychiatric disorders, which may contribute to increased risk (Mann, 2003). As such, information will be presented on the neuroanatomical, neurobiological, and neuropsychological correlates of self-directed violence (SDV), selected findings regarding conditions of interest (e.g., cerebrovascular accident [CVA]), and theoretical links to concepts (e.g., executive dysfunction) frequently discussed and associated with impairment and disability. This chapter will conclude with a brief discussion

TABLE 5.1

Key terms with definitions

Key term	Definition
Neuroanatomy	The anatomy of the nervous system[a]
Neurobiology	Biology of the nervous system[a]
Neuropsychology	Applying the principles of assessment and intervention based upon the scientific study of human behavior as it relates to normal and abnormal functioning of the central nervous system.[b]

[a]Venes et al. (2009).
[b]APPCN (2012).

regarding incorporating the information outlined herein in assessment and treatment practices.

Neuroanatomical Correlates of Suicide

SUICIDAL THOUGHTS AND BEHAVIORS AMONG THOSE WITHOUT NEURODISABILITY

In a recent review of neuropsychological and neuroimaging studies among suicidal individuals, Jollant, Lawrence, Olié, Guillaume, and Courtet (2011) suggested that the most "replicated" and "robust" findings regarding brain regions implicated among those with a history of suicidal behavior included the (1) ventrolateral prefrontal cortex, (2) anterior cingulate gyrus, (3) dorsomedial prefrontal cortex, (4) dorsolateral prefrontal cortex, (5) amygdala, and (6) medial temporal cortex. Based on these findings, Jollant et al. (2011) suggested that a network of brain regions associated with decision-making are likely involved with SDV.

SUICIDAL THOUGHTS AND BEHAVIORS AMONG THOSE WITH NEURODISABILITIES

Research regarding the neuroanatomical correlates among those with suicidal thoughts and/or behaviors is limited. Moreover, existing findings are often inconclusive and/or focused on the neuroanatomical correlates of emotional distress (e.g., depression) versus suicide. As noted in previous chapters, depression is both frequently endorsed among those with neurodisabilities and a risk factor for suicide. As such, increased understanding regarding the neuroanatomical correlates of psychiatric symptoms among those with neurodisabilities may in fact assist with suicide prevention efforts.

Regarding CVA, Carson and colleagues (2000) conducted a systematic review to examine the hypothesis that depression is more commonly associated with left-sided strokes. Forty-eight studies were included in the review, and findings did not support the proposed hypothesis. In fact, the authors found no associations, whether they analyzed articles including all cases of depression, those that only included major depression, or those that examined onset of depression within 1 month of CVA. Despite these seemingly conclusive findings, publications with contradictory results continue to appear in the literature. For example, in exploring the role of expressed emotion in post-stroke depression and the extent to which partner/spouse expressed emotion interacted with lesion laterality in post-stroke depression, Rashid, Clarke, and Rogish (2013) found that left hemisphere stroke survivors reported higher levels of depression than right hemisphere stroke survivors.

In one of the few studies specifically focused on CVA, suicide, and lesion location, Santos, Caeiro, Ferro, and Figueira (2012) assessed the presence of suicidal ideation (SI) among 177 individuals within 4 days post-stroke. Fifteen percent (N = 27) had SI, and six individuals had a suicidal plan. Of the 27 with SI, 85% also endorsed symptoms of acute depression. No differences were found between depressed and nondepressed or suicidal and nonsuicidal individuals in terms of lesion location. The authors noted that this is in contrast to findings by Kishi, Robinson, and Kosier (1996) who found that among those post-CVA, acute suicidal plans were associated with anterior lesions. In the same publication, Kishi et al. (1996) reported that delayed suicidal plans were associated with posterior lesions. Moreover, in examining clinical correlates of stroke, Pohjasvaara, Vataja, Leppävuori, Kaste, and Erkinjuntti (2001) found that at 15 months post-event, SI was correlated with having had a right-sided event. These mixed findings continue to call into question neuroanatomical correlates of psychiatric risk among those with neurodisability, continuing to confirm the insightful summation of British neuropsychiatrist W. A. Lishman half a century ago, that "The simple neurological model, which seeks to relate a defined clinical picture to defined lesions within the central nervous system, is . . . unlikely to prove adequate as a complete explanation" (1973, p. 304).

To further the very limited science regarding the neuroanatomical underpinnings of SI in US military veterans with mild traumatic brain injury (TBI; Yurgelun-Todd et al. (2011) used diffusion tensor imaging to compare 15 individuals with a history of injury to 17 matched healthy controls. Among those with TBI, measures of impulsivity were significantly greater, and total and right cingulum fractional anisotropy were positively correlated with SI and measures of impulsivity (P <0.03). The authors concluded that a significant reduction in fractional anisotropy in frontal white matter tracts in veterans with mild TBI was associated with both impulsivity and suicidality. These findings are notable in that they start to create links between areas of the brain (frontal white matter tracts), behavior known to increase risk for suicide (impulsivity), and suicidality.

Neurobiological Correlates of Suicide

SUICIDAL THOUGHTS AND BEHAVIORS

To the best of our knowledge, the research to date examining the neurobiology of suicidal thoughts and behaviors among those with neurodisability is extremely limited (e.g., Juengst, Kumar, Arenth, & Wagner, 2014). More broadly, serotenergic, noradrenergic, and dopaminergic neurotransmitter systems have been studied in relationship to suicidal behavior across a range of populations (Mann, 2003), with the most consistent findings implicating the serotenergic system. Among those who died by suicide, postmortem binding differences in serotonin transporters and receptors have been identified (Mann, 2003). In addition, low levels of the main metabolite of serotonin have been found in the cerebral spinal fluid of those who have attempted suicide when compared to those without this history who have same psychiatric conditions. Among animal models and human studies, depleted serotonergic function has been shown to increase aggressive behavior (Mann, 2003), a risk factor for suicide.

Recent work supports the role of inflammatory mediators in the pathophysiology of both major depression and suicidal behavior (Serafini et al., 2013). As described by Rook, Lowry, and Raison (2013), "inflammation is a protective mechanism, classically accompanied by pain, heat, redness and swelling, that evolved to remove tissue-damaging stimuli (such as infections) and then initiate the healing process" (p. 46). Although negative feedback mechanisms exist which block inflammation when such processes are no longer needed, findings suggest that both physical and psychological health conditions may in part be related to regulatory mechanism failures. Work in the area of mental health has focused on several cytokines (proteins that act as mediators between cells and play a role in immune system functioning; Serafini et al., 2013). Moreover, Serafini and colleagues (2013) conducted a systematic review regarding the role of inflammatory mediation, major affective disorders, and suicidal behavior, with findings supporting the assertion that inflammation plays a key role in the pathophysiology of suicidal behavior.

A recently published article by Juengst and colleagues (2014) is the first identified by us that specifically explores the link between a member of a group of cytokine (tumor necrosis factor [TNF]) to disinhibition and SI post-TBI. In specific, those with a history of acute moderate to severe TBI had higher cerebral spinal fluid and serum TNF. Moreover, acute and chronic TNF serum levels were significantly associated with disinhibition at 6 months post-TBI. In turn, disinhibition at 6 months was associated with suicide ideation at both 6 and 12 months. The authors conclude that the "preliminary data suggest a biological to behavioral pathway" from TBI to suicide ideation via disinhibition. Interestingly, in 2013, Spalleta et al. investigated the relationship between interleukin (IL)-6 serum levels and psychiatric, neurologic, cognitive, and functional outcomes following acute ischemic stroke. Based on the results, the authors suggested that "at least in the acute phase of stroke, [inflammation] could play an important role in the onset of apathetic amotivational and somatic symptoms of depression, such as loss of appetite and sleep disorders, resulting in higher disability and poorer outcome of stroke patients" (p. 261).

There is also a small literature regarding neurotransmitters and psychiatric conditions of interest (e.g., depression) among those with neurodisabilities. Specifically, the studies suggest that changes secondary to an event (TBI) or disease process (multiple sclerosis [MS]) alter neurotransmitter production and delivery both acutely and chronically thereby contributing to the development of psychiatric symptoms (Silver, Hales, & Yudofsky, 2008). For example, Mayberg et al. (1988) looked at cortical S2 serotonin receptor binding and its relationship to depression among those with a history of CVA and found that "biochemical responses of the brain may be different depending on which hemisphere is injured and that some depressions may be a consequence of the failure to up regulate serotonin receptors" post-CVA (p. 937).

Neuropsychological Impairments and Suicide

FINDINGS IN THE GENERAL POPULATION AND OTHER CLINICAL GROUPS

As noted by Homaifar, Bahraini, Silverman, and Brenner (2012a), "executive functioning refers to a set of higher-order mental activities primarily governed by the frontal lobes" (Lezak, Howieson, & Loring, 2004; McDonald, Flashman, & Saykin, 2002) including initiation, planning, and self-regulation of goal-directed behavior" (Berger & Posner, 2000, pp. 3–5). Executive functioning allows for individuals to engage and direct subordinate mental activities to resolve everyday problems. Sequelae commonly associated with frontal lobe damage include increased impulsivity and aggression and decreased decision-making ability and concept formation, all of which are associated to some extent with deficits in self-regulation (Dyer, Bell, McCann, & Rauch, 2006; Kim, 2002; Marson, Dreer, Krzywanski, Huthwaite, Devivo, & Novack, 2005; Salmond & Sahakian, 2005).

Researchers have linked executive dysfunction, as measured by performance on neuropsychological measures, to suicidal behavior among individuals without brain damage (Dougherty, Mathias, Marsh, & Jager, 2005; Jollant et al., 2005; Keilp et al., 2001). Using the Iowa Gambling Test (IGT; Bechara, Damasio, Damasio, & Anderson, 1994), a computerized measure of decision-making, Jollant et al. (2005) investigated executive functioning in those with a history of violent and nonviolent suicide attempts, those with affective disorders, and healthy comparison subjects. Differences in performance were noted both between those with histories of suicide attempts and healthy controls, and between those with a history of violent suicide attempts and affective controls; in both cases, those who attempted suicide demonstrated poorer executive dysfunction. Performance on the IGT (Bechara, Damasio, Damasio, & Anderson, 1994) was also positively associated with anger expression on the State Trait Anger Expression Inventory (STAXI-2) (Spielberger, 1999). Interestingly, Jollant et al. (2005) did not find a relationship between impulsivity, as measured by the Barratt Impulsiveness Scale, a self-report measure, and the IGT (Bechara et al., 1994), thereby highlighting a potential disconnect between an individual's self-appraisal of impulsive behaviors versus a more objective measure.

Similarly, using the Immediate and Delayed Memory Test (Dougherty, Marsh, & Mathias, 2002), a modified continuous performance test designed to measure impulsive characteristics, Dougherty et al. (2002) distinguished between groups of individuals with varying histories of suicidality. Specifically, impulsive responses increased with the number of suicide attempts (Jollant et al., 2005). Finally, Keilp et al. (2001) employed neuropsychological measures often used in general clinical practice, including the Wisconsin Card Sorting Test (WCST; Heaton, Chelune, Talley, Kay, & Curtiss, 1993), a measure of concept formation that is believed to be linked to the prefrontal cortex. Among high-lethality suicide attempters, low-lethality attempters, depressed control subjects, and comparison subjects they found that "failure to maintain set" (an individual's inability to employ a previously successful strategy) on the WCST (Heaton et al., 1993) differentiated between high-lethality attempters and all other groups. In a follow-up study, Keilp et al. (2013) found that "past attempters' poorer performance on the Stroop tasks and memory/working memory measures was not a function of depression severity or suicide ideation," (p. 8). The authors suggest that such deficits are a "relatively independent" marker of suicide risk. Moreover, in the review by Jollant et al. (2011) mentioned earlier, the neuropsychological functions noted in Table 5.2 were discussed as being

TABLE 5.2

Examples of neuropsychological functions implicated in those with suicidal behavior

Neuropsychological function	As measured by
Higher attention to specific emotional stimuli	Time to respond to emotional content (e.g., emotionally charged words or pictures)
Impaired decision-making	Performance on ecologically valid measures of decision making
Lower problem-solving abilities	Performance on problem-solving tasks
Reduced verbal fluency	Ability to rapidly think of words
Non-attention and decreased concentration	Performance of measures of attention and continuous performance

From Jollant et al. (2011).

implicated in those with suicidal behavior. It is important to note that many with neurodisability demonstrate impaired cognition on neuropsychological measures; therefore, it may be difficult to extrapolate the above-stated findings to those with such conditions. That being said, organic damage secondary to neurodisability results in impairments (e.g., executive dysfunction) and associated behaviors (e.g., impulsivity) believed to increase risk for suicide thereby highlighting potential mechanisms for increased self-destructive violent behaviors in these populations.

FINDINGS IN THOSE WITH NEURODISABILITIES WITH A FOCUS ON EXECUTIVE FUNCTIONING

Although existing research among those with neurodisability disease certainly supports the relationship between depressed mood and suicidal thoughts and behaviors, it is also likely that impairments such as executive dysfunction contribute to the increased risk. Among the eight types of neurodisability addressed in this book, the relationship between executive dysfunction and suicide may be particularly salient for those with a history of TBI. As such, this condition will be used to highlight neuropsychological correlates associated with suicidal behavior which may be relevant for individuals coping with other types of neurodisability (e.g., CVA).

A TBI can result in focal and/or diffuse brain damage, which impacts cognitive and emotional functioning (Bivona et al., 2008; Levine et al., 2005; Lezak et al., 2004; Sherer, Hart, Whyte, Nick, & Yablon, 2005). Moreover, research has demonstrated that the majority of moderate and severe TBIs result in diffuse, rather than focal, structural damage associated with impairments in the areas of attention, memory and learning, executive function, language and communication, visual-spatial skills, and processing speed (Lezak et al., 2004). Additional neuropsychiatric manifestations include decreased self-awareness (Sherer et al., 2005), increased aggression (Oquendo et al., 2004; Sabaz et al., 2014), and personality change. The frontal lobes are particularly vulnerable to damage secondary to their location near bony protuberances inside the skull (Bigler, 2007), and injuries involving the frontal lobes and related subcortical structures often result in executive dysfunction (McDonald et al., 2002).

Impulsivity is another common sequela of TBI. Such injuries can result in a "predisposition toward rapid, unplanned reactions to internal or external stimuli without regard to the negative consequences of these reactions to the individual or to others" (Moeller, Barratt, Dougherty, Schmitz, & Swann, 2001, p. 1784). Impulsivity appears to be a multifaceted construct that requires multiple modes of assessment (Dougherty, Mathias, Marsh, & Jager, 2005). A variety of laboratory behavioral measures have been utilized to measure different aspects of impulsivity, including (1) reward-directed paradigms, where impulsivity is defined as preference for a smaller-sooner over a larger-later reward, and (2) rapid-decision paradigms, where impulsivity is defined as either premature or disinhibited responding (Moeller et al., 2001; Dougherty et al., 2005). Impulsivity among those with a history of TBI has been found using both reward-directed paradigms and rapid-decision paradigms (Fork et al., 2005).

Research also suggests a relationship between TBI and aggression (Oquendo et al., 2004; Baguley, Cooper, & Felmingham, 2006), the cause of which appears multifaceted. Some suggest that a history of TBI can exacerbate preexisting aggressive tendencies (Dyer et al., 2006). Disinhibition of aggression following TBI has also been found to be related to impairments in emotional regulation and impulse control. Such impairments commonly occur after damage to the frontal lobes (Dyer et al., 2006). As with impulsivity, inconsistencies exist in the conceptualization and measurement of aggression (Suris et al., 2004); however, two forms of aggression, are frequently discussed. These include premeditated and impulsive aggression, the latter reflecting the type of aggression most often observed in those with TBI.

Despite the theoretical connections among TBI, executive dysfunction, and suicide, limited original research has been conducted in this area. Using self-report measures, Mann, Waternaux, Haas, and Malone (1999) identified an association between suicide risk and TBI in that those with a history of TBI had higher aggression and impulsivity factor scores. In looking at psychiatrically hospitalized individuals with major depression, Oquendo et al. (2004) found increased suicidal behavior in those with higher levels of aggression. In their study, aggression was also identified as a risk factor for sustaining a TBI. Moreover, those with TBI endorsed higher levels of aggression post-injury, thereby suggesting that this increase was at least in part related to their TBI. Individuals with a loss of consciousness of greater than 5 minutes were excluded from participating in this study.

Homaifar and colleagues (2012b) explored the relationship between executive dysfunction and suicidal behavior in two groups of participants: veterans with TBI ($n = 18$) and a history of at least one suicide attempt versus veterans with TBI and no history of suicide attempts ($n = 29$). Measures included the IGT, Immediate and Delayed Memory Test, WCST, and Lifetime History of Aggression scale. Between individuals with and without histories of one or more suicide attempts, only the perseverative errors score on the WCST differed significantly. More recently, members of this team examined the relationship between executive dysfunction as a multidimensional construct (i.e., decision-making, impulsivity, aggression, concept formation) and suicide attempt history in a high-risk sample of veterans with moderate to severe TBI (Brenner et al., 2015). Findings suggested that veterans with a history of both suicide attempts and TBI demonstrated unique decision-making challenges (poor performance on the IGT) thereby suggesting that this group may benefit from specialized interventions focused on overall distress reduction and means safety.

The relationship between executive dysfunction and SI has also been peripherally looked at among those with Huntington's disease (HD). Anderson and colleagues (2010) examined obsessive/compulsive symptoms in HD. More than 27% of the 1,642 individuals reported significant obsessive/compulsive symptoms. Those with obsessive/compulsive symptoms exhibited significantly greater psychiatric symptoms (i.e., depressed mood, SI, aggression, delusions, and audiovisual hallucinations), and, for those with the more severe obsessive/compulsive symptoms, there was a trend toward performing more poorly on the Stroop Color Word Interference task ($F = 5.57$, df $= 1$, $p = 0.02$).

Conclusion

Scant research has explored neuroanatomical, neurobiological, or neuropsychological correlates of suicidal thoughts and behavior after neurodisability. Incorporating findings to date regarding neuropsychological and neuroimaging findings from among other clinical populations, Jollant et al. (2011) present a three-step process (see Figure 5.1) in which neurocognitive dysfunction results in suicidal crises. Underlying proposed cognitive dysfunction includes "altered modulation of value attribution" ("including sensitivity to social environment and impaired risk

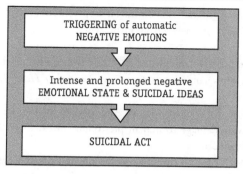

FIGURE 5.1 Three-step suicidal process.
From Jollant et al. (2011).

processing and decision making") and "impaired regulations of emotional and cognitive responses" ("including impaired problem solving abilities, verbal fluency, and increased self-focus," which facilitate acts in emotional contexts (including "diminished response inhibition") (Jollant et al., 2011, p. 332). This model could be the driver for future research investigating the mechanisms of suicide among people with neurodisability. For a further discussion regarding possible implications of the presented model as it pertains to clinical suicide prevention efforts in those with TBI and/or posttraumatic stress disorder, see Nazem et al. (2014).

Implications for Clinicians

1. The onset of neurodisability can predispose individuals to suicidal thoughts and/or behaviors, while at the same time decreasing their ability to cope with psychosocial stressors.
2. Simple neurological models that try to link lesions in specific regions of the brain to clinical presentation may be of limited utility.
3. Findings from cohorts with and without a history of neurodisabilty suggest that executive dysfunction (e.g., aggression, impulsivity, poor decision-making) may increase risk for suicidal behaviors.

References

Anderson, K. E., Gehl, C. R., Marder, K. S., Beglinger, L. J., Paulsen, J. S.; Huntington's Study Group. (2010). Comorbidities of obsessive and compulsive symptoms in Huntington's disease. *Journal of Nervous and Mental Diseases, 198*(5), 334–338. doi: 10.1097/NMD.0b013e3181da852a

Association of Postdoctoral Programs in Clinical Neuropsychology (APPCN). (2012). *Definition of clinical neuropsychology.* Retrieved from http://www.appcn.org/definitionofclinicalneuropsychology

Baguley, I. J., Cooper, J., & Felmingham, K. (2006). Aggressive behavior following traumatic brain injury: How common is common? *Journal of Head Trauma Rehabilitation, 21*(1), 45–56.

Bechara, A., Damasio, A. R., Damasio, H., & Anderson, S. W. (1994). Insensitivity to future consequences following damage to human prefrontal cortex. *Cognition, 50*(1-3), 7–15. doi: 10.1016/0010-0277(94)90018-3

Berger, A., & Posner, M. I. (2000). Pathologies of brain attentional networks. *Neuroscience and Behavioral Review, 24*(1), 3–5. doi: 10.1016/S0149-7634(99)00046-9

Bigler, E. D. (2007). Anterior and middle cranial fossa in traumatic brain injury: Relevant neuroanatomy and neuropathology in the study of neuropsychological outcome. *Neuropsychology, 21*(5), 515–531.

Bivona, U., Ciurli, P., Barba, C., Onder, G., Azicnuda, E., Silvestro, D., . . . Formisano, R. (2008). Executive function and metacognitive self-awareness after severe traumatic brain injury. *Journal of the International Neuropsychological Society, 14*(5), 862–868. doi: 10.1017/S1355617708081125

Brenner, L. A., Bahraini, N., Homaifar, B. Y., Monteith, L. L., Nagamoto, H., Dorsey-Holliman, B., & Forster, J. E. (2015). Executive functioning and suicidal behavior among veterans with and without traumatic brain injury. *Archives of Physical Medicine and Rehabilitation, 96*(8), 1411–1418. doi:10.1016/j.apmr2015.04.0100

Carson, A. J., MacHale, S., Allen, K., Lawrie, S. M., Dennis, M., House, A., & Sharpe, M. (2000). Depression after stroke and lesion location: A systematic review. *Lancet, 356*(9224), 122–126. doi: 10.1016/S0140-6736(00)02448-x

Dougherty, D. M., Marsh, D. M., & Mathias, C. W. (2002). Immediate and delayed memory tasks: A computerized behavioral measure of memory, attention, and impulsivity. *Behavior Research Methods, Instruments, & Computers, 34*(3), 391–398.

Dougherty, D. M., Mathias, C. W., Marsh, D. M., & Jager, A. A. (2005). Laboratory behavioral measures of impulsivity. *Behavior Research Methods, 37*(1), 82–90.

Dougherty, D. M., Mathias, C. W., Marsh, D. M., Papageorgiou, T. D., Swann, A. C., & Moeller, F. G. (2004). Laboratory measured behavioral impulsivity relates to suicide attempt history. *Suicide and Life-Threatening Behavior, 34*(4), 374–385. doi: 10.1521/suli.34.4.374.53738

Dyer, K. F., Bell, R., McCann, J., & Rauch, R. (2006). Aggression after traumatic brain injury: Analysing socially desirable responses and the nature of aggressive traits. *Brain Injury, 20*(11), 1163–1173. doi: 10.1080/02699050601049312

Fork, M., Bartels, C., Ebert, A. D., Grubich, C., Synowitz, H., & Wallesch, C. W. (2005). Neuropsychological sequelae of diffuse traumatic brain injury. *Brain Injury, 19*(2), 101–108. doi:10.1080/02699050410001726086

Heaton, R. K., Chelune, G. J., Talley, J. L., Kay, G. G., & Curtiss, G. (1993). *Wisconsin scoring test manual: Revised and expanded.* Odessa, FL: Psychological Assessment Resources.

Homaifar, B. Y., Bahraini, N., Silverman, M. M., & Brenner, L. A. (2012a). Executive functioning as a component of suicide risk assessment: Clarifying its role in standard clinical applications. *Journal of Mental Health Counseling, 34*(2), 110–120.

Homaifar, B. Y., Brenner, L. A., Forster, J. E., & Nagamoto, H. (2012b). Traumatic brain injury, executive functioning, and suicidal behavior: A brief report. *Rehabilitation Psychology, 57*(4), 337–341. doi: 10.1037/a0030480

Jollant, F., Bellivier, F., Leboyer, M., Astruc, B., Torres, S., Verdier, R., . . . Courtet, P. (2005). Impaired decision making in suicide attempters. *American Journal of Psychiatry, 162*(2), 304–310.

Jollant, F., Lawrence, N. L., Olié, E., Guillaume, S., & Courtet, P. (2011). The suicidal mind and brain: A review of neuropsychological and neuroimaging studies. *World Journal of Biological Psychiatry. 12*(5), 319–339. doi: 10.3109/15622975.2011.556200

Juengst, S. B., Kumar, R. G., Arenth, P. M., & Wagner, A. K. (2014). Exploratory associations with Tumor Necrosis Factor-α, disinhibition and suicidal endorsement after traumatic brain injury. *Brain, Behavior, and Immunity, 41*, 134–143. http://dx.doi.org/10.1016/j.bbi.2014.05.020

Keilp, J. G., Sackheim, H. A., Brodsky, B. S., Oquendo, M. A., Malone, K. M., & Mann, J. J. (2001). Neuropsychological dysfunction in depressed suicide attempters. *American Journal of Psychiatry, 158*(5), 735–741. doi: 10.1176/appi.ajp.158.5.735

Keilp, J. G., Gorlyn, M., Russell, M., Oquendo, M. A., Burke, A. K., Harkavy-Friedman, J., & Mann, J. J. (2013). Neuropsychological function and suicidal behavior: Attention control, memory and executive dysfunction in suicide attempt. *Psychological Medicine, 43*(3), 539–551. doi: 10.1017/S0033291712001419

Kim, E. (2002). Agitation, aggression, and disinhibition syndromes after traumatic brain injury. *NeuroRehabilitation, 17*(4), 297–310.

Kishi, Y., Robinson, R. G., & Kosier, J. T. (1996). Suicidal plans in patients with stroke: Comparison between acute-onset and delayed-onset suicidal plans. *International Psychogeriatrics, 8*(4), 623–632. doi: 10.1017/S1041610290002931

Levine, B., Black, S. E., Cheung, G., Campbell, A., O'Toole, C., & Schwartz, M. L. (2005). Gambling task performance in traumatic brain injury: Relationships to injury severity, atrophy, lesion location, and cognitive and psychosocial outcome. *Cognitive and Behavioral Neurology, 18*(1), 45–54.

Lezak, M. D., Howieson, D. B., & Loring, D. W. (2004). *Neuropsychological assessment* (4th ed.). New York: Oxford University Press.

Lishman, W. A. (1973). The psychiatric sequelae of head injury: A review. *Psychological Medicine, 3*(3), 304–318.

Mann, J. J. (2003). Neurobiology of suicidal behavior. *Nature Reviews. Neuroscience. 4*(10), 819–828.

Mann, J. J., Waternaux, C., Haas, G. L., & Malone, K. M. (1999). Toward a clinical model of suicidal behavior in psychiatric patients. *American Journal of Psychiatry, 156*(2), 181–189.

Marson, D. C., Dreer, L. E., Krzywanski, S., Huthwaite, J. S., Devivo, M. J., & Novack, T. A. (2005). Impairment and partial recovery of medical decision-making capacity in traumatic brain injury: A 6-month longitudinal study. *Archives of Physical Medicine and Rehabilitation, 86*(5), 889–895. doi: 10.1016/j.apmr.2004.09.020

Mayberg, H. S., Robinson, R. G., Wong, D. F., Parikh, R., Bolduc, P., Starkstein, S. E., . . . Wagner, H. N. (1988). PET imaging of cortical S2 serotonin receptors after stroke: Lateralized changes and relationship to depression. *American Journal of Psychiatry, 145*(8), 937–943.

McDonald, B. C., Flashman, L. A., & Saykin, A. J. (2002). Executive dysfunction following traumatic brain injury: Neural substrates and treatment strategies. *NeuroRehabilitation, 17*(4), 333–344.

Moeller, F. G., Barratt, E. S., Dougherty, D. M., Schmitz, J. M., & Swann, A. C. (2001). Psychiatric aspects of impulsivity. *American Journal of Psychiatry, 158*(11), 1783–1793. doi: 10.1176/appi.ajp.158.11.1783

Nazem, S., Lonnquist, E., Monteith, L. L., & Brenner, L. A. (2014). Traumatic brain injury (TBI) and post-traumatic stress disorder (PTSD) as risk factors for suicidal thoughts and behaviors. In T. J. Hudzik & K. Cannon (Eds.), *Suicide: Phenomenology and biology.* New York: Springer.

Oquendo, M. A., Friedman, J. H., Grunebaum, M. F., Burke, A., Silver, J. M., & Mann, J. J. (2004). Suicidal behavior and mild traumatic brain injury in major depression. *Journal of Nervous and Mental Disease, 192*(6), 430–434.

Pohjasvaara, T., Vataja, R., Leppävuori, A., Kaste, M., & Erkinjuntti, T. (2001). Suicidal ideas in stroke patients 3 and 15 months after stroke. *Cerebrovascular Diseases, 12*(1), 21–26.

Rashid, N., Clarke, C., & Rogish, M. (2013). Post-stroke depression and expressed emotion. *Brain Injury, 27*(2), 223–238. doi: 10.3109/02699052.2012.129287

Rook, G. A., Lowry, C. A., & Raison, C. L. (2013). Microbial 'old friends', immunoregulation and stress resilience. *Evolution, Medicine, and Public Health, 2013*(1), 46–64.

Sabaz, M., Simpson, G. K., Walker, A., Rogers, J., Gillis, I., & Strettles, B. (2014). Prevalence, comorbidities and predictors of challenging behaviour among a cohort of community-dwelling adults with severe traumatic brain injury: A multi-centre study. *Journal of Head Trauma Rehabilitation, 29*, E19–E30.

Salmond, C. H., & Sahakian, B. J. (2005). Cognitive outcome in traumatic brain injury survivors. *Current Opinion in Critical Care, 11*(2), 111–116.

Santos, C. O., Caeiro, L., Ferro, J. M., & Figueira, M. L. (2012). A study of suicidal thoughts in acute stroke patients. *Journal of Stroke and Cerebrovascular Diseases, 21*(8), 749–754. doi: 10.1016/j.strokecerebrovasdis.2011.04.001

Serafini, G., Pompili, M., Elena Seretti, M., Stefani, H., Palermo, M., Coryell, W., & Girardi, P. (2013). The role of inflammatory cytokines in suicidal behavior: A systematic review. *European Neuropsychopharmacology, 23*(12), 1672–1686. doi:10.1016/j.euroneuro.2013.06.0022202000

Sherer, M., Hart, T., Whyte, J., Nick, T. G., & Yablon, S. A. (2005). Neuroanatomic basis of impaired self-awareness after traumatic brain injury: Findings from early computed tomography. *Journal of Head Trauma and Rehabilitation, 20*(4), 287–300.

Silver, J. M., Hales, R. E., & Yudofsky, M. B. A. S. (2008). Neuropsychiatric aspects of traumatic brain injury. In M. B. A. S. Yudofsky & R. E. Hales (Eds.), *Essentials of neuropsychiatry and behavioral neurosciences* (pp. 223–274). Arlington, VA: American Psychiatric Association.

Spalletta, G., Cravello, L., Imperiale, F., Salani, F., Bossù, P., Pichetto, L., . . . Cacciari, C. (2013). Neuropsychiatric symptoms and interleukin-6 serum levels in acute stroke. *The Journal of Neuropsychiatry and Clinical Neurosciences, 25*(4), 255–263.

Spielberger, C. D. (1999). *State-Trait Anger Expression Inventory-2.* Odessa, FL: Psychological Assessment Resources.

Suris, A., Lind, L., Emmett, G., Borman, P. D., Kashner, M., & Barratt, E. S. (2004). Measures of aggressive behavior: Overview of clinical and research instruments. *Aggression and Violent Behavior, 9*(2), 165–227. doi: 10.1016/S1359-1789(03)00012-0

Venes, D., Biderman, A., Fenton, B. G., Patwell, J., Enright, A. D., Adler, E., & Ponser, D. M. (Eds.). (2009). *Taber's cyclopedic medical dictionary*. Philadelphia, PA: F. A. Davis Company.

Yurgelun-Todd, D. A., Bueler, C. E., McGlade, E. C., Churchwell, J. C., Brenner, L. A., & Lopez-Larson, M. P. (2011). Neuroimaging correlates of traumatic brain injury and suicidal behavior. *Journal of Head Trauma and Rehabilitation, 26*(4), 276–289. doi: 10.1097/HTR.obo13e31822251dc

6 Epidemiology, Risk, and Protective Factors for Suicide after Neurodisability

Introduction

A growing number of studies have addressed the prevalence of suicidal thoughts and behaviors after neurodisability, as well as associated risk factors. The literature comprises a mixture of population-based, cohort, case-control, and case series studies. In this chapter, the epidemiology of suicide, suicide attempts, and suicide ideation (SI) will be outlined. The clinical issues of suicide notes and the possibility of "passive suicide" after spinal cord injury (SCI) will both be briefly highlighted in the section addressing suicide. The following section will detail current understanding of risk factors for suicidal thoughts and behaviors. To assist readability, risk factors are grouped into five domains (see Table 6.1), following Simpson and Tate (2007). The first three of these domains can be considered distal and the latter two proximal risk factors for suicidal thoughts and behaviors (Dennis et al., 2011). The final section of the chapter will then address protective factors.

TABLE 6.1

Distal and proximal risk factors for suicidal thoughts and behaviors

Domains		Risk factors
DISTAL RISK FACTORS	Demographic	Sex
		Age at onset
		Education
	Premorbid	History of family fragmentation
		History of family mental illness
		Lifetime history of substance abuse
		Previous history of injury/illness (e.g., prior stroke)
	Clinical	*Characteristics of Neurodisability*
		- Mechanism of injury
		- Severity of injury
		- Variant of condition (e.g., different types of stroke, multiple sclerosis, epilepsy)
		Course of Neurodisability
		Impact of onset/diagnosis
		Impact of disease progression
		Time post onset
		Impairment and Functional status
		Cognitive impairment
		Functional limitations
PROXIMAL RISK FACTORS	Mental Health Conditions/Symptoms	Presence of any psychiatric condition including depression, substance abuse, or post traumatic stress disorder
		Aggression
		Impulse control problems
	Psychosocial	Religious affiliation
		Living situation (living alone, living with others)
		Marital status

Epidemiology of Suicidal Thoughts and Behaviors

SUICIDE

Nonprogressive Conditions

Suicide after cerebrovascular accident (CVA) is almost double the risk for the general population, based on two Danish population-based studies (see Table 6.2). This elevated risk was consistent across all diagnostic categories of CVA (i.e., subarachnoid

TABLE 6.2

Risk of suicidal thoughts and behaviors after neurodisability

Condition	Analysis	Elevated risk for suicide	Elevated risk for suicide attempts	Elevated risk for SI
Nonprogressive				
Cerebrovascular accident	Unadjusted	1.8[1], 2.8[2]	-	2.1[3]
Spinal cord injury	Unadjusted	4.4[4], 4.5[5], 4.7[6], 4.9[7], 5.7[8], 3.0[9]	-	-
Traumatic brain injury	Unadjusted	2.1[10], 2.4[11], 2.9[12],		-
	Adjusted	3.3[13], 4.0[14], 3.0[15]	3.0[18], 4.5[19]	1.6[18]
		1.4[16,V], 1.9[17]	2.8[18], 2.4[19]	
Progressive				
Amyotrophic lateral sclerosis	Unadjusted	5.8[20]	-	-
Epilepsy	Unadjusted	-	-	2.2[25]
	Adjusted	1.9[21]	4.4[24]	2.1[24]
	Meta-analysis	3.3[22], 5.1[23]	-	-
Huntington's disease	Meta-analysis	2.9[26]	-	-
Multiple sclerosis	Unadjusted	1.8[27], 2.1[28], 2.3[29]	-	-
Parkinson's disease	Unadjusted	5.3[30]	-	-
Parkinson's disease	Meta-analysis	2.5[31]	-	-
+ deep brain stimulation	Adjusted	12.6[32]		

Note. Study by first author, date. **CVA:** [1]Teasdale, 2001a; [2]Waern, 2002; [3] Fuller-Thompson, 2012; **SCI:** [4]Soden, 2000; [5]Hartkopp, 1997; [6]Lidal, 2007; [7]DeVivo, 1991; [8]Hagen, 2010; [9]Cao, 2014; **TBI:** [10]Harrison-Felix, 2012; [11]Ventura, 2010; [12]Harrison-Felix, 2009; [13]Fazell, 2014; [14]Teasdale, 2001b; [15]Fralick, 2016; [16]Brenner, 2011; [17]Madsen, 2018; [18]Ilie, 2014; [19]Silver, 2001; **ALS:** [20]Fang, 2008; **Epilepsy:** [21]Christensen, 2007; [22]Bell, 2009; [23]Harris, 1997; [24]Scott, 2010; [25]Tellez-Zenteno, 2007 **HD:** [26]Harris, 1994; **MS:** [27]Stenager, 1992; [28]Brønnum-Hansen, 2005; [29]Fredrikson, 2003; **PD:** [30]Kostic, 2010; [31]Harris, 1994; **PD+ Deep Brain Stimulation:** [32]Voon, 2008

[V] risk estimate for military Veterans.

haemorrhage, intracerebral hemorrhage, cerebral ischemia, and CVA of unknown origin) (Teasdale & Engberg, 2001a). Two smaller case-controlled studies have also been published (Waern et al., 2002; Webb et al., 2012).

Suicide risk among adults with SCI is 4–5 times greater than the general population (see Table 6.2). This elevated risk is reported across all levels of neurological impairment (incomplete and complete paraplegia and tetraplegia). Studies documenting risk have been reported from the United States, Sweden, Denmark, and Australia (see Table 6.2).

Studies have found that suicide risk is elevated between 1.5 and 4 times for traumatic brain injury (TBI) among both civilians and military veterans, respectively (see Table 6.2). This risk is observed not only after severe TBI but also mild. For example, the risk for suicide after concussion is elevated between 1.8 and 3 times greater than the general population (Brenner, Ignacio, & Blow, 2011; Fralick, Hassan, Burke, Mostofsky, & Karsies, 2018; Fralick, Thiruchelvam, Tien, & Redelmeier, 2016; Teasdale & Engberg, 2001b). One possible confounding factor for elevated suicide after TBI is the high rate of comorbid psychiatric disorders, particularly depression and substance abuse. However, in a Swedish population study, people with TBI without any psychiatric disorders still had an elevated risk of suicide compared to the general population (Fazel, Wolf, Pllas, Lichtenstein, & Långström, 2014; see Table 6.2).

The great majority of studies across CVA, SCI, and TBI have focused on risk estimates. However, four studies used the data to generate estimated rates of suicide. Two of these are based on small samples (SCI, TBI) and need to be treated with caution, but rates of suicide are an important metric for communicating the level of suicide risk (see Table 6.3).

Progressive Conditions

The risk of suicide is also elevated after progressive neurodisability. Elevated suicide risk has been found for amyotrophic lateral sclerosis (ALS) based on the only population-based study conducted to date (Fang et al., 2008), and this contrasts with earlier negative findings in the meta-analysis by Harris and Barraclough (1994). One complication in determining suicide rates after ALS is the advent of physician-assisted suicide, with two studies (Albert et al., 2005; Veldink, Wokke, van der Wal, Vianney de Jong, & van den Berg, 2002) reporting that a small number of patients availed themselves of this option. The issue of physician-assisted suicide will be discussed further in Chapter 13.

In epilepsy, a large meta-analysis of 74 studies (Bell, Gaitatzis, Bell, Johnson, & Sander, 2009) found a threefold elevated risk of suicide associated with epilepsy. This risk of suicide was particularly elevated among the subgroup of people with temporal lobe epilepsy. A more detailed breakdown of the findings from Bell et al.

TABLE 6.3

Estimated annualised rates of suicide after neurodisability

Country	Type	Rate after neurodisability	General population rate	Comment
Denmark[1]	All CVA	83 per 100,000	45 per 100,000	Significant difference (38, 95%CI 27, 49)
United States[2]	All SCI	59.2 per 100,000	12.3 per 100,000	Not tested
	Paraplegia	54.3 per 100,000		
	Quadriplegia	64.5 per 100,000		
United Kingdom[3]	All SCI	62.5 per 100,000	12.2 per 100,000	Not tested
Pooled data, three studies[4]	All TBI	112 per 100,000	25 per 100,000 males aged 25–44	Aggregated three studies

CVA, cerebrovascular accident; SCI, spinal cord injury; TBI, traumatic brain injury.

[1]Teasdale & Engberg, 2001a; [2]Charlifue & Gerhart, 1991; [3]Savic et al., 2017; [4]Fleminger et al., 2003

(2009) are provided as part of Appendix 1. Independent of this meta-analysis, a population-based case-control study found the risk for suicide after epilepsy remained elevated even after excluding those with a history of psychiatric illness and adjusting for socioeconomic factors (Christensen, Vestergaard, Mortensen, Sidenius, & Agerbo, 2007).

Due to the relative scarcity of Huntington's disease (HD), there have been a range of challenges in determining a reliable estimate of the suicide risk after HD. The current best estimate (3 times the general population) was produced from a meta-analysis (see Table 6.2). Due to the relative scarcity, studies have reported on deaths identified over long time frames (e.g., 1920–1997, Baliko, Csala, & Czopf, 2004) with related concerns about the reliable confirmation of the causes of death (e.g., Di Maio et al., 1993; Schoenfeld et al., 1984) and are often based on patient membership in registries which may or may not be representative of the HD population. Only one report on suicides has been produced since the mid-1990s, when direct testing for the mutation became widely available. In a large cross-national study, Almquist, Bloch, Brinkman, Craufurd, & Hayden (1999) found five suicides (among 4,527 test participants, 100 centers, 22 countries), all from the group with the mutation/an increased risk; however, data on suicides, suicide attempts, and psychiatric hospitalization were aggregated, so no specific risk-related ratios were calculated.

National population studies of people with multiple sclerosis (MS) have found almost double the rate for suicide compared to the general population (see Table 6.2). This is consistent with results from an early meta-analysis (H&B, 1994). All studies have provided a global risk estimate only, with no breakdown of risk by MS subtype (i.e., relapsing remitting, secondary progressive, primary progressive, progressive relapsing).

In contrast to the other diagnostic groups, most studies investigating elevated suicide among people with Parkinson's disease (PD) have not found an elevated risk (Stenager et al., 1992; Gale, Braidwood, Winter, & Martyn, 1999; Myslobodsky, Lalonde, & Hicks, 2001; Juurlink, Herrmann, Szalai, Kopp, & Redelmeier, 2004). The reliability of the higher standard mortality ratio (SMR) reported by Kostic et al. (2010) needs to be treated with caution given the small sample size ($n = 102$), with the SMR calculated on only two suicides. Stronger evidence for risk can be found among patients with PD who underwent deep brain stimulation. A large international multicenter survey found the risk of suicide among patients with PD who had undergone subthalamic nucleus deep brain stimulation was greater than for the general population in the first year following surgery (matched against age, sex, and country rates; Voon et al., 2008). While the risk decreased over the ensuing 2 years, it was still significantly elevated in the fourth year after surgery.

Not every study has found evidence for elevated risk of suicide. In CVA, Webb et al. (2012) found that the increased risk of suicide disappeared after controlling for clinical depression (set against a living comparison group). After TBI, a small number of studies have also found no evidence of elevated risk. The reasons for nonsignificant results may reflect a limited sample size (e.g., Lewin, Marshall, & Roberts, 1979; McMillan & Teasdale, 2007; McMillan, Teasdale, Weir, & Stewart, 2011) with a corresponding lack of power, or limited sample composition, with a sample in a US study comprising teenagers and children injured before the age of 21 years and including participants as young as 10 years of age (Shavelle, Strauss, Whyte, Day, & Yu, 2001). Overall, however, the growing weight of research supports the link between neurodisability and elevated suicide risk.

SUICIDE NOTES

The presence of suicide notes has been recorded in some studies. Suicide notes are an important source of clinical information (either written, audio, or digital). They constitute the only first-person source of information about the motivation for the death (Berman & Samuel, 1993; Leenars, 2008). There are references to the presence of suicide notes after TBI (11%, 9/85, Achte, Lonnqvist, & Hillbom, 1971; 38%, 3/8, Tate, Simpson, Flanagan, & Coffey, 1997), MS (38%, 19/50, Stenager et al., 2011), and HD (11%, 1/9, Lipe, Schultz, & Bird, 1993). However, no analysis of the content of such notes has been published, and this is an important area for future research.

PASSIVE MEANS OF SUICIDE AFTER SPINAL CORD INJURY

In the case of SCI, an important question has been whether severity of neurologic impairment presents a barrier to suicide. In reviewing the literature, deaths have been documented among people with both paraplegia and tetraplegia (incomplete and complete) by diverse means. One study provided a breakdown of methods by level of neurologic injury (Soden et al., 2000). Among the small number of deaths (n = 15: 5 paraplegia, 10 tetraplegia), people with both paraplegia and tetraplegia used gunshot to the head (3/15 deaths) and overdose (3/15 deaths). The other means included carbon monoxide poisoning, drowning (tetraplegia, 7/15 deaths), and hanging (paraplegia, 1 death) with the means of one death unknown. These data illustrate that most suicides after SCI occurred by the same methods observed in the general public; however, one reported suicide involved disconnection from a ventilator (Charlifue & Gerhart, 1991).

The further possibility that some people with severe functional limitations due to SCI end their lives by "passive" means—that is, through self-neglect (e.g., refusal to follow medical advice or treatment)—has been raised (Macleod, 1988; DeVivo, Black Richards, & Stover, 1991; Charlifue & Gerhart, 1991; Kennedy, Rogers, Speer, & Frankel, 1999). Such behavior could be fatal, resulting from common medical complications such as septicemia or urinary tract infections (Hartkopp, Brønnum-Hansen, Seidenschnur, & Biering-Sørensen, 1998; Charlifue & Gerhart, 1991). These concerns were linked to concepts in broader suicidology that various self-destructive behaviors constituted indirect means of suicide (e.g., Farberow, 1980).

Despite these concerns, there is growing documentation of suicide among people with the most severe SCI (American Spinal Injury Association [ASIA] level A, complete tetraplegia) dying from suicide at rates equivalent to those of people with less severe injuries (Hartkopp et al., 1998; Soden et al., 2000; Kennedy & Garmon-Jones, 2017). Furthermore, mortality due to all causes including septicemia has continued to decline over the past two decades while the risk of suicide alone has risen (Soden et al., 2000). In the absence of systematic research, current evidence suggests that people with even the most severe levels of SCI have been able to find an active means of ending their lives. However, the possibility of deaths occurring due to neglect that have not been documented as suicide cannot be discounted.

SUICIDE ATTEMPTS

As outlined in Chapter 3, suicide attempts are the strongest predictor of eventual suicide. In contrast to deaths by suicide and SI, much less information is available about suicide attempts across all neurodisability conditions. Furthermore, understanding the prevalence is also complicated by some reports that do not always clearly distinguish among suicides and suicide attempts, referring to "suicide attempts among which some ended in deaths" (e.g., De Vivo et al., 1991, SCI; Farrer, Opitz, & Reynolds, 1986, HD; Kalinin & Polyanskiy, 2005, epilepsy; Patten et al., 2005, MS; Soulas et al., 2008, PD). In reviewing suicide attempts across neurodisability, very limited data are available on suicide attempts after SCI (Charlifue & Gerhart, 1991; McCullumsmith et al., 2015) or PD (Soulas et al., 2008; Nazem et al., 2008). Moreover, no survey data on suicide attempts after CVA or ALS could be located.

Nonprogressive Conditions

In the evidence to date of increased risk associated with TBI, two population studies have found the risk of suicide attempts was between 2 and 3 times greater than the general population after controlling for a range of demographic, illness, and mental health covariates (see Table 6.2). The one major limitation of the study by Silver, Kramer, Greenwald, & Weissman (2001), however, was that the date of the TBI was not known; therefore, it could not be determined whether the suicide attempts occurred prior or subsequent to the TBI. Elevated rates of attempts have also been found among veterans with TBI from the Iraq and Afghanistan conflicts in comparison to the general veteran population (Fonda et al., 2017).

In findings from a rehabilitation cohort, participants with TBI in the US National Institute on Disability and Rehabilitation Research (NIDRR) Traumatic Brain Injury Model Systems reported a 4.3% rate of pre-injury lifetime attempts (195/4,515) (Fisher et al., 2016). Within the same cohort, rates of suicide attempts within the previous year remained consistently between 1.1% and 1.7% at the 1-, 2-, 5-, and 10-year post-injury time-points (Fisher et al., 2016).

Progressive Conditions

The largest study addressing suicide attempts after epilepsy drew on cross-national data from 14 World Mental Health surveys (Scott et al., 2010). Epilepsy was associated with an elevated risk of suicide attempts among people with SI and a suicide plan after adjusting for demographic, other disease, and mental health variables (see Table 6.2). Some other smaller scale studies that document suicide attempts after epilepsy have also been published (Hara, Akanuma, Adachi, Hara, Koutroumanidis, 2009; Hawton, Fagg, & Marsack, 1980; Mendez, Lanska, Manon-Espaillat, & Burnstine, 1989).

There are limited data about suicide attempts among people with HD. A Huntington Study Group project found a 9.5% lifetime rate of suicide attempts among 1,941 participants from the 43 participating centers (Wetzell et al., 2011).

Two population-based studies (each involving a single province) examined suicide attempts among people with MS. In comparing hospital admission codes for people with MS to those of the general population in Nova Scotia over a 3-year period, Fisk, Morehouse, Brown, Skedgel, & Murray (1998) found that people with MS had 3 times the number of admissions for suicide attempts. In contrast, in a single county of Denmark, no significantly increased risk for suicide attempts was observed among people with MS in comparison to the general population. However, the authors acknowledge that the results must be viewed with caution due to the relatively small population involved (Stenager et al., 2011).

SUICIDE IDEATION

SI is clinically significant, both as an indicator of psychological distress and a warning sign of the increased likelihood of more severe suicidal behavior. Data about SI are found in research that focuses specifically on SI per se, from broader suicide studies, and from studies of depression which report symptom-based data including SI items. The rates of SI vary with definition and the time frame (last week, last year, lifetime) over which it is measured. There is little published about SI after SCI (Bombadier, Richards, Krause, Tulsky, & Tate, 2004; Wu & Chan, 2007).

Nonprogressive Conditions

Studies into SI have been reported for CVA and TBI, but not for SCI (see Table 6.2). The one population-based study for CVA found that a 15.2% cumulative lifetime frequency of SI among stroke survivors was double the odds ratio (OR 2.07) in comparison to the general population (see Table 6.2).

Two longitudinal studies provide useful information about the course of SI after CVA, with SI appearing in both the acute and chronic phases post-injury at rates between 7% and 14% at the acute (i.e., 3 months) and chronic (i.e., >12 months) phases post CVA (Pohjasvaara, Vataja, Leppävuori, Kaste, & Erkinjuntti, 2001; Kishi, Kosier, & Robinson, 1996a). Kishi et al. (1996a) suggested that acute suicidality is more closely linked to primary injury to the brain, but this effect gradually dissipates over the first year post-stroke, whereas suicide plans observed in the chronic phase are more likely to reflect responses to secondary psychosocial stressors (Kishi, Robinson, & Kosier, 1996b).

SI is significantly higher among adolescents with TBI at almost double the rate for the general population (see Table 6.2). An Australian population-based study also found that adults with TBI reported a significantly higher level of SI over the previous 12 months than did adults without TBI (Anstey et al., 2004), but no risk statistics were calculated. Similar to CVA, SI has been observed in both the acute and chronic phases post-TBI, with mixed severity of TBI (mild–severe) ranging from 16% to 30% (Jorge, Robinson, & Arndt, 1993; Seel & Kreutzer, 2003; Simpson & Tate, 2002; Sliwinski, Gordon, & Bogdany, 1998; Tsaousides, Cantor, & Gordon, 2011). The one longitudinal study conducted to date has found a cumulative prevalence of SI of 25% over the first year post-injury, almost 7 times greater than the rate expected for the general population (Mackelprang et al., 2014).

Progressive Conditions

Limited data are available on SI after ALS (Clarke, McLeod, Smith, Trauer, & Kissane, 2005; Palmieri et al., 2010), with most attention focused on the issue of the wish to end life, particularly among patients in the final phase of the disease (Albert et al., 2005; Veldink et al., 2002; Ganzini, Silveira, & Johnston, 2002). Two population-based studies have found that people with epilepsy are twice as likely to report a lifetime history of SI compared to the general population (Scott et al., 2010; Tellez-Zenteno, Patten, Jetté, Williams, & Wiebe, 2007), with a smaller study by Jones et al. (2003) finding the prevalence of current SI at 12.2%.

In a study from the Huntington Study Group database, Wetzel et al. (2011) discovered a lifetime history of SI of 26.5% among the 1,941 participants. Furthermore, a total of 19% reported current SI. In an earlier report from the same database, Paulsen, Hoth, Nehl, & Stierman (2005) found an overall 17.5% rate of SI, but only 1.3% of this group had a suicide plan.

Limited information is available on the prevalence of SI among people with MS, with the available evidence suggesting levels around 30% (Feinstein, 2002, 28.6%; Turner, Williams, Bowen, Kivlahan, & Haselkorn, 2006, 29.4%; Viner, Patten, Berzins, Bulloch, & Feist, 2014, 22.1%). In PD, researchers have also documented death intent (thoughts about dying, not wanting to live) as well as more explicit SI. Studies have found current levels of SI around 7–11%, with combined rates of SI/death ideation ranging from 14.4% to 30% (Leentjens, Marinus, Van Hilten, Lousberg, & Verhey, 2003; Nazem et al., 2008; Kummer, Cardoso, Teixeira, 2009; Kostic et al., 2010).

Risk Factors for Suicidal Thoughts and Behaviors

Evidence of risk factors for suicidal thoughts and behaviors have been documented across all five domains proposed by Simpson and Tate (2007). However, the domains tested and the strength of the evidence varies across suicide, suicide attempts, and SI. For suicide, most data on risk are available for demographic (age and sex) and clinical (time following onset) domains, due largely to the retrospective nature of this research (see Table 6.4). Among this research, no substantive studies have been published on risk factors for suicide after HD or PD. Next, there are very limited data on risk factors for suicide attempts across any of the types of neurodisability. The small number of studies that do exist all identify higher levels of post-onset comorbid mental health issues as the key risk factor (e.g., Simpson & Tate, 2005).

The most comprehensive models testing risk factors for suicidal thoughts and behaviors have been conducted in the area of SI, in part because it is logistically easier to study this group (see Table 6.5). The two exceptions are SCI and ALS. For SCI, this is due to the broader lack of studies documenting SI, which would provide the opportunity to identify risk factors. For ALS, as already flagged, the issue of risk factors is subsumed within the broader considerations in relation to physician-assisted suicide (see Chapter 13).

Demographic Factors

AGE

Across all neurodisability groups for which data were available, a younger age of onset was associated with elevated risk of suicide compared to the general population. This risk was observed for CVA, SCI, ALS, and MS (see Table 6.4). Across these four conditions, the elevated risk disappeared with onset at later ages, typically from 60 years and older (MS, SCI) and a decade later for ALS and CVA (see Figure 6.1). In contrast, the risk of suicide appears to be constant across the adult age span for both TBI and epilepsy. To date, there have been no age-related risk factors identified for suicide attempts or SI.

SEX

There has been an elevated risk for both males and females compared to the general population (CVA, SCI, TBI, ALS, epilepsy, MS). Studies that have tested sex within a neurodisability condition have found that males have a significantly higher rate of suicide compared to females, but this appears to simply reflect the baseline difference between males and females in the general population (CVA, MS; see Table 6.4). To date, there have been no sex-related risk factors identified for suicide attempts or SI.

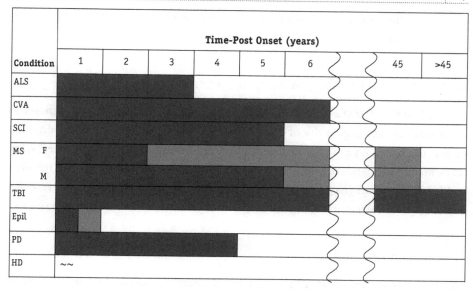

FIGURE 6.1 Years of elevated risk for death by suicide post onset by condition.

Premorbid Factors

Two studies from independent research groups found that a clinical variable (prior history of CVA) was a significant risk factor for longer term SI (15 months post CVA, Pohjasvaara et al., 2001; Kishi et al., 1996b) in multivariate analyses. No other data on premorbid risk factors for suicide thoughts and behaviors across the other types of neurodisability could be identified.

One longitudinal study of SI during the first year post-TBI found that premorbid histories of bipolar disorder, low educational level (less than completing a high school education), and a premorbid history of a suicide attempt were predictors of SI in the first year post-injury (Mackelprang et al., 2014).

Clinical Factors

Clinical risk factors for suicidal thoughts and behaviors include the neurodisability caused by a suicide attempt (SCI, TBI), the severity of the condition, the time post-onset, the course of the condition, the presence of cognitive impairments, and other clinical features.

NEURODISABILITY CAUSED BY A SUICIDE ATTEMPT

For TBI and SCI, if the injury occurred as the result of a suicide attempt, then the individuals are at a higher risk of dying by suicide. In the case of TBI, a sevenfold increase (6.9; 95% CI, 3.2–14.8; Teasdale & Engberg, 2001b) has been documented, with an estimated incidence of 1 out of every 130 TBIs due to a suicide attempt. In relation to SCI, some reports have suggested that between 0% and 6.8% of injuries were the result of suicide attempts (Kennedy & Garmon-Jones, 2017; Stanford et al., 2007).

SEVERITY OF CONDITION

In a multivariate hazard analysis, severe brain injury (as defined by the ICD codes for lesion) resulted in almost double the suicide risk (hazard 1.67; 95% CI, 1.36–2.06) compared to concussion (Teasdale & Engberg, 2001b). Severity of injury was also identified as a risk factor for suicide after SCI (Cao et al., 2014).

TIME POST-ONSET

Varying times post-onset are associated with heightened suicide risk. The time period of elevated risk for most groups (CVA, SCI, ALS, MS) lies within the first 6 years post-onset, with the highest elevation in the first 1–2 years. For PD, elevated risk of suicide has been measured up to 4 years post-neurosurgery for subthalamic nucleus deep brain stimulation (Voon et al., 2008). In contrast, some groups present a uniformly chronic risk over long periods post-onset (TBI, epilepsy, MS; see Table 6.4).

COURSE OF THE CONDITION

The influence of the course of neurodisability on suicidal thoughts and behaviors can occur both among nonprogressive (e.g. recurrent CVA, TBI) and progressive conditions. Among nonprogressive conditions, a recent meta-analysis in CVA (Bartoli et al., 2017) found that recurrent stroke was a risk factor for SI (OR 1.77, $p<0.001$). Among progressive conditions, data from the Huntington Study Group found that the highest risk of current SI occurred in the stage immediately preceding a confirmed diagnosis of HD (Paulsen et al., 2005). People identified as having motor abnormalities on neurological exam associated with the onset of HD had significantly higher levels of SI compared to people with normal results or people with a confirmed diagnosis (Paulsen et al., 2005). The elevated risk around the time of onset has also been highlighted by other authors (Di Maio et al., 1993; Schoenfeld et al., 1984). Furthermore, there were significant differences in SI related to the progression of the disease, with people at stage 2 (total functional capacity score of 7–10, Unified Huntington's Disease Rating Scale; Shoulson et al., 1989), the stage associated with the loss of independence, having significantly higher levels of SI compared to people at Stage 1 or Stages 3–5 (Paulsen et al., 2005).

COGNITIVE IMPAIRMENTS

Overall, there are limited data about any increase in risk associated with post-onset cognitive impairments. To some degree, the absence of such research may be because the widespread nature of cognitive impairments across all types of neurodisability can reduce its sensitivity. Also, in some cases, the use of global measures of cognition (such as the Mini-Mental State Examination [MMSE]) may not have the required sensitivity to detect the impairments that are present.

In CVA, a recent meta-analysis (Bartoli et al., 2017) found that cognitive impairment was a risk factor for SI in stroke (Standardized mean difference −0.22, $p = 0.03$). Among individual studies, Kishi et al. (1996a) found that the presence of cognitive impairment (as measured by the MMSE) was one of three independent predictors of the presence of a suicide plan in the acute phase post-CVA (3 months post; see Table 6.4). As outlined in Chapter 5, there is some limited neuroanatomical and neuropsychological data to suggest that executive impairments may contribute to increased suicide risk after TBI (Brenner et al., 2015; Homaifar, Brenner, Forster, & Nagamoto, 2012), but the exploratory nature of these studies means that much more research will be needed to better understand such links.

FUNCTIONAL IMPAIRMENTS

In CVA, a recent meta-analysis (Bartoli et al., 2017) found that disability was a risk factor for SI in stroke (standardized mean difference 0.58, $p = 0.01$). In MS, self-reported bladder and bowel symptoms and difficulties with speaking and swallowing almost trebled the risk of SI (Viner et al., 2014). These variables remained significant even after depression was controlled for. However, the authors caution that endorsement of the SI item (item 9 on the Patient-Health Questionnaire-9) can also reflect concerns about disease-related mortality and therefore be nonspecific to SI.

TABLE 6.4

Risk factors associated with increased risk of suicide

	Variable	Cerebrovascular accident	Spinal cord injury	Traumatic brain injury	Amyotrophic lateral sclerosis	Epilepsy	Multiple sclerosis
Demographic	Younger age at onset	Younger onset elevated (<60), extends older for females[1,2]	Younger onset elevated risk (<50)[3,4]	Constant elevated risk across age span[8]	Younger onset elevated risk (<60)[5]	Constant, younger onset elevated risk (<18)[9]	Younger onset elevated risk (<40), extends older for females[6,7]
	Sex	Both sex elevated risk compared to general population; Male with CVA significantly higher than female with CVA[2]	Both sex elevated risk compared to general population[3,4]	Both sex elevated risk compared to general population[8]	Both sex elevated risk compared to general population[5]	Both sex elevated risk compared to general population[9]	Both sex elevated risk compared to general population; Male with MS significantly higher than female with MS[7]
Clinical	Time-post onset	Elevated risk within first 6 years, decreases with time post-stroke[1,2]	Elevated risk within first 5 years[3,4]	No specific time period, elevated risk throughout[8,10]	Elevated risk within first 3 years[5]	Elevated risk within first year, especially first six months[9]	Elevated risk within first 2 years (F), 5 years (M)[6,7], up to 45 years post-diagnosis[11]
	Injury due to suicide attempt	~	Increased risk	Increased risk	~	~	~
	Other	~	Injured from fall, complete neurologic lesion[12]	~	~	~	More severe disability, late stage (chronic-progressive)[13]

Mental Health	Mental health issue	~	Depressive symptoms, alcohol, symptoms of aggression[12]	Depression,[14] substance misuse[8]	~	Affective disorder, schizophrenia, anxiety, alcohol, other mental health disorder[9]	~
	Prior SA/SI	~	~	Yes (SA and SI)	~	Yes (SA and SI)	Yes (SA and SI)
	Miscell-aneous	~	Non-Catholic religious preference[12]	~	~	~	~
Psychosocial		~	~	~	Married/cohabiting vs. single[5]	Marital status, labor market status, residence, absence from work[9]	Unemployed financial stress[13]

SA, suicide attempt; SI, suicide ideation; M, male; F, female.

[1]Stenager et al. (1998); [2]Teasdale & Engsberg (2001a); [3]Soden et al. (2000); [4]DeVivo et al. (1991) and Fang et al. (2008); [6]Stenager et al. (1992); [7]Fredrikson et al. (2003); [8]Teasdale and Engsberg (2001b); [9]Christensen et al. (2007); [10]Achte et al. (1971); [11]Brønnum-Hansen et al. (2005); [12]Charlifue et al. (1991); [13]Berman and Samuel (1993); [14]Fazel et al. (2014).

TABLE 6.5

Independent risk factors of suicide ideation

	CVA	TBI	HD	MS	PD
Outcome					
Outcome	Suicide plan present vs absent[1,2]	SI present vs absent[3,4]	SI present vs absent[5]	SI present vs absent[6]	Death thought or SI present vs absent[7-9]
Predictors					
Demographic	-	-	-	-	-
Premorbid	Pre-injury alcohol abuse[2]	-	-	-	-
Clinical	Cognitive impairment[1]	-	-	-	-
Mental Health Comorbidities/ Symptoms	Depression[1]	Hopelessness[3], Post-injury psychiatric history[3], Worthlessness[4]	Depression/ Anxiety[5], aggression[5], Past or current history of alcohol abuse[5]	Current depression[6], Lifetime diagnosis of alcohol abuse[6]	Depression[7-9], Psychosis[7], Hopelessness[7]
Psychosocial	Limited social functioning[1]	-	-	Living alone[6]	-

CVA, cerebrovascular accident; TBI, traumatic brain injury; HD, Huntington's disease; MS, multiple sclerosis; PD, Parkinson's disease; SI, suicide ideation.

[1] Kishi (1996a); [2] Kishi (1996b); [3] Simpson and Tate (2002); [4] Wood et al. (2010); [5] Wetzel (2011); [6] Feinstein (2002); [7] Kostic (2010); [8] Kummer (2009); [9] Nazem (2008).

Mental Health Comorbidities

In documenting mental health comorbidities, some studies have focused on specific disorders such as depression, substance abuse, anxiety, and so forth. In other studies, a global descriptor of psychopathology has been employed.

The risk of suicide is elevated in the presence of comorbid psychopathology in the two conditions for which there are data (TBI, epilepsy). Furthermore, the risk of suicide remained elevated once the analyses controlled for comorbid psychopathology, evidence that the presence of neurodisability made a unique contribution to suicide risk (Christensen et al., 2007; Fazel et al., 2014). Although the presence of suicide risk among people with TBI but no comorbid psychiatric disorder was significantly elevated in comparison with the general population (adjusted OR between 2.4 and

3.1), the presence of comorbid depression or substance abuse significantly increased the suicide risk (AOR 17.6 and 15.6, respectively) (Fazel et al., 2014).

Suicide risk was found to be elevated among people with epilepsy who had a global history of mental illness (Nilsson, Ahlbom, Farahmand, Åsberg, & Tomson, 2002) or specific comorbid mental health disorders (affective disorder, schizophrenia, anxiety, chronic alcohol use, or other mental health disorders) in comparison to the general population (Christensen et al., 2007). In the latter study, the category of affective disorders was associated with a significantly higher risk compared to the other mental health disorders (Christensen et al., 2007). Furthermore, although males and females with epilepsy but no psychiatric disease had a significantly increased suicide risk compared to the general population (adjusted risk ratio 1.81 for males, 2.50 for females), the risk was significantly higher in the presence of comorbid psychiatric disease (adjusted risk ratio 9.86 for males, 23.60 for females) (Christensen et al., 2007).

Post-onset and/or current mental health comorbidities have been identified as a risk factor for suicide attempts in TBI (Simpson & Tate, 2002), epilepsy (Jones et al., 2003), MS (Berman & Samuel 1993), and people who underwent deep brain stimulation for PD (Voon et al., 2008). Comorbidities included depression (Jones et al., 2003; Berman & Samuel 1993; Voon et al., 2008), a post-onset history of emotional distress (Simpson & Tate, 2002), a manic episode (Jones et al., 2003), substance abuse (Simpson & Tate, 2005), or SI (Simpson & Tate, 2002) compared to the comparator groups employed across the four studies.

A number of risk factors for SI have been identified. In a longitudinal study of SI during the first year post-TBI, elevated scores on the Patient Health Questionnaire (eight items minus the SI item) were the strongest predictor of subsequent SI over nine time points during the first year post-injury (Mackelprang et al., 2014). Two cross-sectional studies employing multivariate regression analyses found that worthlessness (Wood et al., 2010; OR 1.91), hopelessness (Simpson & Tate, 2002, OR 8.7), and a post-injury history of psychiatric disorder/emotional distress (OR 5.5) were all independent predictors of post-injury SI.

One study with an HD sample tested a model of demographic, clinical, and psychopathological risk factors for SI over the previous 30 days (Wetzel et al., 2011). Two psychopathological variables were identified as significant individual predictors. These were higher depression/anxiety scores (OR 1.11; 95% CI, 1.10, 1.13) and aggression (OR 1.04; 95% CI, 1.02, 1.06).

Risk factors for SI after MS were tested in a multivariate model by Feinstein (2002). Results found the model had 75% sensitivity, 90% specificity, and 85.7% classification accuracy in predicting SI among people with MS. Independent predictors included current depressive symptoms and a lifetime diagnosis of alcohol abuse.

In PD, three multivariate regression analyses all identified the presence of co-morbid mental health issues as having the strongest association with SI, including depression (Kostic et al., 2010; Kummer et al., 2009; Nazem et al., 2008), presence of psychosis (Kostic et al., 2010), and increasing hopelessness (as measured by the Beck Hopelessness Scale; Kostic et al., 2010). Quantifying the level of risk, Kummer et al. (2009) found that depression accounted for 58% (Nagelkerke R^2) of the variance in SI and Nazem et al. (2008) found that increasing severity of depressive symptoms alone predicted death/SI (OR 2.76; 95% CI, 1.88, 4.07).

Psychosocial Factors

No studies for suicide or suicide attempts could be identified in which psychosocial factors were investigated as possible risk factors. Poor social functioning and/or related social isolation was identified as a risk factor for SI. Post-CVA, Kishi et al. (1996a) found that a psychosocial (social functioning) variable in combination with psychopathological (depression) and clinical (cognition) variables were significantly associated with the presence of suicide plans in the acute phase (3 months post-CVA, multivariate analysis). After MS, "living alone" made an independent contribution to increased risk of SI in combination with mental health comorbidities (Feinstein, 2002).

Protective Factors for Suicidal Thoughts and Behaviors

In contrast to the research conducted into risk factors, only one or two studies have examined protective factors. Some initial evidence for the existence of protective factors among people with neurodisability have also been found; namely, social support, psychological factors, spirituality, and availability of services. These were derived from the only systematic study of protective factors (Brenner et al., 2009), as well as the handful of other studies across various neurodisability conditions that have made reference to this issue.

PERCEIVED SOCIAL SUPPORT

The availability of perceived social support is the most extensively researched protective factor in the general suicide literature (Graham et al., 2000). In a qualitative study of veterans with TBI, Brenner et al. (2009) found that participants derived support from family, friends, peers, and even pets. Apart from the emotional benefits that the veterans reported from their perceived social support, a secondary outcome was that engaging with supports also flowed through to increased activity, which had a further positive benefit (Brenner et al., 2009). At least one other qualitative study in brain injury has reported similar findings (Kuipers & Lancaster, 2000). After epilepsy, Kalinin et al. (2005) reported on one group of individuals with persistent suicidal ideation ($n = 33$) who did not end their lives. The authors asserted that one reason accounting for this was their sense of debt to family members.

One quantitative study also reported findings in relation to social support. After MS, Turner et al. (2006) found that higher levels of social support, as measured by the Modified Social Support Survey, were significantly correlated with the reduced likelihood of thoughts that a person would be better off dead or likely to harm themselves in some way. However, when added to a multivariate model, the authors did not find that social support was an independent predictor (Turner et al., 2006).

The presence of children is an important element within social support (e.g., USDHHS, 2012). Brenner et al. (2009) found evidence of this, reporting one participant as saying "My son . . . he's the only reason that really keeps me going" (p. 393). Further support can be found in the study of an HD sample (Lipe et al., 1993) in which people who died by suicide were less likely to have children. Despite this, the presence of children does not always act as a protective factor. Several of the clinical accounts of suicide published within the neurodisability literature involved people with children (e.g., TBI, Achte et al., 1971; Tate et al., 1997; CVA, Garden, Garrison, & Jain, 1990). One possible reason for this is that parents who are severely depressed can end up believing that their children would be better off without them.

PSYCHOLOGICAL FACTORS

Having a sense of purpose and a sense of hope are important psychological factors (Brenner et al., 2009). Although sometimes expressed in a religious form, for a number of respondents, purpose was found in some form of meaningful occupation (Brenner et al., 2009). In addition to psychological states, other research has identified the importance of cognitive skills, specifically those related to executive functioning. Cognitive functions such as effective problem-solving have been identified in the general literature as important protective factors that decrease the risk of suicide (Bryan & Rudd, 2006).

Psychological factors also encompass cognitive processes such as executive functioning. Preserved problem-solving capacity is one component of executive function, and effective problem-solving may play a protective role in reducing the sense of hopelessness experienced after neurodisability. In TBI, the presence of limited awareness has also been identified as a possible protective factor.

SPIRITUAL FAITH/RELIGION

Spiritual belief or religious membership is another common protective factor for suicide. For example, in the United States, the high involvement of African Americans in church is identified as a protective factor that helps to account for the lower suicide rates among African American females compared to the overall rates for the United States (Utsey et al., 2008). Spiritual belief and/or links with a religion can have at least three dimensions (Brenner et al., 2009). First, people with spiritual beliefs were often members of a religious community which provided an avenue for social support. Furthermore, faith in god was one avenue for finding a sense of purpose or meaning after a TBI, "he's [God] got something else for me to do" (p. 394). Although not identified in the study by Brenner et al., research in other populations has found the religions with a strong prohibition against suicide (i.e., suicide is prohibited by God) acted as a protective factor.

HEATH SERVICE-RELATED FACTORS

Receiving treatment for mental health conditions, capacity to engage in a therapeutic alliance with mental health staff, and ability to cooperate with treatment are all important service-related protective factors (Bryan & Rudd, 2006; Rudd, 2012; Simpson & Tate, 2007). In the qualitative study, veterans reported positively on several aspects of treatment including access to mental health staff, psychiatric medication, crisis intervention, and longer term therapeutic support (Brenner et al., 2009), results echoed in the earlier qualitative TBI study (Kuipers & Lancaster, 2000).

One of the initial challenges in neurodisability is ensuring that people are identified as needing mental health intervention. In MS, Feinstein (2002) found that, over an 8-year period, one-third of patients who were depressed or displaying suicidal intent did not receive needed treatment (either medication or psychological intervention). However, even with better identification, a number of case reports in the literature highlighted the difficulties in getting some people with neurodisability to engage with mental health support and cooperate with needed treatment (e.g., TBI, Tate et al., 1997; SCI, Bombadier et al., 2004).

Conclusion

Suicide risk was generally elevated by 2–5 times across the various types of neurodisability in comparison to the general population, with the one exception of PD. In a number of conditions, this risk remained elevated after controlling for comorbid mental health conditions. Given these findings, it is not surprising that there is also evidence of an elevated risk of suicide attempts and SI. However, the data on suicide attempts are generally weaker than the data for suicide and SI, and further large-scale studies addressing this issue are required for most neurodisability groups. There is robust evidence for elevated rates of SI after neurodisability in comparison to the general population, and, once again, this risk remains significant after controlling for psychiatric comorbidity.

The strongest evidence for risk factors for suicidal thoughts and behaviors was evident in demographic (age and sex), clinical features and mental health comorbidities. Furthermore, initial qualitative evidence was identified for protective factors. However, these factors need to be tested further to establish their clinical significance in mediating the degree of suicide risk after neurodisability.

Implications for Clinicians

1. Across neurodisability, the risk for suicide is increased for both males and females in comparison to the general population, so it is important to monitor both sexes.

2. Suicide attempts occur at a greater frequency in those with neurodisability than for the general population and are associated with elevated levels of SI. Therefore, if SI is detected, the existence of past or possible future suicidal behavior needs to be taken into account.

3. Across most types of neurodisability, SI follows a recognizable pattern, similar in many aspects to that seen in the general community. However, this pattern does not extend to ALS. In ALS, the intersection between SI and physician-assisted suicide requires a different set of clinical and ethical frameworks, assumptions, and approaches.

4. To date, there is limited research on the potential contribution of cognitive impairments to increased risk of suicidal thoughts and behaviors.

5. Assessment and treatment of mental health comorbidities after neurodisability is a front-line treatment option; however the variation in suicide risk after neurodisability is greater than is accounted for by mental health comorbidities alone. Therefore, simply treating the mental health comorbidities may not extinguish suicide risk in all cases.

References

Achte, K. A., Lonnqvist, J., & Hillbom, E. (1971). Suicides following war brain-injuries. *Acta Psychiatrica Scandinavica*, Suppl, 1–94.

Albert, S. M., Rabkin, J. G., Del Bene, M. L., Tider, T., O'Sullivan, I., Rowland, M. P., & Mitsumodo, H. (2005). Wish to die in end-stage ALS. *Neurology, 65*(1), 68–74.

Almqvist, E. W., Bloch, M., Brinkman, R., Craufurd, D., & Hayden, M. R. (1999). A worldwide assessment of the frequency of suicide, suicide attempts or psychiatric hospitalization after predictive testing for Huntington disease. *American Journal of Human Genetics, 64*(5), 1293–1304.

Anstey, K., Butterworth, P., Jorm, A. F., Chistensen, H., Rodgers, B., & Windsor, T. D. (2004). A population survey found an association between self-reports of traumatic brain injury and increased psychiatric symptoms. *Journal of Clinical Epidemiology, 57*(11), 1202–1209.

Baliko, L., Csala, B., & Czopf, J. (2004). Suicide in Hungarian Huntington's disease patients. *Neuroepidemiology, 23*(5), 258–260.

Bartoli, F., Pompili, M., Lillia, N., Crocamo, C., Salemi, G., Clerici, M., & Carrà, G. (2017). Rates and correlates of suicidal ideation among stroke survivors: A meta-analysis. *Journal of Neurology, Neurosurgery & Psychiatry, 88*, 498–504.

Bell, G. S., Gaitatzis, A., Bell, C. L., Johnson, A. L., & Sander, J. W. (2009). Suicide in people with epilepsy: How great is the risk? *Epilepsia, 50*(8), 1933–1942.

Berman, A. L., & Samuel, L. (1993). Suicide among people with multiple sclerosis. *Journal of NeuroRehabilitation, 7*(2), 53–62.

Bethune, A., Da Costa, L., van Niftrik, C. H. B., & Feinstein, A. (2017). Suicidal ideation after mild traumatic brain injury: A consecutive Canadian sample. *Archives of Suicide Research, 21*(3), 392–402.

Biering-Sørensen, F., Pedersen, W., & Müller, P. G. (1992). Spinal cord injury due to suicide attempts. *Spinal Cord, 30*, 139–144.

Bombadier, C. H., Richards, J. S., Krause, J. S., Tulsky D., & Tate, D. G. (2004). Symptoms of major depression in people with spinal cord injury: Implications for screening. *Archives of Physical Medicine and Rehabilitation, 85*(11), 1749–1756.

Brenner, L. A., Bahraini, N., Homaifar, B. Y., Monteith, L. L., Nagamoto, H., Dorsey-Holliman, B., & Forster, J. E. (2015). Executive functioning and suicidal behavior among veterans with and without traumatic brain injury. *Archives of Physical Medicine and Rehabilitation, 96*(8), 1411–1418. doi:10.1016/j.apmr2015.04.0100

Brenner, L. A., Carlson, N. E., Harrison-Felix, C., Ashman, T., Hammond, F., & Hirschberg, R. E. (2009). Self-inflicted traumatic brain injury: Characteristics and outcome. *Brain Injury, 23*(13-14), 991–998.

Brenner, L. A., Ignacio, R. V., & Blow, F. C. (2011). Suicide and traumatic brain injury among individuals seeking Veterans Health Administration Services *Journal of Head Trauma Rehabilitation, 26*(4), 257–264.

Brønnum-Hansen, H., Stenager, E., Stenager, E. N., & Koch-Henriksen, N. (2005). Suicide among Danes with multiple sclerosis. *Journal of Neurology, Neurosurgery and Psychiatry, 76*(10), 1457–1459.

Bryan, C. J., & Rudd, M. D. (2006). Advances in the assessment of suicide risk. *Journal of Clinical Psychology, 62*, 185–200.

Cao, Y., Massaro, J. F., Krause, J. S., Chen, Y., & Devivo, M. J. (2014). Suicide mortality after spinal cord injury in the United States: injury cohorts analysis. *Archives of Physical Medicine and Rehabilitation, 95*, 230–235.

Charlifue, S. W., & Gerhart, K. A. (1991). Behavioral and demographic predictors of suicide after traumatic spinal cord injury. *Archives of Physical Medicine and Rehabilitation, 72*(7), 488–492.

Christensen, J., Vestergaard, M., Mortensen, P., Sidenius, P., & Agerbo, E. (2007). Epilepsy and risk of suicide: A population-based case-control study. *Lancet Neurology, 6*(8), 693–698.

Clarke, D. M., McLeod, J. E., Smith, G. C., Trauer, T., & Kissane, D. W. (2005). A comparison of psychosocial and physical functioning in patients with motor neurone disease and metastatic cancer. *Journal of Palliative Care, 21*(3), 173–179.

Dennis, J. P., Ghahramanlou-Holloway, M., Cox, D. W., & Brown, G. K. (2011). A guide for the assessment and treatment of suicidal patients with traumatic brain injuries. *The Journal of Head Trauma Rehabilitation, 26*, 244–256.

DeVivo, M. J., Black, K. J., Richards, J. S., & Stover, S. L. (1991). Suicide following spinal cord injury. *Paraplegia, 29*(9), 620–627.

Di Maio, L., Squitieri, F., Napolitano, G., Campanella, G., Trofatter, J. A., & Conneally, P. M. (1993). Suicide risk in Huntington's disease. *Journal of Medical Genetics, 30*(4), 293–295.

Fang, F., Valdimarsdóttir, U., Fürst, C. J., Hultman, C., Fall, K., Sparén, P., & Ye, W. (2008). Suicide among people with amyotrophic lateral sclerosis. *Brain, 131*(10), 2729–2733.

Farberow, N. L. (1980). The many faces of suicide: Indirect self-destructive behavior, classification and characteristics. In N. L. Farberow (Ed.), *The many faces of suicide: Indirect self-destructive behavior, classification and characteristics* (pp. 15–17). New York: McGraw-Hill.

Farrer, L. A., Opitz, J. M., & Reynolds, J. F. (1986). Suicide and attempted suicide in Huntington disease: Implications for preclinical testing of persons at risk. *American Journal of Medical Genetics, 24*(2), 305–311.

Fazel, S., Wolf, A., Pllas, D., Lichtenstein, P., & Långström, N. (2014). Suicide, fatal injuries, and other causes of premature mortality in patients with traumatic injury: A 41-year Swedish population study. *JAMA Psychiatry, 71*(3), 326–333.

Feinstein, A. (2002). An examination of suicidal intent in patients with multiple sclerosis. *Neurology, 59*(5), 674–678.

Fisher, L. B., Pedrelli, P., Iverson, G. L., Bergquist, T. F., Bombardier, C. H., Hammond, F. M., . . . & Zafonte, R. (2016). Prevalence of suicidal behaviour following traumatic brain injury: longitudinal follow-up data from the NIDRR traumatic brain injury model systems. *Brain Injury, 30*, 1311–1318.

Fisk, J. D., Morehouse, S. A., Brown, M. G., Skedgel, C., & Murray, T. J. (1998). Hospital-based psychiatric service utilization and morbidity in multiple sclerosis. *Canadian Journal of Neurological Science, 25*(3), 230–235.

Fonda, J. R., Fredman, L., Brogly, S. B., McGlinchey, R. E., Milberg, W. P., & Gradus, J. L. (2017). Traumatic brain injury and attempted suicide among veterans of the wars in Iraq and Afghanistan. *American Journal of Epidemiology, 186*, 220–226.

Fralick, M., Sy, E., Hassan, A., Burke, M. J., Mostofsky, E., & Karsies, T. (2018). Association of concussion with the risk of suicide: A systematic review and meta-analysis. *JAMA Neurology.* doi:10.1001/jamaneurol.2018.3487

Fralick, M., Thiruchelvam, D., Tien, H. C., & Redelmeier, D. A. (2016). Risk of suicide after a concussion. *Canadian Medical Association Journal, 188*, 497–504.

Fredrikson, S., Cheng, Q., Jiang, G.-X., & Wasserman, D. (2003). Elevated suicide risk among patients with multiple sclerosis in Sweden. *Neuroepidemiology, 22*(2), 146–152.

Fuller-Thomson, E., Tulipano, M. J., & Song, M. (2012). The association between depression, suicidal ideation and stroke in a population-based sample. *International Journal of Stroke, 7*(3), 188–194.

Gale, C. R., Braidwood, E. A., Winter, P. D., & Martyn, C. N. (1999). Mortality from Parkinson's disease and other causes in men who were prisoners of war in the Far East. *Lancet, 354*(9196), 2116–2118.

Ganzini, L., Silveira, M. J., & Johnston, W. S. (2002). Predictors and correlates of interest in assisted suicide in the final month of life among ALS patients in Oregon and Washington. *Journal of Pain and Symptom Management, 24*(3), 312–317.

Garden, F. H., Garrison, S. J., & Jain, A. (1990). Assessing suicide risk in stroke patients: Review of two cases. *Archives of Physical Medicine and Rehabilitation, 71*(12), 1003–1005.

Graham, A., Reser, J., Scuderi, C., Zubrick, S., Smith, M., & Turley, B. (2000). Suicide: An Australian psychological society discussion paper. *Australian Psychologist, 35*, 1–28.

Hagen, E. M., Lie, S. A., Rekand, T., Gilhus, N. E., & Gronning, M. (2010). Mortality after traumatic spinal cord injury: 50 years of follow-up. *Journal of Neurology, Neurosurgery and Psychiatry, 81*(4), 368–373.

Hara, E., Akanuma, N., Adachi, N., Hara, K., & Koutroumanidis, M. (2009). Suicide attempts in adult patients with idiopathic generalized epilepsy. *Psychiatry and Clinical Neurosciences, 63*(2), 225–229.

Harris, E. C., & Barraclough, B. M. (1994). Suicide as an outcome or medical disorders. *Medicine, 73*(6), 281–296

Harris, E. C., & Barraclough, B. (1997). Suicide as an outcome for mental disorders. *British Journal of Psychiatry, 170*(3), 205–228.

Harrison-Felix, C., Kreider, S., Arango-Lasprilla, J. C., Brown, A. W., Dijkers, M., . . . Zasler, N. D. (2012). Life expectancy following rehabilitation: A NIDRR Traumatic Brain Injury Model systems study. *Journal of Head Trauma Rehabilitation, 27*(6), E69–E80.

Harrison-Felix, C., Whiteneck, G., Jha, A., DeVivo, M. J., Hammond, F. M., & Hart, D. M. (2009). Mortality over four decades after traumatic brain injury rehabilitation: A retrospective cohort study. *Archives of Physical Medicine and Rehabilitation, 90*(9), 1506–1513.

Hartkopp, A., Brønnum-Hansen, H., Seidenschnur, A.-M., & Biering-Sørensen, F. (1997). Survival and cause of death after traumatic spinal cord injury: A long-term epidemiological survey from Denmark. *Spinal Cord, 35*(2), 76–85.

Hartkopp, A., Brønnum-Hansen, H., Seidenschnur, A.-M., & Biering-Sørensen, F. (1998). Suicide in a spinal cord injured population: Its relation to functional status. *Archives of Physical Medicine and Rehabilitation, 79*(11), 1356–1361.

Hawton, K., Fagg, J., & Marsack, P. (1980). Association between epilepsy and attempted suicide. *Journal of Neurology, Neurosurgery and Psychiatry, 43*(2), 168–170.

Homaifar, B. Y., Brenner, L. A., Forster, J. E., & Nagamoto, H. (2012). Traumatic brain injury, executive functioning, and suicidal behavior: A brief report. *Rehabilitation Psychology, 57*(4), 337–341. doi: 10.1037/a0030480

Ilie, G., Mann, R. E., Boak, A., Adlaf, E. M., Hamilton, H., Asbridge, M., . . . Cusimano, M. D. (2014). Suicidality, bullying and other conduct and mental health correlates of traumatic brain injury in adolescents. *PLoS ONE, 9*(4), e94936

Jones, J. E., Hermann, B. P., Barry, J. J., Gilliam, F. G., Kanner, A. M., & Meador, K. J. (2003). Rates and risk factors for suicide, suicidal ideation and suicide attempts in chronic epilepsy. *Epilepsy and Behavior, 4*, 31–38.

Jorge, R. E., Robinson, R. G., & Arndt, S. (1993). Are there symptoms that are specific for depressed mood in patients with traumatic brain injury? *The Journal of Nervous and Mental Disease, 181*(2), 91–99.

Juurlink, D., Herrmann, N., Szalai, J. P., Kopp, A., & Redelmeier, D. A. (2004). Medical illness and the risk of suicide in the elderly. *Archives of Internal Medicine, 164*(11), 1179–1184.

Kalinin, V. V., & Polyanskiy, D. A. (2005). Gender differences in risk factors of suicidal behavior in epilepsy. *Epilepsy and Behavior, 6*(3), 424–429.

Kennedy, P., Rogers, B., Speer, S., & Frankel, H. (1999). Spinal cord injuries and attempted suicide: A retrospective review. *Spinal Cord, 37*(12), 847–852.

Kennedy, P., & Garmon-Jones, L. (2017). Self-harm and suicide before and after spinal cord injury: a systematic review. *Spinal Cord, 55*, 2–7.

Kishi, Y., Kosier, J. T., & Robinson, R. G. (1996a). Suicidal plans in patients with acute stroke. *The Journal of Nervous and Mental Disease, 184*(5), 274–280.

Kishi, Y., Robinson, R. G., & Kosier, J. T. (1996b). Suicidal plans in patients with stroke: Comparison between acute-onset and delayed-onset suicidal plans. *International Psychogeriatrics, 8*(4), 623–634.

Kostić, V. S., Pekmezović, T., Tomić, A., Ječmenica-Lukić, M., Stojković, T., Špica, V., ... Džoljić, E. (2010). Suicide and suicidal ideation. *Journal of the Neurological Sciences, 289*(1), 40–43.

Kuipers, P., & Lancaster, A. (2000). Developing a suicide prevention strategy based on the perspectives of people with brain injuries. *The Journal of Head Trauma Rehabilitation, 15*, 1275–1284.

Kummer, A., Cardoso, F., & Teixeira, A. L. (2009). Suicidal ideation in Parkinson's Disease. *CNS Spectrum, 14*(8), 431–436.

Leenars, A. A. (2008). Suicide: A cross-cultural theory. In F. T. L. Leong & M. M. Leach (Eds.), *Suicide among racial and ethnic minority groups: Theory, research and practice* (pp.13–38). New York: Taylor & Frances.

Leentjens, A. F. G., Marinus, J., Van Hilten, J. J., Lousberg, R., & Verhey, F. R. J. (2003). The contribution of somatic symptoms to the diagnosis of depressive disorder in Parkinson's Disease: A discriminant analytic approach. *Journal of Neuropsychiatry and Clinical Neurosciences, 15*(1), 74–77.

Lewin, W., Marshall, T. F., & Roberts, A. H. (1979). Long-term outcome after severe head injury. *British Medical* Journal, *2*(6204), 1533–1538.

Lidal, I. B., Snekkevik, H., Aamodt, G., Hjeltnes, N., Stanghelle, J. K., & Biering-Sørensen, F. (2007). Mortality after spinal cord injury in Norway. *Journal of Rehabilitation Medicine, 39*(2), 145–151.

Lipe, H., Schultz, A., & Bird, T. D. (1993). Risk factors for suicide in Huntingtons Disease: A retrospective case controlled study. *American Journal of Medical Genetics Part A, 48*(4), 231–233.

Mackelprang, J. L., Bombadier, C. H., Fann, J. R., Temkin, N. R., Barber, J. K., & Dikmen, S. S. (2014). Rates and predictors of suicidal ideation during the first year after traumatic brain injury. *American Journal of Public Health, 104*, e100–e107.

Macleod, A. D. (1988). Self-neglect of spinal injured patients. *Paraplegia, 26*(5), 340–349.

Madsen, T., Erlangsen, A., Orlovska, S., Mofaddy, R., Nordentoft, M., & Benros, M. E. (2018). Association between traumatic brain injury and risk of suicide. *JAMA, 320*, 580–588.

McCullumsmith, C. B., Kalpakjian, C. Z., Richards, J. S., Forchheimer, M., Heinemann, A. W., Richardson, E. J., ... & Fann, J. R. (2015). Novel risk factors associated with current suicidal ideation and lifetime suicide attempts in individuals with spinal cord injury. *Archives of Physical Medicine and Rehabilitation, 96*, 799–808.

McMillan, T. M., & Teasdale, G. M. (2007). Death rate is increased for at least 7 years after head injury: A prospective study. *Brain, 130*(10), 2520–2527.

McMillan, T. M., Teasdale, G. M., Weir, C. J., & Stewart, E. (2011). Death after head injury: The 13 year outcome of a case control study. *Journal of Neurology, Neurosurgery and Psychiatry, 82,* 931–935.

Mendez, M. F., Lanska, D. J., Manon-Espaillat, R., & Burnstine, T. H. (1989). Causative factors for suicide attempts by overdose in epileptics. *Archives of Neurology, 46*(10), 1065–1068.

Myslobodsky, M., Lalonde, F. M., & Hicks, L. (2001). Are patients with Parkinson's Disease suicidal? *Journal of Geriatric Psychiatry and Neurology, 14*(3), 120–124.

Nazem, S., Siderowf, A. D., Duda, J. E., Brown, G. K., Have, T. T., Stern, M. B., & Weintraub, D. (2008). Suicidal and death ideation in Parkinson's disease. *Movement Disorders, 23*(11), 1573–1579.

Nilsson, L., Ahlbom, A., Farahmand, B. Y., Åsberg, M., & Tomson, T. (2002). Risk factors for suicide in epilepsy: A case control study. *Epilepsia, 43*(6), 644–651.

Palmieri, A., Sorarù, G., Albertini, E., Semenza, C., Vottero-Ris, F., D'Ascenzo, C., . . . Angelini, C. (2010). Psychopathological features and suicidal ideation in amyotrophic lateral sclerosis patients. *Neurological Sciences, 31*(6), 735–740.

Patten, S. B., Francis, G., Metz, L. M., Lopez-Bresnahan, M., Chang, P., & Curtin, F. (2005). The relationship between depression and interferon beta-1a therapy in patients with multiple sclerosis. *Multiple Sclerosis, 11*(2), 175–181.

Paulsen, J. S., Hoth, K. F., Nehl, C., & Stierman, L.; Huntington Study Group. (2005). Critical periods of suicide risk in Huntington's disease. *American Journal of Psychiatry, 162*(4), 725–731.

Pohjasvaara, T., Vataja, R., Leppävuori, A., Kaste, M., & Erkinjuntti, T. (2001). Suicidal ideas in stroke patients 3 and 15 months after stroke. *Cerebrovascular Disease, 12*(1), 21–26.

Savic, G., DeVivo, M. J., Frankel, H. L., Jamous, M. A., Soni, B. M., & Charlifue, S. (2017). Long-term survival after traumatic spinal cord injury: a 70-year British study. *Spinal Cord, 55,* 651.

Schoenfeld, M., Myers, R. H., Cupples, A., Berkman, B., Sax, D. S., & Clark, E. (1984). Increased rate of suicide among patients with Huntington's disease. *Journal of Neurology, Neurosurgery and Psychiatry, 47*(12), 1283–1287.

Scott, K. M., Hwang, I., Chiu, W.-T., Kessler, R. C., Sampson, N. A., Angermeyer, M., . . . Florescu, S. (2010). Chronic physical conditions and their association with first onset of suicidal behaviour in the world mental health surveys. *Psychosomatic Medicine, 72*(7), 712–719.

Seel, R. T., & Kreutzer, J. S. (2003). Depression assessment after traumatic brain injury: An empirically based classification method. *Archives of Physical Medicine and Rehabilitation, 84*(11), 1621–1628.

Shavelle, R. M., Strauss, D., Whyte, J., Day, S. M., & Yu, Y. L. (2001).Long-term causes of death after traumatic brain injury. *Archives of Physical Medicine and Rehabilitation, 80*(7), 510–516.

Shoulson, I., Kurlan, R., Rubin, A., Goldblatt, D., Behr, J., Miller, C., . . . & Plumb, S. (1989). Assessment of functional capacity in neurodegenerative movement disorders: Huntington's disease as a prototype. In T.L. Munsat (Ed.), *Quantification of Neurologic Deficit* (pp. 271–283). Boston: Butterworths.

Silver, J. M., Kramer, R., Greenwald, S., & Weissman, M. (2001). The association between head injuries and psychiatric disorders: Findings from the New Haven NIMH Epidemiologic Catchment Area study. *Brain Injury, 15*(11), 935–945.

Simpson, G. K., & Tate, R. L. (2002). Suicidality after traumatic brain injury: Demographic, injury and clinical correlates. *Psychological Medicine, 32*(4), 687–697.

Simpson, G. K., & Tate, R. L. (2005). Clinical features of suicide attempts after TBI. *The Journal of Nervous and Mental Disease, 193*(10), 680–685.

Simpson, G. K., & Tate, R. L. (2007). Suicidality in people surviving a traumatic brain injury: Prevalence, risk factors and implications for clinical management. *Brain Injury, 21*(13-14), 1335–1351.

Sliwinski, M., Gordon, W. A., & Bogdany, J. (1998). The Beck Depression Inventory: Is it a suitable measure of depression for people with traumatic brain injury? *Journal of Head Trauma Rehabilitation, 13*(4), 40–46.

Soden, R. J., Walsh, J., Middleton, J. W., Craven, M. L., Rutkowski, S. B., & Yeo, J. D. (2000). Causes of death after spinal cord injury. *Spinal Cord, 38*(10), 604–610.

Soulas, T., Gurruchaga, J.-M., Palfi, S., Cesaro, P., Nguyen, J.-P., & Fénelon, G. (2008). Attempted and completed suicides after subthalamic nucleus stimulation for Parkinson's disease. *Journal of Neurology, Neurosurgery and Psychiatry, 79*(8), 952–954.

Stanford, R. E., Soden, R., Bartrop, R., Mikk, M., & Taylor, T. K. F. (2007). Spinal cord and related injuries after attempted suicide: Psychiatric diagnosis and long-term follow-up. *Spinal Cord, 45*(6), 437–443.

Stenager, E. N., Jensen, B., Stenager, M., Stenager, K., & Stenager, E. (2011). Suicide attempts in multiple sclerosis. *Multiple Sclerosis Journal, 17*(10), 1265–1268.

Stenager, E. N., Madsen, C., Stenager, E., & Boldsen, J. (1998). Suicide in patients with stroke: Epidemiological study. *British Medical Journal, 316*(7139), 1206–1210.

Stenager, E. N., & Stenager, E. (1992). Suicide and patients with neurologic diseases: Methodologic problems. *Archives of Neurology, 49*(12), 1296–1303

Stenager, E. N., Stenager, E., Koch-Henriksen, N., Brønnum-Hansen, H., Hyllested, K., Jensen, K., & Bille-Brahe, U. (1992). Suicide and multiple sclerosis: An epidemiological investigation. *Journal of Neurology, Neurosurgery & Psychiatry, 55*(7), 542–545.

Tate, R., Simpson, G., Flanagan, S., & Coffey, M. (1997). Completed suicide after traumatic brain injury. *Journal of Head Trauma Rehabilitation, 12*(6), 16–28.

Teasdale, T. W., & Engberg, A. W. (2001a). Suicide after a stroke: A population study. *Journal of Epidemiology and Community Health, 55*(12), 863–866.

Teasdale, T. W., & Engberg, A. W. (2001b). Suicide after traumatic brain injury: A population study. *Journal of Neurology, Neurosurgery & Psychiatry, 71*(4), 436–440.

Tellez-Zenteno, J. F., Patten, S. B., Jetté, N., Williams, J., & Wiebe, S. (2007). Psychiatric comorbidity in epilepsy: A population-based analysis. *Epilepsia, 48*(12), 2336–2344.

Tsaousides, T., Cantor, J. B., & Gordon, W. A. (2011). Suicidal ideation following traumatic brain injury: Prevalence rates and correlates in adults living in the community. *Journal of Head Trauma Rehabilitation, 26*(4), 265–275.

Turner, A. P., Williams, R. M., Bowen, J. D., Kivlahan, D. R., & Haselkorn, J. K. (2006). Suicidal ideation in multiple sclerosis. *Archives of Physical Medicine and Rehabilitation, 87*(8), 1073–1078.

US Department of Health and Human Services (USDHHS), Office of the Surgeon General and National Action Alliance for Suicide Prevention. (2012). *2012 National strategy for suicide prevention: Goals and objectives for action.* Washington, DC: HHS.

Utsey, S. O., Giesbrecht, N., Hook, J., & Stanard, P. M. (2008). Cultural, sociofamilial, and psychological resources that inhibit psychological distress in African Americans exposed to stressful life events and race-related stress. *Journal of Counseling Psychology, 55,* 49–62.

Veldink, J. H., Wokke, J. H., van der Wal, G., Vianney de Jong, J. M. B., & van den Berg, L. H. (2002). Euthanasia and physician-assisted suicide among patients with amyotrophic lateral sclerosis in the Netherlands. *New England Journal of Medicine, 346*(21), 1638–1644.

Ventura, T., Harrison-Felix, C., Carlson, N., DiGuiseppi, C., Gabella, B., Brown, A., . . . Whiteneck, G. (2010). Mortality after discharge from acute care hospitalization with traumatic brain injury: A population-based study. *Archives of Physical Medicine and Rehabilitation, 91*(1), 20–29.

Viner, R., Patten, S. B., Berzins, S., Bulloch, A. G., & Fiest, K. M. (2014). Prevalence and risk factors for suicidal ideation in a multiple sclerosis population. *Journal of Psychosomatic Research, 76,* 312–316.

Voon, V., Krack, P., Lang, A. E., Lozano, A. M., Dujardin, K., Schüpbach, M., . . . Speelman, J. D. (2008). A multicentre study on suicide outcomes following subthalamic stimulation for Parkinson's disease. *Brain, 131*(10), 2720–2728.

Waern, M., Rubenowitz, E., Runeson, B., Skoog, I., Wilhelmson, K., & Allebeck, P. (2002). Burden of illness and suicide in elderly people: Case-control study. *British Medical Journal, 324*(7350), 1355–1358.

Webb, R. T., Kontopantelis, E., Doran, T., Qin, P., Creed, F., & Kapur, N. (2012). Suicide risk in primary care patients with major physical diseases: A case-control study. *Archives of General Psychiatry, 69*(3), 256–264.

Wetzel, H. H., Gehl, C. R., Dellefave–Castillo, L., Schiffman, J. F., Shannon, K. M., Paulsen, J. S.; Huntington Study Group. (2011). Suicidal ideation in Huntington disease: The role of comorbidity. *Psychiatry Research, 188*(3), 372–376.

Wood, R. L., Williams, C., & Lewis, R. (2010). Role of alexithymia in suicide ideation after traumatic brain injury. *Journal of the International Neuropsychological Society, 16,* 1108–1114.

Wu, M.-Y., & Chan, F. (2007). Psychosocial adjustment patterns of persons with spinal cord injury. *Disability and Rehabilitation, 29*(24), 1847–1857.

II Suicide Prevention after Neurodisability

7   Screening for Suicide Risk

Introduction

The first part of this book focused on defining neurodisability and suicide and exploring what theory and neurobiology can tell us about the etiology of the problem. Following this, current evidence about the epidemiology, risk factors, and protective factors were detailed. The second part of the book, starting with this chapter, focuses on suicide prevention.

Suicide prevention is a multifaceted activity. The early identification and assessment of suicide risk is an important initial step in the prevention and management of suicidal behavior (Marušič et al., 2009). A positive finding arising from screening should trigger a fuller suicide risk assessment. In healthcare more generally, screening for many different types of physical or mental health conditions is a common clinical strategy. Screening can potentially identify any history of the clinical issue targeted, as well as the presence of current symptoms (Bahraini & Brenner, 2013). This chapter will provide the rationale for screening for suicide risk, the clinical delivery of screening, issues in the implementation and efficacy of screening, and screening for suicide risk after neurodisability.

Rationale for Screening

The rationale for screening is that the presence of suicide risk is often not spontaneously reported by clients or is underidentified by clinical staff (Druss & Pincus, 2000; Ganzini et al., 2013; Gould et al., 2005). Once clinically meaningful risk has been detected, evidence-informed treatments can be initiated to address suicidal thoughts and behaviors as well as comorbid mental health problems (Druss & Pincus, 2000; Gould et al., 2005). Moreover, as suicidal distress is typically associated with identifiable risk factors, some of which are modifiable (e.g., depression), additional strategies can be employed to address these potential drivers of suicidal behavior (Gould et al., 2005).

Suicidal thoughts and behaviors are often conceptualized as lying along a continuum of growing intensity, and so screening increases the prospect of being able to intervene at the earliest possible moment along that continuum to reduce the level of suicidal distress and the potential danger for self-directed violence. The importance of considering screening among members of the general population is reflected in the recommendation from the 2012 US National Strategy for Suicide Prevention (USDHHS, 2012) that healthcare systems, insurers, and clinicians screen for mental health needs, including suicidal thoughts and behaviors (Objective 5.3).

One example of the possible benefits, but also of the scale of the challenge in conducting screening, is provided in a recent US study. Simon et al. (2013) examined subsequent deaths by suicide among 84,418 outpatients from Washington or Idaho who completed 207,265 Patient Health Questionnaire-9 (PHQ-9) depression questionnaires during a visit to a primary care or mental health provider. There was a 0.03% cumulative risk of suicide death over the following year among patients who reported no suicide ideation (SI; thoughts of death or self-harm, item 9 on the PHQ-9 Depression Questionnaire) compared to a 0.3% cumulative risk of death among patients who reported thoughts of death or self-harm "nearly every day." Although self-reported ideation was a predictor of death by suicide, it should also be noted that approximately one fifth of the attempts and one fifth of the suicide deaths occurred among the 70% of individuals who responded "not at all"; thereby highlighting the need to identify risk via multiple modalities (Simon et al., 2013).

Clinical Delivery of Screening

Screening approaches may be broadly targeted at a population level (e.g., all people with neurodisability) or at people within various types of neurodisability identified as being of clinical concern (i.e., emotionally distressed and/or displaying a number of risk factors associated with elevated suicide risk). Whichever the focus, the screening strategy needs to be grounded in a clear underlying definition of suicidal behavior (Brown, 2000; Bryan & Rudd, 2006). For example, to ask clients about thoughts of dying, an item included in some suicide measures, is not the same as asking about intent to end one's life. Standardized definitions of SI and suicide attempts have been delineated in Chapter 3. Clinical questions or observations conducted as part of screening need to be consistent with these definitions.

Screening can comprise various activities ranging from eliciting information as part of a broader health/clinical interview, through to the use of various validated measures. Starting with the clinical interview, asking a patient about SI is the most direct method for assessing imminent risk of self-directed violence (Druss & Pinkus, 2000). However, Olfson, Weissman, Leon, Sheehan, and Farber (1996) have pointed out the difficulties of asking such a question without adequate context. One alternative is to ask about suicide within the framework of broader questions about other high-risk symptom clusters (e.g., sleep disturbance, mood disturbance, feelings of guilt; Cooper-Patrick, Crum, & Ford, 1994), but this more extensive approach can be time-consuming. Another option is to provide self-administered screening inventories that identify patients at risk for mental disorders (e.g., Spitzer et al., 1994; Broadhead et al., 1995) and then follow-up more closely with patients who have responded to items that are flagged as needing further investigation (when endorsed). Self-administration of computer-based screening tools provides another option, although some users have seen this process as perfunctory and disrespectful (Ganzini et al., 2013).

Several measures have been employed as suicide screening instruments, with the scope of the clinical content varying widely. Screening instruments can focus solely on suicidal behaviors, such as lifetime and current history of ideation and/ or attempts (e.g., Scale for Suicide Ideation, Beck, Kovacs, & Weissman, 1979; Suicide Behaviors Questionnaire, Cotton & Range, 1993; Suicidal Ideation Questionnaire, Reynolds, 1988), suicide risk factors and suicidal behaviors (e.g., Suicide Probability Scale; Cull & Gill, 1988; Suicide Risk Screen, Eggart, Thompson, & Herting, 1994), or screens for mental health conditions that in-clude an SI item (e.g., PHQ-9 Depression Questionnaire; Spitzer, Kroenke, & Williams, 1999).

One example of a broad screening approach is the use of the SAD PERSONS, a brief measure of suicide risk (Hockberger & Rothstein, 1988). The acronym signifies 10 key risk factors; namely, sex (male), age (younger than 20 or older than 45 years), depression, previous attempts, ethanol abuse, rational thinking loss, social support lacking, organized plan for suicide, no spouse or not living with relations, and sick-ness/poor physical health. Risk is calculated by scoring 1 point for each factor that is present (0–10), and bands of risk have been generated (0–2 low; 3–4 moderate; 5–6 high risk; 7–10 very high risk of suicide). Proper psychometric validation of SADS PERSONS is lacking (Bech & Awata, 2009).

Despite this, the possibility for introducing the SAD PERSONS to neurodisability has been suggested (Wasserman et al., 2008). However, it is yet to be tested, and there are some reasons for caution. First, two items may lead to underestimates of risk. Although the relatively larger numbers of male versus female deaths by suicide that exist in the general population are also maintained after neurodisability, therefore lending support to gender as a risk factor, the concern is that both sexes have a similar quantum of elevated risk in relation to the general population (as outlined in Chapter 6), and therefore both sexes need to be monitored. Second, the SAD PERSONS identifies under 20 and over 45 as the two age-related areas at elevated risk; however, as outlined in Chapter 6, for a number of neurodisability groups the standardized mortality ratios are elevated across all age groups under 50 or 60, once again increasing the possibility of underestimating risk. On the other hand, two items refer to the presence of organic brain damage and the loss of health. All people with neurodisability could be classified as scoring on these items, thereby potentially inflating the level of risk as well as reducing the discriminatory value for the screen to identify true positives.

Different service contexts (e.g., hospitals, community agencies, sole therapists) will influence the selection of the most appropriate screening strategy. Whatever form the screening takes (whether as a question in a clinical interview or through the administration of a validated measure), there is a danger that if the process becomes too mechanistic or bureaucratic, this potentially can reduce the reliability of responses provided by the clients being screened (Ganzini et al., 2013). In a study investigating client accounts of undergoing mental health assessment, veterans were more likely to report a positive experience if they (1) had sufficient time to respond to the questions, (2) perceived that the clinician conducting the assessment was genuine, and (3) were provided with a rationale and the goals of the assessment (Taylor, Hawton, Fortune, & Kapur, 2009).

Issues in the Implementation of Screening

Several issues arise in the therapeutic delivery of screening and possible harms that might be caused. Whether by clinical question or screening measure, the therapeutic delivery of the screening is important to consider. In a qualitative study, Ganzini and colleagues (2013) interviewed US military veterans about their experiences of having participated in suicide screening. Deriving from their analysis of the veterans' responses, the authors have proposed four domains that require consideration in the implementation of screening: namely (1) the therapeutic relationship within which the screening is undertaken, (2) the importance of empathy/genuineness, (3) the communication approach, and (4) the information that should be delivered to provide context for the screening (see Ganzini et al., 2013).

Perceived potential harms include the possibility that asking people about suicide increases the risk that people will attempt suicide. In relation to this concern, if handled sensitively, an interview which includes the issue of suicide is more likely to be beneficial and decrease the degree of suicidal distress (Graham et al., 2000). In the United States, suicide and mental health screening has been investigated among adolescents in high school (e.g., Gould et al., 2005). The authors found no iatrogenic risks associated with screening, but instead some lessening of the intensity of SI, presumably related to the opportunity it provided for participants to share their feelings (Gould et al., 2005).

Harms may also arise from overscreening. US military veterans may be exposed to multiple screening occasions as they access different providers and progress through different service settings. The veterans reported that they found this to be repetitive, annoying, frustrating, and a waste of time and that it reflected a lack of communication among service providers (Ganzini et al., 2013).

The Efficacy of Screening

Evidence for the efficacy of screening is most commonly demonstrated by reference to sensitivity and specificity of detection rates in correctly identifying individuals who have a history or current levels of suicidal thoughts or behaviors. A number of the screening instruments referred to in this chapter have relatively low specificity (in the range of .50 to .70). Gaynes et al. (2004) raise a cautionary note about the logistics of screening for suicide, highlighting the relatively poor positive predictive values that screening tools with typical levels of sensitivity (e.g., 0.80) and specificity (e.g., 0.70) achieve and the associated large numbers of false positives generated. Furthermore, the criterion standard against which detection rates are often calibrated is a retrospective history of suicide, with few screening measures tested prospectively and tested against the gold standard of a structured clinical interview (Shaffer et al., 2004). Finally, there is limited evidence for the longer term impact of screening on suicide mortality rates (Gaynes et al., 2004) due to the low base rate for suicide. In considering screening for suicidal thoughts and behaviors after neurodisability, it will be useful to keep some of these considerations from the broader litera-ture in mind.

Screening for Suicide Risk after Neurodisability

In response to the findings of elevated suicide after neurodisability, screening is one of the most frequently suggested front-line responses. Screening for suicide has been proposed for cerebrovascular accident (CVA; Fuller-Thompson, Tulipano, & Song, 2012), epilepsy (Pompili, Girardi, Tatarelli, Angeletti, & Tatarelli, 2006; Robertson, 1997), Huntington's disease (HD; Wetzel et al., 2011), multiple sclerosis (MS; Turner, Williams, Bowen, Kivlahan, & Haselkorn, 2006; Gaskill, Foley, W., Kolzet, & Picone, 2011), Parkinson's disease (PD; Voon et al., 2008), traumatic brain injury (TBI; Breshears, Brenner, Harwood, & Gutierrez, 2010; Simpson & Tate, 2007; Wasserman et al., 2008), and spinal cord injury (SCI; Soden et al., 2000; Kennedy, Rogers, Speer, & Frankel,1999). Despite these calls, there has been little discussion about how any such screening should be implemented.

The first question that arises is who should be screened. There are at least three options: (1) all people with neurodisability (e.g., either stand-alone or as part of a broader screen for mental health problems), (2) particularly high risk subgroups (e.g., people with neurodisability and comorbid substance abuse), or (3) those with neurodisability and with a known history of suicidal thoughts or behavior. In terms of screening the whole population, one suggestion has been to expand mental health screening to include suicide risk. For example, in the context of HD, Wetzel and colleagues (2011) suggested that screening for psychiatric conditions targeting all people with HD but with a specific emphasis on those with comorbid mental health conditions (e.g., depression, substance abuse, etc.) might be a useful approach and could incorporate an item or clinical question about SI.

One measure designed specifically for conducting population-based mental health screening could play such a role. The clinician-rated Health of the Nation Outcome Scale includes an item on SI, and a validated version for neurodisability has been developed (Health of the Nation Outcome Scale-Acquired Brain Injury; Coetzer & Du Toit, 2001; Fleminger et al., 2005). An alternative to screening across the whole population is to be more selective.

Another option is to target those more specifically with depression, given the strong correlation documented between depression and suicidal thoughts and behaviors after neurodisability (see Chapter 6). Going down this avenue, two pos-sible approaches are to use a depression screen or a full depression measure. In regards to the first of these approaches, the limited empirical investigation conducted to date has found that depression screens produced only modest results in detecting suicide risk after neurodisability. Among US veterans with MS, the 2-question depression screen (depression and anhedonia items from the PHQ-9; US Preventative Services Task Force, 2002) displayed only marginal sensitivity and specificity in identifying individuals who had reported SI in the 2 previous weeks (65.6% and 79.9%, respectively), although stronger results were found for persistent SI (88.6% and 71.2%, respectively; Turner et al., 2006, p. 1077).

An alternative approach would be to employ full depression scales rather than depression screens. Evidence for the usefulness of the PHQ-9 has been demonstrated in a cohort of people admitted to hospital with complicated mild to severe TBI (Mackelprang et al., 2014). However, Hackett, Hill, Hewison, Anderson, and House (2010) have reported results among people with CVA that raise similar concerns about the possible underidentification of cases. Data collected in two longitudinal studies of depression after CVA (New Zealand, United Kingdom) were analyzed. Up to 28% of participants who did not meet case criteria for depression as defined either by a full psychological distress scale (General Health Questionnaire-28; Bridges & Goldberg, 1986) or a single-item depression screen (Wing, Cooper, & Sartorius, 1974) still reported symptoms including worthlessness, hopelessness, or SI (Hackett et al., 2010).

Reinforcing this finding from another perspective, the predictive power of the individual symptoms of the PHQ-9 in predicting the presence of a major depressive disorder among people with SCI has been examined (Bombadier, Richards, Krause, Tulsky, & Tate, 2004). The SI item (thoughts of death) was only a marginally significant predictor of major depressive disorder. Specifically, the SI item had a low positive predictive value (41.1%) indicating that a large proportion of people reporting this item did not have major depression.

These findings reinforce the general observation made in respect of TBI (Wasserman et al., 2008; Simpson, Tate, Whiting & Cotter, 2011) and MS (Sadovnick, Eisen, Ebers, & Paty, 1991) that suicide is not always secondary to a diagnosed depressive disorder. Therefore, targeting depression alone (either through a depression screen or full depression scale) *will not* identify everyone who has SI. For example, Hackett et al. (2010) concluded that if the presence of clinical depression was the threshold for triggering the administration of a suicide screen, 3 in 10 participants with CVA reporting SI would have potentially not have received clinical attention.

In the absence of an existing screening program, several options have been highlighted that could be introduced, ranging from key clinical questions to suicide screens, SI questionnaires, depression screens, mental health screens, and depression questionnaires (e.g., Caine & Schwid, 2002, MS; Fuller-Thompson et al., 2012, CVA; Jones et al., 2003, epilepsy). If the screening is implemented as an expansion of existing depression screens, Hackett et al. (2010) have suggested that this could be achieved by adding one or more items on suicide. In the case of full depression measures, not every depression measure used in the field of neurodisability has an item for SI (e.g., Hospital Anxiety and Depression Scale; Zigmond & Snaith, 1983; Depression Anxiety Stress Scale; Lovibond & Lovibond, 1995). If a full depression measure is already employed, then ensuring that positive responses on any SI items are followed-up (Desseilles, Gosselin, & Peroud, 2013), even if overall depression scores do not meet a case level for intervention, is important.

The timing of screening has also been canvassed. Elevated suicide risk during high-risk transition periods has been identified in the broader suicide prevention literature (Brenner & Barnes, 2012). This concept has found application in the field of neurodisability. Authors have flagged certain crisis points within the natural course of neurodisability during which suicide risk may be increased and screening indicated. These have included the confirmation of diagnosis and times of disease progression in MS (Stenager et al., 1992), early post-injury and during the rehabilitation phase in SCI (Soden et al., 2000), during the first year after diagnosis in ALS (Fang et al., 2008), pre- and post-surgery in epilepsy (Pompili et al., 2006), and among people with early-onset (i.e., >50 years of age) CVA (Teasdale & Engberg, 2001a; Stenager, Madsen, Stenager, & Boldsen, 1998). In contrast, some conditions display a chronicity of suicide risk that persists for decades without specific time periods of elevated risk (e.g., TBI; Teasdale & Engberg, 2001b; Achte, Lonnqvist, & Hillbom, 1971). In these circumstances, adding a suicide screen to any routine mental health assessments that are conducted may be the preferred option.

To be conducted effectively, the approach to screening is ideally conducted systemically as defined by policy and procedures (whether at the clinical practice, agency/unit level, or service system level; Marušič et al., 2009) rather than left to the personal initiative and judgment of individual clinicians. Universal screening may be justified given the high rates of current SI reported after most types of neurodisability (see Chapter 6). If universal screening is not viable, then targeting at-risk groups (e.g., people with depression, substance abuse, other mental health problems) is likely to be the best option.

An important question is to ask who conducts any such screening. Although enquiring about SI is considered mandatory in psychiatric consultations, it is seldom part of traditional medical or neurological assessment (Paulsen, Hoth, Nehl, & Stierman, 2005), and to this we could add rehabilitation. Psychologists, social workers, nurses, or other staff with mental health training could potentially conduct any such screening. Staff need to be able to manage any needs or adverse events arising from screening questions, although the limited evidence available suggests that such adverse effects are rare. For example, in the administration of the self-report Beck Scale for Suicide (Beck et al., 1979) to 172 outpatients with TBI, only three participants reported distress in response to the items (Simpson & Tate, 2002). Whatever approach is taken to screening, a clear corollary is that policies and procedures are established to guide appropriate service-level responses to positive cases.

When Suicide Is Identified as an Issue

The identification of a person as having suicidal thoughts or recent behaviors may arise from the results of screening or may arise within the context of some other routine clinical interaction with the client (e.g., the person discloses his or her feelings to a nurse on an inpatient ward or to an allied health member of staff during a therapy session) or the client's family and friends (i.e., informed by a family member of the client making comments such as "I would be better off dead" at home). However identified, it is then important to ensure that the client has the opportunity to see a mental health professional for a suicide risk assessment and, if needed, treatment.

It can be useful to first establish whether the issue of suicidal thoughts and behaviors is known to any mental health staff that is part of a treating team (e.g., asking the client, "Have you told anyone else that you have been feeling this way? Thinking of this? If so, who?"). In some cases, the staff member will have the competencies to conduct a suicide risk assessment. In those cases where this involves a referral, some clients will be quite willing to attend an appointment to address the reasons for their suicidal distress. Depending on the intensity of the clients' suicidal distress, this might involve remaining with the person (or ensuring someone else does) until the person can be seen. In cases where the client might be reluctant to attend an appointment, it might be possible to organize a joint interview involving the staff member to whom the disclosure was made and a suitable mental health professional.

Conclusion

Screening has been recommended as an important element of suicide prevention across all eight neurological conditions. However, there has been little exploration of how the screening might be conducted or examination of the results from conducting a screening. Given this absence of evidence, a range of possible approaches to screening people with neurodisability for suicide risk have been outlined. A positive finding of some degree of suicidal risk should trigger a suicide risk assessment. The content and processes for conducting such an assessment are the subject of the next chapter.

Implications for Clinicians

1. Screening is a commonly recommended option for the early detection of the presence of suicide risk after neurodisability

2. Screening can either be conducted among all clients of an agency or service, or, if that is not logistically possible, can be targeted to people with known risk factors (e.g., people with a history of SI, people with recent onset of MS).

3. Screening is likely to work best if it is part of existing routines in clinical practice and can take the form of a question about SI as part of a brief clinical interview, the administration of a validated suicide screening measure, or a suicide item contained in a depression measure.

4. Particularly in the context of clinical interviews, the use of language in asking about suicidal thoughts and behaviors needs to be consistent with standardized definitions.

5. Implementation of screening programs necessitates having policies and procedures in place to outline the clinical response to be taken following a positive screen.

6. A positive suicide screen should be followed by a more sensitive secondary screen or a suicide risk evaluation.

References

Achte, K. A., Lonnqvist, J., & Hillbom, E. (1971). Suicides following war brain-injuries. *Acta Psychiatrica Scandinavica*, Suppl, 1–94.

Bahraini, N., & Brenner, L. A. (2013). Screening for TBI and persistent symptoms provides opportunities for prevention and intervention. *Journal of Head Trauma Rehabilitation, 28*(3), 223–226.

Bech, P., & Awata, S. (2009). Measurement of suicidal behaviour with psychometric scales. In D. Wasserman & C. Wasserman (Eds.), *Oxford textbook of suicidology and suicide prevention: A global perspective* (pp. 305–311). New York: Oxford University Press.

Beck, A. T., Kovacs, M., & Weissman, A. (1979). Assessment of suicidal intention: The Scale for Suicide Ideation. *Journal of Consulting and Clinical Psychology, 47*(2), 343–352.

Bombadier, C. H., Richards, J. S., Krause, J. S., Tulsky D., & Tate, D. G. (2004). Symptoms of major depression in people with spinal cord injury: Implications for screening. *Archives of Physical Medicine and Rehabilitation, 85*(11), 1749–1756.

Brenner, L. A., & Barnes, S. M. (2012). Facilitating treatment engagement during high-risk transition periods: A potential suicide prevention strategy. *American Journal of Public Health* 102, Supplement 1, S12–S14.

Breshears, R. E., Brenner, L. A., Harwood, J. E., & Gutierrez, P. M. (2010). Predicting suicidal behavior in veterans with traumatic brain injury: The utility of the personality assessment inventory. *Journal of Personality Assessment, 92*(4), 349–355.

Bridges, K. W., & Goldberg, D. P. (1986). The validation of the GHQ-28 and the use of the MMSE in neurological in-patients. *The British Journal of Psychiatry, 148*(5), 548–553.

Broadhead, W. E., Leon, A. C., Weissman, M. M., Barrett, J. E., Blacklow, R. S., Gilbert, T. T., . . . Higgins, E. S. (1995). Development and validation of the SDDS-PC screen for multiple mental disorders in primary care. *Archives of Family Medicine, 4*(3), 211–219.

Brown, G. K. (2000). *A review of suicide assessment measures for intervention research with adults and older adults.* Retrieved from http://www.suicidology.org/c/document_library/get_file?folderId= 235& name=DLFE-113.pdf.

Bryan, C. J., & Rudd, M. D. (2006). Advances in the assessment of suicide risk. *Journal of Clinical Psychology, 62*(2), 185–200.

Caine, E. D., & Schwid, S. R. (2002). Multiple sclerosis, depression, and the risk of suicide. *Neurology, 59*(5), 662–663.

Coetzer, R., & Du Toit, P. L. (2001). HoNOS—ABI: A clinically useful outcome measure? *Psychiatric Bulletin, 25*(11), 421–422.

Cooper-Patrick, L., Crum, R. M., & Ford, D. E. (1994). Identifying suicidal ideation in general medical patients. *Journal of the American Medical Association, 272*(22), 1757–1762.

Cotton, C. R., & Range, L. M. (1993). Suicidality, hopelessness, and attitudes toward life and death in children. *Death Studies, 17*(2), 185–191.

Cull, J. G., & Gill, W. S. (1988). *Suicide probability scale.* Los Angeles, CA: Western Psychological Services.

Department of Veterans Affairs/ Department of Defense. (2013). *Clinical practice guideline for assessment and management of patients at risk for suicide.* Retrieved from https://www.healthquality.va.gov/guidelines/MH/srb/VADODCP_suiciderisk_full.pdf

Desseilles, M., Gosselin, N., & Perroud, N. (2013). Assessing suicide ideations in Traumatic Brain Injury (TBI) patients by using depression scales. *Journal of Head and Trauma Rehabilitation, 28*(2), 149–150.

Druss, B., & Pincus, H. (2000). Suicidal ideation and suicide attempts in general medical illnesses. *Archives of Internal Medicine, 160*(10), 1522–1526.

Eggert, L. L., Thompson, E. A., & Herting, J. R. (1994). A measure of adolescent potential for suicide (MAPS): Development and preliminary findings. *Suicide and Life-Threatening Behavior, 24*(4), 359–381.

Fang, F., Valdimarsdóttir, U., Fürst, C. J., Hultman, C., Fall, K., Sparén, P., & Ye, W. (2008). Suicide among people with amyotrophic lateral sclerosis. *Brain, 131*(10), 2729–2733.

Fleminger, S., Leigh, E., Eames, P., Langrell, L., Nagraj, R., & Logsdail, S. (2005). HoNOS—ABI: A reliable outcome measure of neuropsychiatric sequelae to brain injury? *Psychiatric Bulletin, 29*(2), 53–55.

Fuller-Thomson, E., Tulipano, M. J., & Song, M. (2012). The association between depression, suicidal ideation and stroke in a population-based sample. *International Journal of Stroke, 7*(3), 188–194.

Ganzini, L., Denneson, L. M., Press, N., Bair, M. J., Helmer, D. A., Poat, J., & Dobscha, S. K. (2013). Trust is the basis for effective suicide risk screening and assessment in veterans. *Journal of General Internal Medicine, 28*(9), 1215–1221.

Gaskill, A., Foley, F. W., Kolzet, J., & Picone, M. A. (2011). Suicidal thinking in multiple sclerosis. *Disability and Rehabilitation, 33*(17-18), 1528–1536.

Gaynes, B. N., West, S. L., Ford, C. A., Frame, P., Klein, J., & Lohr, K. N. (2004). Screening for suicide risk in adults: A summary of the evidence for the US Preventive Services Task Force. *Annals of Internal Medicine, 140*(10), 822–835.

Gould, M. S., Marrocco, F. A., Kleinman, M., Thomas, J. G., Mostkoff, K., Cote, J., & Davies, M. (2005). Evaluating iatrogenic risk of youth suicide screening programs: A randomized controlled trial. *JAMA, 293*(13), 1635–1643.

Graham, A., Reser, J., Scuderi, C., Zubrick, S., Smith, M., & Turley, B. (2000). Suicide: An Australian psychological society discussion paper. *Australian Psychologist, 35*(1), 1–28.

Hackett, M. L., Hill, K. M., Hewison, J., Anderson, C. S., & House, A. O. (2010). Stroke survivors who score below threshold on standard depression measures may still have negative cognitions of concern. *Stroke, 41*(3), 478–481.

Hockberger, R. S., & Rothstein, R. J. (1988). Assessment of suicide potential by nonpsychiatrists using the SAD PERSONS score. *Journal of Emergency Medicine, 6*, 99–107.

Jones, J. E., Hermann, B. P., Barry, J. J., Gilliam, F. G., Kanner, A. M., & Meador, K. J. (2003). Rates and risk factors for suicide, suicidal ideation and suicide attempts in chronic epilepsy. *Epilepsy and Behavior, 4*, 31–38.

Kennedy, P., Rogers, B., Speer, S., & Frankel, H. (1999). Spinal cord injuries and attempted suicide: A retrospective review. *Spinal Cord, 37*(12), 847–852.

Lovibond, S. H., & Lovibond, P. F. (1995). *Depression Anxiety Stress Scales (DASS).* Sydney, Australia: Psychology Foundation of Australia.

Mackelprang, J. L., Bombadier, C. H., Fann, J. R., Temkin, N. R., Barber, J. K., & Dikmen, S. S. (2014). Rates and predictors of suicidal ideation during the first year after traumatic brain injury. *American Journal of Public Health, 104*, e100–e107.

Marušič, A., Jurišić, B., Kozel, D., Mirjanič, M., Petrović, A. (2009). Early detection of mental ill-health, harmful stress and suicidal behaviours. In D. Wasserman & C. Wasserman (Eds.), *Oxford textbook of suicidology and suicide prevention: A global perspective* (pp. 543–550). New York: Oxford University Press.

Olfson, M., Weissman, M. M., Leon, A. C., Sheehan, D. V., & Farber, L. (1996). Suicidal ideation in primary care. *Journal of General Internal Medicine, 11*(8), 447–453.

Paulsen, J. S., Hoth, K. F., Nehl, C., & Stierman, L.; the Huntington Study Group. (2005). Critical periods of suicide risk in Huntington's disease. *American Journal of Psychiatry, 162*(4), 725–731.

Pompili, M., Girardi, P., Tatarelli, G., Angeletti, G., & Tatarelli, R. (2006). Suicide after surgical treatment in patients with epilepsy: A meta-analytic investigation. *Psychological Reports, 98*(2), 323–338.

Reynolds, W. M. (1988), *Suicidal Ideation Questionnaire (SIQ): Professional manual*. Odessa, FL: Psychological Assessment Resources.

Robertson, M. M. (1997). Suicide, parasuicide and epilepsy. In J. Engel Jr. & T. A. Pedley (Eds.), *Epilepsy: A comprehensive textbook* (pp. 2141–2151). Philadelphia, PA: Lippincott-Raven.

Sadovnick, A. D., Eisen, K., Ebers, G. C., & Paty, D. W. (1991). Cause of death in patients attending multiple sclerosis clinics. *Neurology, 41*(8), 1193–1196.

Shaffer, D., Scott, M., Wilcox, H., Maslow, C., Hicks, R., Lucas, C. P., . . . Greenwald, S. (2004). The Columbia SuicideScreen: Validity and reliability of a screen for youth suicide and depression. *Journal of the American Academy of Child & Adolescent Psychiatry, 43*(1), 71–79.

Simon, G. E., Rutter, C. M., Peterson, D., Oliver, M., Whiteside, U., Operskalski, B., & Ludman, E. J. (2013). Does response on the PHQ-9 Depression Questionnaire predict subsequent suicide attempt or suicide death? *Psychiatric Services, 64*(12), 1195–1202.

Simpson, G. K., & Tate, R. L. (2002). Suicidality after traumatic brain injury: Demographic, injury and clinical correlates. *Psychological Medicine, 32*(4), 687–697.

Simpson, G. K., & Tate, R. L. (2007). Suicidality in people surviving a traumatic brain injury: Prevalence, risk factors and implications for clinical management. *Brain Injury, 21*(13-14), 1335–1351.

Simpson, G. K., Tate, R. L., Whiting, D. L., & Cotter, R. E. (2011). Suicide prevention after traumatic brain injury: A randomized controlled trial of a program for the psychological treatment of hopelessness. *Journal of Head Trauma Rehabilitation, 26*(4), 290–300.

Soden, R. J., Walsh, J., Middleton, J. W., Craven, M. L., Rutkowski, S. B., & Yeo, J. D. (2000). Causes of death after spinal cord injury. *Spinal Cord, 38*(10), 604–610.

Spitzer, R. L., Kroenke, K., Williams, J. B.; Patient Health Questionnaire Primary Care Study Group. (1999). Validation and utility of a self-report version of PRIME-MD: The PHQ primary care study. *JAMA, 282*(18), 1737–1744.

Spitzer, R. L., Williams, J. B., Kroenke, K., Linzer, M., Verloin deGruy, F., Hahn, S. R., . . . Johnson, J. G. (1994). Utility of a new procedure for diagnosing mental disorders in primary care: The PRIME-MD 1000 study. *Journal of the American Medical Association, 272*(22), 1749–1756.

Stenager, E. N., Madsen, C., Stenager, E., & Boldsen, J. (1998). Suicide in patients with stroke: Epidemiological study. *British Medical Journal, 316*(7139), 1206–1210.

Stenager, E. N., Stenager, E., Koch-Henriksen, N., Brønnum-Hansen, H., Hyllested, K., Jensen, K., & Bille-Brahe, U. (1992). Suicide and multiple sclerosis: An epidemiological investigation. *Journal of Neurology, Neurosurgery & Psychiatry, 55*(7), 542–545.

Taylor, T. L., Hawton, K., Fortune, S., & Kapur, N. (2009). Attitudes towards clinical services among people who self-harm: Systematic review. *British Journal of Psychiatry, 194*(2), 104–110.

Teasdale, T. W., & Engberg, A. W. (2001a). Suicide after a stroke: A population study. *Journal of Epidemiology and Community Health, 55*(12), 863–866.

Teasdale, T. W., & Engberg, A. W. (2001b). Suicide after traumatic brain injury: A population study. *Journal of Neurology, Neurosurgery & Psychiatry, 71*(4), 436–440.

Turner, A. P., Williams, R. M., Bowen, J. D., Kivlahan, D. R., & Haselkorn, J. K. (2006). Suicidal ideation in multiple sclerosis. *Archives of Physical Medicine and Rehabilitation, 87*(8), 1073–1078.

US Department of Health and Human Services (HHS), Office of the Surgeon General, & National Action Alliance for Suicide Prevention. (2012). *2012 National strategy for suicide prevention: Goals and objectives for action.* Washington, DC: HHS.

US Preventative Services Task Force. (2002). *Screening for depression: Recommendations and rationale.* Rockville, MD: Agency for Healthcare Research and Quality.

Voon, V., Krack, P., Lang, A. E., Lozano, A. M., Dujardin, K., Schüpbach, M., . . . Speelman, J. D. (2008). A multicentre study on suicide outcomes following subthalamic stimulation for Parkinson's disease. *Brain, 131*(10), 2720–2728.

Wasserman, L., Shaw, T., Vu, M., Ko, C., Bollegala, D., & Bhalerao, S. (2008). An overview of traumatic brain injury and suicide. *Brain Injury, 22*(11), 811–819.

Wetzel, H. H., Gehl, C. R., Dellefave–Castillo, L., Schiffman, J. F., Shannon, K. M., Paulsen, J. S.; Huntington Study Group. (2011). Suicidal ideation in Huntington disease: The role of comorbidity. *Psychiatry Research, 188*(3), 372–376.

Wing, J., Cooper, J., & Sartorius, N. (1974). *Measurement and classification of psychiatric symptoms: An instruction manual for the PSE and Catego Program.* Cambridge, UK: Cambridge University Press.

Zigmond, A. S., & Snaith, R. P. (1983). The hospital anxiety and depression scale. *Acta Psychiatrica Scandinavica, 67*(6), 361–370.

8 Suicide Risk Assessment ·

Introduction

Clinicians become aware that assessment of suicide risk may be needed secondary to various circumstances. It could be a positive result arising from a routine screening for suicide risk (see Chapter 7) or arise from direct interaction with a client who discloses suicidal thoughts and/or behaviors or who has other aspects of his or her presentation (e.g., acute psychological distress) that give rise to the question about whether he or she might also be at risk for suicide. Alternatively, it may be other staff or third parties, such as family members or friends of the client, who alert the clinician to the issue.

The clinical response involves undertaking a suicide risk assessment. As an aid to conducting such assessments, the SMART checklist for neurodisability is introduced. The SMART checklist is an aide-memoire, highlighting key clinical features of a client's presentation that need to be explored in making a judgment about the severity and imminence of suicide risk. Suicide risk assessments are often a dynamic process, and the clinical information is best collected through a multifaceted approach which occurs over one or more therapeutic encounters depending on the circumstances. Such an approach can comprise a mix of (1) clinical interviews,

(2) validated measures, (3) monitoring for warning signs, and (4) checking with other sources (e.g., review of medical files, speaking to family members).

The unpredictability of suicide and implications for assessment will be addressed and the limited literature about assessment among various types of neurodisability will be outlined, followed by the introduction of the SMART checklist. The multifaceted approaches to collecting the data proposed by the checklist will then be described. Following this, a matrix is presented that guides the formulation of the level of suicide risk both in terms of severity (high, intermediate, low) and temporality (acute, chronic) based on a synthesis of the gathered information. Finally, some of the pragmatic issues that arise in the conduct of suicide risk assessment will be highlighted.

Unpredictability of Suicide and Implications for Assessment

Good assessment is a key starting point for quality treatment and management in suicide prevention. Decision-making algorithms or models have been used to structure such suicide risk assessments. However, even the best of information will not reliably predict suicide at the level of specific individuals (Fowler, 2012; Department of Veterans Affairs [DVA/DoD], 2013). Referencing the work of Pokorny (1983, 1993), Simon (2012) has stated that "A standard of care does not exist for prediction of suicide" (p. 3). Extrapolating from this universally accepted fact, the DVA/DoD (2013) clinical guidelines conclude that current approaches to both risk assessment and treatment therefore need to comprise an amalgam of the best available evidence complemented by clinical experience and common sense.

There are three implications that arise from this state of the evidence. First, given that suicide risk assessments do not have strong positive predictive power in identifying the individuals who do end their lives, assessments are likely to result in false positives, but, as Rudd and colleagues (2006) observe, "it is preferable to err on the side of caution when dealing with such a [potentially] devastating outcome" (p. 256). Second, a multifaceted assessment approach is warranted rather than adhering to a single-strand assessment approach. Third, it is important to understand that even if implementing the world's best practice and in spite of our best efforts, there is always the possibility that a client will end his or her life (Hendin, 2006). Despite this, suicide is a relatively rare event, and so we should be able to approach an assessment with the belief that, in the great majority of cases, the people we assess will survive their current suicidal crisis.

Literature on Suicide Risk Assessment in Neurodisability

To the best of our knowledge, across the eight neurological conditions addressed in this book, there has only been detailed discussion of suicide risk assessment among those with epilepsy or traumatic brain injury (TBI). Jones and colleagues (2003) have proposed that the Mini-International Neuropsychiatric Interview (developed by Sheehan et al., 1998) would be a suitable assessment tool for people with epilepsy. It incorporates the assessment of 10 Axis I disorders combined with a suicidality module which collects data on five items (ranging from "think you would be better off dead" through to "attempts suicide" over the past month, plus an additional item asking about lifetime history of suicide attempts). The items are weighted so that endorsing a more severe item contributes a higher score to the overall total. The total score from the six items is then used to classify suicide risk as low, medium, or high. Drawing on the work of Jacobs, Brewer, and Klein-Benheim (1999), the authors also explore clinical features of the Axis I disorders that might lead to low, medium, or high ratings of suicide risk. In a later review, Verroti and colleagues (2008) cover much of the same ground but focus their guide for physicians. The concern with this approach is that it may not give sufficient weight to a range of other factors that also mediate suicide risk. Apart from these standardized approaches, some practice options that can help inform the conduct of a suicide risk assessment for people with TBI have been outlined in a detailed clinical discussion by Dennis, Ghahramanlou-Holloway, Cox, and Brown (2011) and will be highlighted later in the chapter.

Introducing the SMART Checklist for Neurodisability

The target population for the SMART checklist is adults with neurodisability who have sufficient cognitive capacity to participate in clinical assessments and who display suicidal thoughts or behavior, with or without a diagnosed mental health condition. The broader evidence base for the SMART checklist includes clinical guidelines (i.e., National Institute for Health and Clinical Excellence, 2011; DVA/DoD Clinical Guidelines, 2013) as well as the general suicide prevention research literature. However, the SMART checklist has not been empirically tested. The SMART elements are outlined in Box 8.1. All sample questions provided in the tables and text boxes have been used in actual clinical assessments of suicide risk among clients with neurodisability experiencing suicidal distress.

BOX 8.1
SMART SUICIDE RISK ASSESSMENT CHECKLIST

SMART Checklist for Neurodisability

S Suicide state and history	Intent, Ideation, Plan, Preparatory Behavior, Attempt, History of thoughts/behaviors, Warning signs
M Mental state (current)	Intoxication, Hallucinations or Delusions, Agitation
A Assess psychological features	Executive impairment, Hopelessness, Aggression, Ambivalence, Anguish
R Risk and protective factors	Risk factors: Sex, age at injury/onset, severity of condition/time since onset, presence of depression, substance use disorders or other mental health conditions
	Protective factors: Social support, sense of purpose/future-oriented hopefulness, religion/spirituality, able to access and engage in mental health treatment
T Time-frame	How imminent is any action? Are the stressors acute or chronic?

S: SUICIDAL STATE AND HISTORY

The core of evaluating suicide risk is the determination of the current suicidal state. Information is needed about the presence of suicidal intent, the nature of any suicidal ideation (SI), the existence of a suicide plan, any preparatory behaviors taken to implement the plan, any immediate occurrence of self-directed violence, and any current attempts as well as any previous history of suicidal thoughts and/or behaviors (see Box 8.2). Warning signs should be evaluated, as well as monitored in an ongoing manner. See further discussion in this chapter under Monitoring for Warning signs.

Intent

Suicidal intent may be either explicit (e.g., a client stating "I want to die") or implicit (e.g., a client engaging in preparatory behaviors). It is important to distinguish self-violence with underlying suicidal intent from nonsuicide self-directed violence (SDV; e.g., cutting behavior; see Chapter 3). The DVA/DoD clinical guidelines observe that, in the latter, the individuals do not wish to die but instead use the behavior as a means of coping that produces transient relief from psychological distress (DVA/DoD, 2013, p. 14). Although not suicidal, these behaviors are still clinically serious because they can lead to injury or accidental death.

BOX 8.2
SUICIDE STATE AND HISTORY

Domain	Sample questions
Presence of suicide intent	"Are you thinking about suicide at the moment?" If yes "Can you tell me about those thoughts?"
Frequency, Intensity and Duration (F-I-D)[a]	"How often do you think about suicide?" "How strong are those thoughts?" "How long do they last?" "Are you able to control these thoughts?"
Plan	"Have you thought about ways of killing yourself (harming yourself; trying to end your life)?"
Preparatory behavior (Has the person started to take some steps to act on their plan?)	If yes, "Have you done anything about this plan?"
Attempt (Has the person already done something to injure themselves?)	"You seem very distressed at the moment, and have had some suicidal thoughts. Have you done anything to hurt yourself?"
Prior history (Does the person have a history of previous suicide thoughts or behaviors?)	"Have you ever thought of suicide (tried to end your life) before?" "If so, what happened?" "How did you get through?"
Warning signs	"What thoughts or feelings have you noticed before you start thinking about suicide?"

[a] Rudd (2012).

There are some limited data on the strength of intent to die in suicide attempts after neurodisability. In TBI, Simpson and Tate (2005) used the relevant item on the Beck Scale for Suicide Ideation (1991) to measure intent to die for each suicide attempt, as reported retrospectively by study participants. The strength of intent to die among post-injury suicide attempts was significantly stronger than the intent to die among pre-injury suicide attempts. Furthermore, in line with previous research, Simpson and Tate (2005) found no correlation between the strength of the intent to die, as measured on the Beck Scale for Suicide Ideation (1991), and the lethality of the attempt, as measured by the Lethality of Suicide Attempts Rating Scale (Smith et al., 1984). The important clinical consideration here is that simply because a suicide attempt was of low lethality, this should not lead to the inference that the individual was not serious about trying to die. Minden and colleagues (1987) reported that 2 of 10 lifetime suicide attempts made by people with multiple sclerosis (MS) involved moderate intent and moderate lethality.

Ideation

The continuum of SI can start with more generic thoughts about "life not worth living" and "being better off dead" as precursors to more specific thoughts about killing oneself and making suicide plans. The strength of SI across this continuum can range from mild fleeting thoughts through to people who become preoccupied with such thoughts. Therefore, the frequency, intensity, and duration (or F-I-D; see Rudd, 2012) of SI are important aspects to assess.

Plans

The presence of a suicide plan is generally a flag signifying an increased level of risk in comparison to a person expressing SI only. In cases in which clients have admitted to the existence of a plan, it is important to listen to the person describe his or her plan. This provides the opportunity to evaluate how well developed their plan may be (If they are talking of hanging, have they thought about where they will do it and how they will hang themselves?; If overdose, have they been thinking about how many tablets they might need?). It is also important to think about how realistic the plan is in the context of their impairments (e.g., if they are thinking of deliberately crashing a car, do they still have their licence? Can they physically drive?; If hanging, do they have the fine motor skills to tie a slip knot?). The degree of lethality of the means of suicide that a person is contemplating also needs to be considered (e.g., the difference between using a gun and deciding to cut one's wrists). Objectively, wrist cutting has a low level of lethality. This is therefore important information in making plans for the person's safety. It is also important to find out whether the person sees the method he or she has chosen as having a high degree of lethality.

Preparatory Behaviors

The next level of escalation arises if the person has started to act on his or her plan, also termed *preparatory behavior* (Bryan & Rudd, 2006). Examples of preparatory behavior observed in people with neurodisability have included handing over financial affairs to a family member, researching suicide methods on the Internet, starting to hoard tablets, finding a length of hose to attempt carbon monoxide poisoning, practising tying nooses with a rope, and buying heroin to attempt an overdose.

Attempts

It is important to ensure that the person has not already made an attempt at the point of the clinical interaction (e.g., has already taken an overdose of medication). In such circumstances, emergency medical help will be immediately required. In seeking to understand any past history of suicide attempts, it is important to gather as much information as is suitable and clinically appropriate. Research within neurodisability has found that up to half of people who have made an index attempt will go on to make one or more further attempts (see Chapter 6). Furthermore, Joiner (2005) highlights the risk that preparatory behaviors and/or attempts can desensitize clients toward future suicidal behavior, including death (see Chapter 4).

History

Collecting data about previous history is important in formulating understanding about the chronicity of suicidal thoughts and behaviors as well as in identifying examples of previous coping (see Box 8.2). However, caution needs to be exercised that any such exploration is not exacerbating the client's current levels of distress.

M: MENTAL STATE

A client's current mental state will also influence the determination of risk. Mental health state refers to acute symptoms of underlying conditions, namely intoxication, hallucinations, or psychomotor agitation. If the client is exhibiting suicidal thoughts or behaviors while intoxicated due to alcohol or drugs (licit or illicit), then keep the individual safe and under observation while sobering up. Once sober, then conduct an assessment, particularly assessing the role of the substance abuse in relation to suicide risk. If the client is reporting hallucinations or appears delusional, a psychiatric assessment may be important. For example, there are documented cases of people dying by suicide during postictal psychotic episodes, particularly those associated with temporal lobe epilepsy or complex partial seizures (Fukuchi et al., 2002; Mendez & Doss, 1992). Finally, clients who are displaying psychomotor agitation (e.g., they find it difficult to sit during an assessment interview, show other signs of physiological arousal) may be at particular risk (see the later description of anguish). In contrast to these acute presentations, current or past mental health conditions are addressed as a risk factor (the R in SMART).

A: ASSESS PSYCHOLOGICAL FEATURES

Five psychological features to be considered include the presence of executive impairments, hopelessness, aggression, ambivalence, and anguish.

Executive impairment

Impaired executive function resulting in inflexible or "concrete" thinking, ineffective problem-solving, and impulsivity may increase suicide risk (see Table 8.1; also Chapter 5). Inflexible or concrete thinking is commonly observed among people with frontal pathology. Similarly, in non–brain damaged populations, Shneidman (1989) has also documented a constriction of cognition, described as "a tunnelling of vision" that can be observed among people experiencing suicidal distress. The following statements made by clients with neurodisability illustrate this constriction: "She meant all the world to me," "He was my whole life" (in the context of a relationship break-up); "I've got nothing left to live for" (in the context of multiple losses); "If I can't walk or ride a motorbike by 2 years post-injury, I will kill myself" (in the context of the loss of physical capacity). If there is a rigidity in adhering to such constricted cognitive precepts which are driving the suicidal distress, then it becomes a clinical priority to work to generate alternative solutions or find other ways to reduce the intensity of such thoughts.

Ineffective problem-solving has been identified as a mediating factor for increased suicide risk within non–brain damaged populations (see Chapter 4). Impairments in problem-solving are commonly observed across many different types of neurodisability. Information can be collected during an interview about problems that have high salience and, particularly if there is a history of failed attempts at solving such problems, with the failures causing substantive levels of distress or lowered self-esteem (e.g., seeing self as a failure).

Homaifar, Bahraini, Silverman, and Brenner (2012) describe impulsivity "as a failure to inhibit or problems with disinhibition" (p. 114) and go on to suggest that assessment of this construct should include evaluation of previous behaviors (see Table 8.1). For suicide risk assessments in general, the following questions to assess impulsivity have been devised and could also be useful for neurodisability: "(1) Do you consider yourself an impulsive person? (2) Why or why not? (3) When have you felt out of control in the past? (4) What did you do that you thought was out of control? (5) What did you do to help yourself feel more in control? (6) When you're feeling out of control, how long does it usually take for you to recover?" (Rudd et al., 2006, p. 59).

Hopelessness

Hopelessness can be the end result of the tunnelling of vision or ineffective problem-solving. Whatever the etiology, the sense of being trapped, of there being no way out from the current distress, can result in suicide being perceived as the

TABLE 8.1

Brief tips for evaluation and intervention of executive functioning as it relates to suicidal thoughts and behaviors

Executive functioning component	Sample questions to augment a suicide risk assessment	What to listen For	Intervention
Impulsivity	When you're feeling out of control, how long is it before you feel like you have to act on your thoughts?	A coping strategy that would take too long to reduce feelings of being out of control (e.g., if it takes 5 minutes before they feel they must act on their thoughts, then coping via watching a 2-hour movie may not be the best choice)	Coping strategies should be tailored to produce immediate gratification (e.g., calling a loved one or playing with a pet)
Insight	How much do you think that others would be better off if you were gone? Does this happen regardless of whether you feel like they value you?	Lack of awareness of the impact their suicide would make on others and/or their value to others	Helping patients identify triggers that contribute to their problems with insight (e.g., an argument with a spouse that makes them feel devalued)
Thinking process	How would you cope during a suicidal crisis? What if that doesn't work?	Degrees of concreteness inflexible thinking	Once coping strategies are identified, trouble-shooting with patients (e.g., visiting a friend makes things better, what happens if the friend is busy?)

From Homaifar et al. (2012).

only alternative. Hopelessness might be expressed in relation to the person ("I will never be able to solve this"), the world ("I will never get the help I need"), or the future ("Because of the injury, my life is over; I have no future").

Aggression

In the general population, a convergence of neurobiological, genetic, and clinical evidence suggest that trait aggression is an important factor associated with increased risk of suicide (Mann, Waternaux, Haas, & Malone, 1999). Epilepsy, Huntington's disease, Parkinson's disease after deep brain stimulation, and TBI are all known to be associated with increased aggressive behavior (Kwan & Brodie, 2001; Rosenblatt & Leroi, 2000; Sabaz, Simpson, Walker, Rogers, Gillis, & Strettles, 2014). However, little is currently known about the relationships among intrapersonal aggression, neurodisability, and suicide.

If interpersonal aggression is an identified issue, it is important to be mindful of the potential link between violence and suicide (Malphurs & Cohen, 2005). Although these events are uncommon, regional rates in homicide/suicides across the United States range from 1% to 20% of all homicides, with the national average at 5% (Cohen, Llorente, & Eisdorfer, 1998). Homicide/suicides most frequently occur within a family context and involve firearms (Cohen et al., 1998). The time gap between the homicide and suicide is usually a matter of minutes or hours, although longer time frames have been reported (Cohen et al., 1998). To the best of our knowledge, there have been two case examples of homicide/suicide associated with neurodisability reported in the literature (Blumer et al., 2002; Tate, Simpson, Flanagan, & Coffey,1997). The prevalence of increased aggression among some types of neurodisability means that this possibility needs to be ruled out as part of the risk assessment, either *indirectly* (identify this is an issue during the course of the interview) or *directly* through asking: "Do you also feel like harming someone else? If yes, do you feel like trying to kill that person before you die?"

Ambivalence

In addition to impairments of executive function, clinician assessment needs to be mindful of the presence of either ambivalence or anguish. Most people who display suicidal thoughts or behaviors have mixed feelings about ending their life (Rudd, 2012; see also Chapter 3). They therefore still have reasons for living. It is important to try identify signs of ambivalence during an assessment because these are important features in the treatment of people who are suicidal. The signs of ambivalence may be identified from what a person says or in some action he or she takes.

Ambivalence could also be present in the degree to which the possibility of discovery or rescue was left open in any previous suicide attempts (Weisman & Worden, 1974). In addition, identifying protective factors (see Chapter 6) is also a departure point for exploring the level of ambivalence.

Anguish

Unbearable mental anguish (Michel, Valach, & Waeber, 1994) or psychological pain (Shneidman, 1989) creates a "press" or movement toward suicide (Shneidman, 1992). The function of suicide as an escape from or cessation of pain is a central tenet to a number of the theories described in Chapter 4. The agitation and distress associated with such pain is described as "perturbation" (Shneidman, 1992), a state greater than motor agitation alone, having a linked possibility to action.

R: RISK FACTORS AND PROTECTIVE FACTORS

Ascertaining the presence of risk factors enables the identification of clients who have an increased likelihood of suicidal behavior and require closer monitoring, intervention, and support (Schecter & Maltsberger, 2007). However, the presence of suicide risk factors is not necessarily indicative of the degree of suicide risk in a particular individual (Powell, Geddes, Hawton, Deeks, & Goldacre, 2000; Mann et al., 1999). Current knowledge about suicide risk factors after neurodisability was outlined in Chapter 6 and provides the starting point for this domain of the SMART checklist (demographic, premorbid, injury, comorbid mental health, and psychosocial factors). In addition, initial tables or lists of suicide risk factors have been proposed for certain neurodisability groups, including epilepsy (Jones et al., 2003, Verrotti et al., 2008), people with Parkinson's disease who have had deep brain stimulation (Voon et al., 2008), and TBI (Simpson & Tate, 2007). These lists rely heavily upon known risk factors from the general population (e.g., Bryan & Rudd, 2006) and clinical experience within the specific diagnostic group. A precis of the important risk factors to target after neurodisability is included in Box 8.1.

Protective factors play an important countervailing role to risk factors. Protective factors can include previous examples of successful coping in difficult or challenging times. During a suicide risk assessment, it is possible to identify such factors through direct and indirect means. As the assessment proceeds, information indicative of protective factors is often disclosed (*indirect means*); the clinician can take note of any such references and, at a suitable point, inquire about such factors in greater detail. (e.g., "What is currently stopping you from taking steps to harm yourself? Taking steps to end your life? Have you been through a crisis [distress] like this before? If yes, what happened at that time? How did you get through? If a person has not experienced a crisis of similar magnitude in the past, then one can ask: "Have there been other times in your life which have been hard? When there was a crisis? When things were really bad for you? If yes, what happened at that time?" Rudd (2012) also recommends asking people (toward the end of an interview) "Can you identify your reasons for living (what is keeping you alive right now?)."

T: TIMEFRAME

Building an understanding of the imminence of possible suicidal behavior is crucial in shaping the clinical response (e.g., is someone at such acute risk that they need to be admitted to a hospital?). Stressors or triggers (also known as "tipping points") often provide the clues to understanding the cause and underlying motivation of a suicidal crisis (Bryan & Rudd, 2006). This will help to inform the development of a safety plan for the client (see Chapter 10).

Stressors can be acute (e.g., the recent loss of a job) or chronic (e.g., the cumulative effect of long-term unemployment). In relation to antecedent circumstances, participants with TBI who were interviewed about their past history of suicide attempts reported depression/hopelessness, relationship breakdown or conflict, social isolation, the pressure of multiple stressors, instrumental difficulties (e.g., financial problems), or a more global sense of the negative impact of the injury as tipping points (Simpson & Tate, 2005). In terms of specific triggers, participants reported arguments, a partner leaving, an impulsive response to an acute stressor (e.g., negative feedback from work), or the ready availability of means.

In the case of epilepsy, one study reported triggers for the most recent attempt prior to the study (Hara et al., 2009). Triggers included relationship break-ups or conflict ($n = 3$), other family mental health issues ($n = 2$; e.g., mother's suicide), non-specific family issues ($n = 1$), and self-discontinuation of antidepressant medication ($n = 1$; fluoxetine). Among 200 patients undergoing deep brain stimulation for PD, the four reported post-surgery suicide attempts were all triggered by home/family conflict (Soulas et al., 2008).

Some limited data are available about the possible role of testing as a trigger suicide attempts in Huntington's disease (HD) (Almqvist et al., 1999). Although some earlier accounts have been provided, the study by Almqvist and colleagues captured data after direct testing for the mutation was available (though some participating centers were still reporting patients who had undertaken a linkage analysis) and so provides information most likely to apply to the contemporary experience of people with HD. Data on the means of suicide were not available.

Almqvist and colleagues (1999) suggested that the receipt of the results rather than the gradual onset of symptoms/formal diagnosis was the decisive trigger for the attempt in a majority of cases they documented. Among the 21 individuals who made suicide attempts, 17 had the mutation or were at increased risk. Ten attempts occurred within 6 months of the receipt of the results, with 15/21 attempts occurring within the first year. At the time of the attempts, 10 were asymptomatic, with another 8 either possibly or probably affected, and only 3 having a confirmed diagnosis (Almqvist et al., 1999), suggesting that the receipt of the results rather than the gradual onset of symptoms/formal diagnosis was the decisive trigger for the attempt in a majority of cases. However, the authors caution about placing too much weight on the findings due to problems with reliable data collection at a number of the participating centers.

A Multifaceted Approach to Gathering Clinical Data for the Suicide Risk Assessment

Gathering the SMART checklist data is best undertaken through a multifaceted approach that includes conducting clinical interviews, administering validated assessment measures, monitoring for warning signs, and other sources. Each has a role to play and can provide complementary information. Levels of suicide distress can fluctuate, with some people displaying suicidal thoughts and behaviors over extended periods of time. Therefore, assessment is often an ongoing rather than a "once-off" process, drawing upon all these four elements.

THE CLINICAL INTERVIEW

The clinical interview is the fundamental instrument for assessing suicide risk (Schecter & Maltsberger, 2009; Dennis et al., 2011; Rudd, 2012). The goal of such interviews is to collect the specific information needed to form a clinical judgment about the degree of suicide risk. Schechter and Maltsberger (2007) highlight the importance of balancing the dual processes of seeking to gather objective data about the level of suicide risk while listening and being responsive to the subjective experiences and distress communicated by the individual. Through the interview, the clinician can provide reassurance and normalize the distress being experienced by the person who is suicidal (Rudd, 2012).

In balancing these two imperatives, a suicide risk assessment will rarely proceed in an orderly stepwise process. Dennis et al. (2011) have suggested that some thought be given to sequencing, highlighting the importance of establishing rapport before asking sensitive questions around suicidal state. With this caveat, a flexible approach can be taken in the order within which the key elements (e.g., of the SMART checklist) are addressed, allowing the interviewer to be responsive to issues presented.

The clinical interview may play other important clinical functions in addition to the primary goal of ascertaining suicide risk, laying the groundwork for therapy (Rudd, 2012). This groundwork can include promoting engagement and contributing to the establishment of a therapeutic alliance (Rudd, 2012). It also provides an opportunity to enhance motivation within the client, join in initial problem-solving, and foster treatment adherence (Schecter & Maltsberger, 2009). Finally, seeking views from family, friends, or clinicians and not simply the client alone is also recommended as part of the assessment process (Dennis et al., 2011).

An alternate strategy is to use a structured clinical interview like the Columbia Suicide-Severity Rating Scale (Posner et al., 2011) which assesses for both SI and suicidal self-directed violence. The measure is now recommended by major US government agencies as an adjunct measure to be employed in clinical trials to monitor for suicidal thoughts and behaviors. However, the validity of the measure among populations with neurodisability is yet to be investigated.

VALIDATED MEASURES

Clinical rating scales can be a useful adjunct to the clinical interview in suicide risk assessment (Homaifar, Matarazzo, & Wortzel, 2013). However, authors have universally warned against relying on the results from administration of such scales in reliably predicting suicide risk. For example, Beck and Steer (1991) warn about setting cutoff scores on the Beck Scale for Suicide Ideation as a means for judging the severity of suicide risk. Extending this, Cochrane-Brinks and colleagues (2000) also cautioned against the use of strict cutoff scores on such scales to dictate decisions about admission to a hospital among people undergoing a suicide assessment risk in emergency departments. Such warnings about reliance on scales have been echoed by authors writing in the field of neurodisability (e.g., Wasserman et al., 2008; Jones et al., 2003).

Some measures suggested for inclusion in suicide risk assessments after neurodisability have been completed by people with TBI. The Personality Assessment Inventory (Breshears, Brenner, Harwood, & Gutierrez, 2010) and the Beck Scale for Suicide Ideation (Beck & Steer, 1991) have both been evaluated for their ability to predict a history of suicidal behavior. Breshears et al. (2010) examined the existing cutoffs of the Suicide Potential Index and found that a higher cutoff score than recommended for the general population significantly strengthened the sensitivity while preserving strong sensitivity in predicting suicidal behavior. Even though retrospective, the Personality Assessment Inventory was administered prior to the suicidal behavior, thereby providing invaluable evidence of the predictive ability of the Suicide Potential Index. One challenge with the Personality Assessment Inventory is its length, which limits the clinical contexts within which it might be administered.

Homaifar, Matarazzo, and Wortzel (2013) recommend the use of the Beck Scale for Suicide Ideation. Simpson and Tate (2002) found that the odds of a history of suicide attempts among people with TBI a Beck Scale for Suicide Ideation score greater than or equal to 9 was almost 5 times greater than people with low or no SI. However, in this study, the suicidal behavior was retrospective, often with extended latency periods between the administration of the measure and the suicidal behavior. No suicide risk scales or other measures (e.g., single-item scales) have been tested prospectively for their predictive power, nor are there records in the literature of scales used as part of clinical management of suicidal behaviors after neurodisability. One caution with the Beck Scale for Suicide Ideation is that if the full scale is administered, it includes some explicit questions about SI which can be distressing to some clients.

Homaifar, Matarazzo, and Wortzel (2013) also recommend the use of the Beck Hopelessness Scale. Hopelessness has clinical significance as a stronger predictor of suicide than depression per se (Beck, Brown, & Steer, 1989). Moreover, not everyone who experiences hopelessness is clinically depressed. The Beck Hopelessness Scale (Beck & Steer, 1988) is a reliable and valid measure of hopelessness that has been used in several neurodisability groups (see Chapters 4 and 6) and, within those groups, was found to be a significant predictor of elevated SI.

Other scales that have been proposed for neurodisability groups but are yet to be tested include the Positive and Negative Suicide Ideation Inventory (PANSI; Muehlenkamp, Gutierrez, Osman, & Barrios, 2005) for TBI (Wasserman et al., 2008); the Suicide Index Scale (Beck, Schuyler, & Herman, 1974) and Index of Potential Suicide (Zung, 1974) for CVA (Garden, Garrison, & Jain, 1990); the Mini International Neuropsychiatric interview suicide module (Sheehan et al., 1998) for epilepsy (Jones et al., 2003), and the Rorsharch (Exner, 2002) in ALS (Palmieri et al., 2010).

Finally, Homaifar, Matarazzo, and Wortzel (2013) recommend the use of the Reasons for Living Inventory (RLI). Asking about reasons for living can be an important prompt for identifying protective factors (Bryan & Rudd, 2006), and the RLI (Linehan, Goodstein, Nielsen, & Chiles, 1983) is a validated tool for gathering information about this clinical area. One caution to keep in mind is the length of the RLI; the brief version might be a better alternative to administering the full measure.

In the light of the number of possible scales that could be administered, Homaifar and colleagues (2013) have recommended the Beck Scale for Suicide Ideation (Beck & Steer, 1991), the Beck Hopelessness Scale (Beck & Steer, 1988), and the RLI (Linehan et al., 1983). Each measure has its strengths, limitations, and challenges in administration, so Homaifar and colleagues (2013) recommend some preparatory work in evaluating the relevance of the scales for each clinical context, and certainly some practice in administration would be important before trying to introduce these instruments into a suicide risk assessment.

Given the questions surrounding the application of risk factors from the general population to neurodisability groups, suicide assessment scales that place significant weight on such risk factors may have uncertain reliability for immediate application to neurodisability without testing. In the meantime, scales that focus more narrowly on SI may have the advantage of being less influenced by the confounds associated with risk factors. However, SI alone is not a robust predictor of eventual suicide compared to more broad-based risk assessment approaches in the general population, and this is also likely to be the case after neurodisability. Detailed reviews of the content and validity of suicide risk assessment measures are available (Brown, 2000; Bech & Awata, 2009).

MONITORING FOR WARNING SIGNS

Warning signs are important indicators of imminent suicidal behavior for which a prompt clinical response is recommended. Despite the eponymous term, these lists typically include both signs (observable behaviors) and symptoms (self-reported well-being) with many predominantly listing symptoms of depression. In the general population, one challenge in applying this clinical concept is that many sets of warning signs have been published on the Internet and in other literature, but the empirical basis for many of the signs is unclear.

To help counter this, the following authoritative definition explains warning signs as

> the earliest detectable sign that indicates heightened risk for suicide in the near-term (i.e., within minutes, hours, or days). A warning sign refers to some feature of the developing outcome of interest (suicide) rather than to as distinct construct (e.g., risk factor) that predicts or may be causally related to suicide. (Rudd et al., 2006, p. 258)

In 2006, a consensus panel of international experts delineated a list of warning signs (Rudd et al., 2006). These signs have been included within the US National Suicide Prevention Plan (US Department of Health and Human Services [USDHHS], 2012). The consensus group proposed a two-tiered response, with the top three signs needing an immediate response and a further set of signs for which seeking support from a mental health counselor was recommended (see Box 8.3).

BOX 8.3

WARNING SIGNS FOR THE GENERAL POPULATION

Warning Signs of Suicide
- Talking about wanting to die
- Looking for a way to kill oneself
- Talking about feeling hopeless or having no purpose
- Talking about feeling trapped or being in unbearable pain
- Talking about being a burden to others
- Increasing the use of alcohol or drugs
- Acting anxious, agitated, or reckless
- Sleeping too little or too much
- Withdrawing or feeling isolated
- Showing rage or talking about seeking revenge
- Displaying extreme mood swings

The more of these signs a person shows, the greater the risk of suicide. Warning signs are associated with suicide but may not be what causes a suicide.

If someone you know exhibits warning signs of suicide:

- Do not leave the person alone
- Remove any objects that could be used in a suicide attempt
- Call a Suicide Prevention Lifeline
- Take the person to an emergency room or seek help from a medical or mental health professional

From USDHHS (2012).

The clinical value of warning signs lies in their dynamic nature (i.e., reflecting the fluctuating intensity of suicide risk) compared to the static property of many risk factors (e.g., age, sex). Furthermore, many risk factors are not modifiable (e.g., past history of suicide attempts) compared to warning signs, which can always be targeted for clinical treatment and/or require clinical decision-making. In addition, risk factors are normally assessed by health or mental health professionals. In contrast, both lay people and staff can identify warning signs. And, further to the importance of lay people, research has found that up to 25% of patients at risk of suicide do not tell clinicians but do tell family, thus reinforcing the important role that social networks can play in the early warning of suicide (Simon, 2012).

The warning signs approach can be applied to the field of neurodisability (Dennis et al., 2011). Examples of "warning signals" have been listed in epilepsy (Jones et al., 2003; Pompili, Girardi, & Tatarelli, 2006) (see Box 8.4). There may also be sufficient evidence to propose an additional warning sign specific to neurodisability, namely the distress people experience in response to a recent diagnosis of MS and HD (Stenager et al., 1992; Paulsen, Hoth, Nehl, Stierman, & the Huntington Study Group, 2005); recent neurosurgery in the cases of epilepsy or PD (Bell, Gaitatzis, Bell, Johnson, & Sander, 2009; Voon et al., 2008), or in response to recent progression of the disease (MS, Stenager et al., 1992). Proactive monitoring can take place as part of regular clinical follow-up (Soden et al., 2000), but particularly when patients are at these key time points.

BOX 8.4
EXAMPLES OF SUGGESTED WARNING SIGNALS OR SCREENING FOR
SUICIDE RISK IN EPILEPSY

Common Warning Signals for Suicide in Epilepsy

- Axis I Disorders (mood disorders, substance abuse, schizophrenia)
- Axis II Disorders (antisocial or borderline personality disorder)
- Prominent feelings of anguish or pain and a wish to escape
- Tendency for risk to be acute
- Compulsive driven quality to the suicidality (Jones et al., 2003)

Assessment of Suicide Risk Pre- and Postsurgery to Reduce Seizures

- Identify the multiple contributing factors
- Conduct thorough psychiatric examination to identify risk factors, protective factors
- Distinguish modifiable from nonmodifiable risk factors
- Ask directly about suicide
- Estimate suicide risk (low, moderate, high)
- Specify treatment setting and plan
- Investigate past and present suicidal ideation, plans, behaviors, intent; hopelessness, anhedonia, anxiety symptoms; reasons for living; associated substance use; homicide ideation
- Look for warning signs: expressing suicidal feelings and bringing up the topic of suicide; giving away prized possessions, settling affairs, making out a will; signs of depression, changes in eating habits, sleeping habits; change of behavior (poor work or school performance); risk-taking behaviors; increased use of alcohol or drugs; social isolation; developing a specific plan for suicide (Pompili et al., 2006)

However, some caution needs to be exercised in utilizing a warning sign approach. The significance of three warning signs listed in Box 8.3 as precursors of suicidal behavior may be confounded by the features of some neurodisability groups. Extreme mood swings, withdrawal or social isolation, and sleeping too little or too much are all commonly observed consequences of neurodisability, whether caused by the underlying neuropathology or as a secondary reaction to the impact of the condition (e.g., Rosenblatt & Leroi, 2000). Therefore, too strong a reliance on these symptoms may increase the number of false positives. Furthermore, although current substance abuse is a risk factor for suicide among a number of neurodisability groups (see Chapter 6), the role of substance abuse in death per se is less certain. In the only investigation that reviewed autopsy data on suicides, Tate and colleagues (1997) found evidence of intoxication (alcohol) at the time of death in only two of a case series of eight people with TBI. Despite these cautions, monitoring for warning signs is an important element to consider in suicide risk assessment among people with neurodisability.

OTHER SOURCES

In addition to clinical interviews, validated measures, and monitoring for warning signs, there are other sources of important information in seeking to assess suicide risk. Medical or agency records are an important source of information about suicide history and past risk factors. For example, Simpson and Tate (2005) found that 1 in 4 people with TBI interviewed did not reveal a history of previous suicide attempts. Finally, family members or staff can be important sources of information about the day-to-day functioning of an individual. One consideration in approaching family members is that of privacy. It is ideal to gain permission from the person being assessed to also speak with other people in their social network. If the person is too severely cognitively impaired to provide valid permission, then the therapist will need to weigh the relative merits of privacy versus the clinical importance of gathering additional assessment information. If there is a proxy decision-maker, then it may be possible to approach that person for further information.

Determining the Level of Suicide Risk

In the process of determining the level of suicide risk, the clinician needs to weigh the information that has been collected from the conduct of the interview and/

or monitoring for warning signs, any knowledge about the history of the client from clinical files, information from any rating or risk assessment scales, and information gathered from close others. The severity of risk is commonly categorized into some configuration of low, moderate, and high (Jacobs et al., 1999; Wortzel, Homaifar, Matarazzo, & Brenner, 2014; DVA/DoD, 2013). As a rule of thumb, a growing number of risk factors would suggest an increasing level of risk (Rudd, 2012). However, there is no simple correlation between the number of risk factors and ultimate suicide (Pokorny, 1983, Powell et al., 2000), and sometimes the severity of a single risk factor can be decisive.

Wortzel and colleagues (2014) advocate for evaluating risk both in terms of severity (high, intermediate, low) and temporality (acute, chronic). Essential clinical features for each level (e.g., "High Acute"—"Suicidal ideation with intent to die by suicide") and indicated actions (e.g., "Typically requires psychiatric hospitalization to maintain safety and aggressively target modifiable factors") are outlined as well as on the Rocky Mountain MIRECC Therapeutic Risk Management Website (http://www.mirecc.va.gov/visn19/trm/docs/RM_MIRECC_SuicideRisk_Table.pdf). Further information about this matrix as a template for determining the level of suicide risk and associated clinical action is provided in Chapter 10.

In the final instance, the determination of the level of suicide risk is a clinical one. Suicide remains an unpredictable and individual decision not captured by statistically generated values of sensitivity and specificity (Beck & Steer, 1991). Therefore, while cutoff scores on assessment scales (Cochrane-Brinks et al., 2000) or more detailed actuarial assessments (Bryan & Rudd, 2006) can complement clinical data, neither are reliable guides as stand-alone approaches. Moreover, there is insufficient evidence to develop a risk estimate stratification for people with neurodisability, and therefore it is important to extrapolate from existing approaches developed for the general population.

Pragmatic Issues in the Assessment of Suicide

A number of pragmatics need to be considered in the assessment of suicide.

CLINICAL INTERVIEW

First, completing a clinical interview may take more than one meeting (Schechter & Maltsberger, 2009), particularly if there is a need to pace the assessment to compensate for cognitive impairments. In such cases, sufficient information will need to have been gathered by the end of the first meeting to be certain that suicidal behavior is not imminent. Next, in conducting the assessment, the clinician's use of language needs to be clear. For example, using terms such as "thinking of killing yourself" or "thinking of ending your life," even though difficult, are unambiguous (Rudd, 2012, p. 59). This is of double importance when clients have significant cognitive impairment.

Even in cases of severe cognitive impairment, it is important to try to ascertain firsthand the views and experiences of the person exhibiting suicidal distress. There is growing experience in compensating for cognitive impairments in the delivery of psychological therapies to people with acquired brain injury. A number of these compensatory cognitive and behavioral strategies are also applicable to the conduct of a suicide risk assessment. A number of the most useful are outlined in Box 8.5.

BOX 8.5
CONDUCTING A SUICIDE RISK ASSESSMENT FOR A PERSON WITH
COGNITIVE IMPAIRMENT DUE TO NEURODISABILITY

- Provide a private, nonthreatening and supportive environment to discuss suicidal distress
- Remain calm, show genuine interest, and listen carefully
- It is important to understand the person's perspective on any recent crises or events that triggered thoughts of suicide
- Adopt a collaborative approach with other care providers, using phrases such as "we can work on this to. . . ."
- Provide accurate summaries of the person's concern's—this can assist the person to remain on track and provide a cue to elicit further information
- Do not avoid terms like "suicide" or "killing oneself" or "ending one's life"; it is important to ensure that the person understands what we are asking
- If the person has cognitive impairments, ensure that questions are framed in plain English and, if necessary, provided in multiple formats (written and verbal)
- Monitor the length of the interview and watch for possible fatigue; take small breaks if needed
- Do not ask too many questions too quickly
- Provide plenty of time for asking questions—the presence of distress in addition to cognitive impairments may increase the person's difficulty in coherently expressing him- or herself

- Write key words or themes from what the person says on paper or a whiteboard to help them keep track of what they are trying to communicate
- Do not try to put words into the person's mouth or finish sentences
- Allow pauses of silence if the person needs time to gather thoughts

Adapted from Dennis et al. (2011); Simpson et al. (2011).

DISCOMFORT EXPERIENCED BY STAFF IN CONDUCTING A SUICIDE RISK ASSESSMENT

In working with people who are suicidal, staff are dealing with an issue that can be both clinically and personally challenging. Personal reactions can include feelings of discomfort, anger, guilt, or anxiety (Rudd, 2012). These feelings can be magnified if the staff person has been through a suicidal crisis himself/herself or has been close to someone who died by suicide. It has been suggested that the negative feelings of workers are the major changeable obstacle to suicide risk assessment (Motto, 1989; Rudd, 2012). These issues can also be exacerbated when a client dies by suicide; the challenges associated with postvention will be addressed in Chapter 10. Some staff seek to reduce their discomfort by minimizing the risk of suicide posed by the client. Thus, there can be a mismatch between the client's report of experiencing unbearable mental anguish in relation to a suicide attempt and the clinicians' attribution of interpersonal communication or manipulation as the key motives (Michel et al., 1994).

It is important for staff to address any such problems because, left unaddressed, this can cause secondary complications when the client senses and reacts to worker's feelings (Motto, 1989). Strategies to help overcome this reluctance on the part of staff can include attending suicide prevention training workshops to become more skilled in dealing with suicide, seeking personal counseling for unresolved emotional issues and always seeking supervision with a senior colleague in clinical work with a suicidal client. If the presenting clinical issues extend beyond an individual's clinical training and skill, then ethical practice dictates that the client should be referred to a suitably qualified clinician. Obviously, any such referral needs to be handled with care and due regard to the client's degree of suicidal distress.

CHALLENGES IN CONDUCTING A SUICIDE RISK ASSESSMENT

By their very nature, suicide risk assessments are often conducted in less than ideal circumstances. A range of challenges increase the difficulty in trying to undertake a thorough assessment. These include a lack of trust, denial of suicidal thoughts or behaviors, lack of self-awareness secondary to cognitive deficits, dual disability, intoxication, the person with suicide risk absconds, and fluctuating level of suicide risk. Various management strategies can be employed to manage these challenges (see Box 8.6).

BOX 8.6
CHALLENGES IN CONDUCTING A SUICIDE RISK ASSESSMENT

If Client Is Intoxicated

1. *Ensure safety*: Intoxication significantly increases risk of self-injury in the short term. Provide a safe detoxification area until a proper assessment of suicide potential can be conducted.

2. *Assess suicide risk*: Do not dismiss risk of a suicide attempt or delay assessment because a person is intoxicated. Commence the assessment based on the person's cognitive abilities, rather than on a specific blood-alcohol level. If initial risk assessment suggests that a more comprehensive assessment is necessary, wait until the person is no longer intoxicated. Given the high prevalence of dual-diagnosis, try to assess all clients for substance use (how often, how much, and how recently), previous psychiatric history, and medications.

3. *Obtain collateral information*: People tend to underreport their substance use, so, wherever possible, obtain collateral history from a family member, partner, or friend. If collateral information is not immediately available, it is always prudent to delay making a decision until all reasonable attempts have been made to obtain such information. Is the person known to an area mental health service? If so, notify the relevant mental health team by phone and consult them regarding the person's management plan/appropriate further action.

Therapeutic Alliance Versus Lack of Trust

Try to reassure the client about confidentiality. Take extra time to build trust—don't try to rush the assessment. Identify other people who the person may trust and liaise with them.

If meeting a person for the first time, refer to the experiences of previous clients (while preserving confidentiality) who have presented and the outcomes that were achieved (e.g., Kuipers & Lancaster, 2000).

Dual Disability

For a person with brain injury and in a psychotic condition, if possible, undertake suicide assessment. Simplify questions and try to just get key information about ideation, plans, and access to means. Check whether there are auditory hallucinations telling them to harm themselves. Link into Mental Health services.

Person with Suicide Risk Absconds

Try to persuade the individual to remain. Locate the worker who has the best relationship with the client. Unless you have assessed the person as lacking competence, do not physically restrain the person. Contact family members/friends who may have influence with the person. Contact the police and document all that has happened in the file.

Level of Risk Keeps Changing

Increase level of monitoring and conduct regular assessments of suicide state. Try to stabilize factors in the person's environment that may be causing risk to fluctuate.

Doing a Suicide Risk Assessment on the Phone

Several difficulties are associated with undertaking assessments over the phone, including the inability to observe the client's nonverbal communication, the client's option of ending the call at any stage, and poor reception or a low battery. It is highly recommended that confirmation of the patient's physical location or a contact number and/or address be obtained at the outset in case it becomes necessary to initiate a welfare check.

Conclusion

Suicide risk assessment is the first step in good management. A suicide risk assessment is best conducted employing a multifaceted approach. The SMART checklist for neurodisability provides an example of the clinical areas that need to be covered in any assessment process.

The following four chapters will delineate treatment approaches, safety planning, and restriction of means. In particular, Chapter 9 will provide an introduction to the current evidence base for suicide prevention; Chapter 10 will outline clinical management approaches that complement evidence-informed interventions; Chapter 11 will review the adaptation of such approaches to cross-cultural contexts; and Chapter 12 will discuss the organizational elements needed to support the assessment and treatment of suicide.

Implications for Clinicians

1. Suicide risk assessment is best conducted using a multifaceted approach.

2. Conducting a clinical interview is part of a frontline assessment response and will provide important information about the severity, risk factors, and imminence of suicide risk.

3. Monitoring for warning signs enables a close watch to be maintained on fluctuating levels of severity of suicidal thoughts and possible behaviors over time.

4. Validated scales such as the Beck Scale for Suicide Ideation (Beck & Steer, 1991) and the Beck Hopelessness Scale (Beck & Steer, 1988) can make an important contribution to the assessment of suicide risk.

5. It is important that the assessment forms the basis for reaching a conclusion about the severity and imminence of the suicide risk.

References

Almqvist, E. W., Bloch, M., Brinkman, R., Craufurd, D., & Hayden, M. R. (1999). A worldwide assessment of the frequency of suicide, suicide attempts, or psychiatric hospitalization after predictive testing for Huntington disease. *The American Journal of Human Genetics, 64*, 1293–1304.

Bech, P., & Awata, S. (2009). Measurement of suicidal behaviour with psychometric scales. In D. Wasserman & C. Wasserman (Eds.), *Oxford textbook of suicidology and suicide prevention: A global perspective* (pp. 305–311). New York: Oxford University Press.

Beck, A. T., Brown, G., & Steer, R. A. (1989). Prediction of eventual suicide in psychiatric inpatients by clinical ratings of hopelessness. *Journal of Consulting and Clinical Psychology, 57*, 309–310.

Beck, A. T., Schuyler, D., & Herman, I. (1974). Development of suicide intent scales. In A. T. Beck, H. L. P. Resnick, & D. J. Lettieri (Eds.), *The prediction of suicide* (pp. 45–56). Bowie, MD: Charles Press.

Beck, A. T., & Steer, R. A. (1988). *Manual for the Beck Hopelessness Scale*. San Antonio, TX: Psychological Corp.

Beck, A. T., & Steer, R. A. (1991). *Manual for the Beck Scale for suicide ideation*. San Antonio, TX: Psychological Corp.

Bell, G. S., Gaitatzis, A., Bell, C. L., Johnson, A. L., & Sander, J. W. (2009). Suicide in people with epilepsy: How great is the risk? *Epilepsia, 50*(8), 1933–1942.

Blumer, D., Montouris, G., Davies, K., Wyler, A., Phillips, B., & Hermann, B. (2002). Suicide in epilepsy: Psychopathology, pathogenesis, and prevention. *Epilepsy and Behavior, 3*, 232–241.

Breshears, R. E., Brenner, L. A., Harwood, J., & Gutierrez, P. M. (2010). Predicting suicidal behaviour in Veterans with traumatic brain injury: The utility of the Personality Assessment Inventory. *Journal of Personality Assessment, 92*, 349–355.

Brown, G. K. (2000). *A review of suicide assessment measures for intervention research with adults and older adults*. Retrieved from http://www.suicidology.org/c/document_library/get_file?folderID=235&name=DLFE-113.pdf.

Bryan, C. J., & Rudd, M. D. (2006). Advances in the assessment of suicide risk. *Journal of Clinical Psychology: In Session, 62*, 185–200.

Cochrane-Brinks, K. A., Lofchy, J. S., & Sakinofsky, I. (2000). Clinical rating scales in suicide risk assessment. *General Hospital Psychiatry, 22*, 445–451.

Cohen, D., Llorente, M., & Eisdorfer, C. (1998). Homicide-suicide in older persons. *American Journal of Psychiatry, 155*, 390–396.

Dennis, J. P., Ghahramanlou-Holloway, M., Cox, D. W., & Brown, G. K. (2011). A guide for the assessment and treatment of suicidal patients with traumatic brain injuries. *Journal of Head Trauma Rehabilitation, 26*, 244–256.

Department of Veterans Affairs/Department of Defense (DVA/DoD). (2013). *Clinical practice guideline for assessment and management of patients at risk for suicide.* Retrieved from https://www.healthquality.va.gov/guidelines/MH/srb/VADODCP_SuicideRisk_Full.pdf

Exner, J. E. (2002). *The Rorschach: A comprehensive system: Vol 1. Basic foundations and principles of interpretation* (4th ed.). New York: Wiley.

Fowler, J. C. (2012). Suicide risk assessment in clinical practice: Pragmatic guidelines for imperfect assessments. *Psychotherapy, 49*, 81–90.

Fukuchi, T., Kanemoto, K., Kato, M., Ishida, S., Yuasa, S., Kawasaki, J., . . . Onuma, T. (2002). Death in epilepsy with special attention to suicide cases. *Epilepsy research, 51*, 233–236.

Garden, F. H., Garrison, S. J., & Jain, A. (1990). Assessing suicide risk in stroke patients: Review of two cases. *Archives of Physical Medicine & Rehabilitation, 71*, 1003–1005.

Hara, E., Akanuma, N., Adachi, N., Hara, K., & Koutroumanidis, M. (2009). Suicide attempts in adult patients with idiopathic generalized epilepsy. *Psychiatry and Clinical Neurosciences, 63*, 225–229.

Hendin, H. (2006). Recognizing a suicide crisis in psychiatric patients. In D. Wasserman & C. Wasserman (Eds.), *Oxford textbook of suicidology and suicide prevention: A global perspective* (pp. 327–331). New York: Oxford University Press.

Homaifar, B. Y., Bahraini, N., Silvermann, M. M., & Brenner, L. A. (2012). Executive functioning as a component of suicide risk assessment: Clarifying its role in standard clinical applications. *Journal of Mental Health Counseling, 34*, 110–120.

Homaifar, B. Y., Matarazzo, B., & Wortzel, H. (2013). Therapeutic risk management of the suicidal Patient: Augmenting clinical suicide risk assessment with structured instruments. *Journal of Psychiatric Practice, 19*, 406–409.

Jacobs, D. G., Brewer, M., & Klein-Benheim, M. (1999). Suicide assessment: An overview and recommended protocol. In D. G. Jacobs (Ed.), *The Harvard Medical School guide to suicide assessment and intervention* (pp. 3–39). San Francisco, CA: Jossey-Bass.

Joiner, T. E. (2005). *Why people die by suicide.* Cambridge, MA: Harvard University Press.

Jones, J. E., Hermann, B. P., Barry, J. J., Gilliam, F. G., Kanner, A. M., & Meador, K. J. (2003). Rates and risk factors for suicide, suicidal ideation and suicide attempts in chronic epilepsy. *Epilepsy and Behavior, 4*, S31–S38.

Kwan, P., & Brodie, M. J. (2001). Neuropsychological effects of epilepsy and antiepileptic drugs. *Lancet, 357*, 216–222.

Kuipers, P., & Lancaster, A. (2000). Developing a suicide prevention strategy based on the perspective of people with brain injuries. *Journal of Head Trauma Rehabilitation, 15*, 1275–1284.

Linehan, M. M., Goodstein, J. L., Nielsen, S. L., & Chiles, J. A. (1983). Reasons for staying alive when you are thinking of killing yourself: The reasons for living inventory. *Journal of Consulting and Clinical Psychology, 51*, 276–286.

Malphurs, J. E., & Cohen, D. (2005). A state-wide case-control study of spousal homicide-suicide in older persons. *The American Journal of Geriatric Psychiatry, 13*, 211–217.

Mann, J. J., Waternaux, C., Haas, G. L., & Malone, K. M. (1999). Towards a clinical model of suicidal behaviour in psychiatric patients. *American Journal of Psychiatry, 156*, 181–189.

Mendez, M. F., & Doss, R. C. (1992). Ictal and psychiatric aspects of suicide in epileptic patients. *International Journal of Psychiatry in Medicine, 22*, 231–237.

Michel, K., Valach, L., & Waeber, V. (1994). Understanding deliberate self-harm: The patient's views. *Crisis, 15*, 172–178.

Minden, S. L., Orav, J., & Reich, P. (1987). Depression in multiple sclerosis. *General Hospital Psychiatry, 9*, 426–434.

Motto, J. A. (1989). Problems in suicide risk assessment. In D. G. Jacobs, & H. N. Brown (Eds.), *Suicide: Understanding and responding: Harvard Medical School perspectives on suicide* (pp. 129–142). Madison, CT: International Universities Press.

Muehlenkamp, J. J., Gutierrez, P. M., Osman, A., & Barrios, F. X. (2005). Validation of the Positive and Negative Suicide Ideation (PANSI) Inventory in a diverse sample of young adults. *Journal of Clinical Psychology, 61*, 431–445.

National Institute for Health and Clinical Excellence. (2011). *Self-harm: Longer-term management*. NICE Clinical Guideline 133. London: Author.

Palmieri, A., Soraru, G., Albertini, E., Semenza, C., Vottero-Ris, F., D'Ascenzo, C., . . . Angelini, C. (2010). Psychopathological features and suicidal ideation in amyotrophic lateral sclerosis patients. *Neurological Sciences, 31*(6), 735–740.

Paulsen, J. S., Hoth, K. F., Nehl, C., & Stierman, L. (2005). Critical periods of suicide risk in Huntington's disease. *American Journal of Psychiatry, 162*, 725–731.

Pokorny, A. D. (1983). Prediction of suicide in psychiatric patients: Report of a prospective study. *Archives of General Psychiatry, 40*, 249–257.

Pokorny, A. D. (1993). Suicide prediction revisited. *Suicide and Life-Threatening Behavior, 23*, 1–10.

Pompili, M., Girardi, P., & Tatarelli, R. (2006). Death from suicide versus mortality from epilepsy in the epilepsies: A meta-analysis. *Epilepsy & Behavior, 9*, 641–648.

Posner, K., Brown, G. K., Stanley, B., Brent, D. A., Yershova, K. V., Oquendo, M. A., . . . Mann, J. J. (2011). The Columbia–Suicide Severity Rating Scale: Initial validity and internal consistency findings from three multisite studies with adolescents and adults. *American Journal of Psychiatry, 168*, 1266–1277.

Powell, J., Geddes, J., Hawton, K., Deeks, J., & Goldacre, M. (2000). Suicide in psychiatric hospital inpatients: Risk factors and their predictive power. *British Journal of Psychiatry, 176*, 266–272.

Rosenblatt, A., & Leroi, I. (2000). Neuropsychiatry of Huntington's Disease and other Basal Ganglia disorders. *Psychosomatics, 41*, 24–30.

Rudd, M. D. (2012). The clinical risk assessment interview. In R. I. Simon, & R. E. Hales (Eds.), *The American Psychiatric Publishing textbook of suicide assessment* (pp. 57–73), Washington DC: American Psychiatric Publishing.

Rudd, M. D., Berman, A. L., Joiner, T. E. Jr., Nock, M. K., Silverman, M. M., Mandrusiak, M., . . . Witte, T. (2006). Warning signs for suicide: Theory, research, and clinical applications. *Suicide and Life-Threatening Behavior, 36*, 255–262.

Sabaz, M., Simpson, G. K., Walker, A., Rogers, J., Gillis, G., & Strettles, B. (2014). Prevalence, co-morbidities and predictors of challenging behaviour among a cohort of community-dwelling adults with severe traumatic brain injury: A multi-centre study. *Journal of Head Trauma Rehabilitation, 29*, E19–E30.

Schecter, M., & Maltsberger, J. T. (2009). The clinical interview as a method in suicide risk assessment. In D. Wasserman & C. Wasserman (Eds.), *Oxford textbook of suicidology and suicide prevention: A global perspective* (pp. 319–325). New York: Oxford University Press.

Sheehan, D. V., Janavs, J., Baker, R., Harnett-Sheehan, K., Knapp, E., Sheehan, M., . . . Bonora, L. I. (1998). MINI-Mini International neuropsychiatric interview-English version 5.0. 0-DSM-IV. *Journal of Clinical Psychiatry, 59*, 34–57.

Shneidman, E. S. (1989). Overview: A multidimensional approach to suicide. In D. G. Jacobs, & H. N Brown (Eds.), *Suicide: Understanding and responding: Harvard Medical School perspectives on suicide* (pp. 1–30). Madison, CT: International Universities Press.

Shneidman, E. S. (1992). What do suicides have in common? Summary of the psychological approach. In B. Bongar (Ed.), *Suicide: Guidelines for assessment, management and treatment* (pp. 3–15). New York: Oxford University Press.

Simon, R. I. (2012). Suicide risk assessment: Gateway to treatment and management. In R. I. Simon, & R. E. Hales (Eds.), *The American Psychiatric Publishing textbook of suicide assessment* (pp. 3–28). Washington, DC: American Psychiatric Publishing.

Simpson, G. K., & Tate, R. L. (2002). Suicidality after traumatic brain injury: Demographic, injury and clinical correlates. *Psychological Medicine, 32*, 687–697.

Simpson, G. K., & Tate, R. L. (2005). Clinical features of suicide attempts after TBI. *The Journal of Nervous and Mental Disease, 193*, 680–685.

Simpson, G. K., & Tate, R. L. (2007). Suicidality in people surviving a traumatic brain injury: Prevalence, risk factors and implications for clinical management. *Brain Injury, 21*, 1335–1351.

Simpson, G. K., Tate, R. L., Whiting, D. L., & Cotter, R. E. (2011). Suicide prevention after traumatic brain injury: A randomized controlled trial of a program for the psychological treatment of hopelessness. *Journal of Head Trauma Rehabilitation, 26*, 290–300.

Smith, K., Conroy, R. W., & Ehler, B. D. (1984). Lethality of suicide attempt rating scale. *Suicide and Life-Threatening Behavior, 14*, 215–242.

Soden, R. J., Walsh, J., Middleton, J. W., Craven, M. L., Rutkowski, S. B., & Yeo, J. D. (2000). Causes of death after spinal cord injury. *Spinal Cord, 38*, 604–610.

Soulas, T., Gurruchaga, J. M., Palfi, S., Cesaro, P., Nguyen, J. P., & Fenelon, G. (2008). Attempted and completed suicides after subthalamic nucleus stimulation for Parkinson's disease. *Journal of Neurology, Neurosurgery & Psychiatry, 79*, 952–954.

Stenager, E. N., Stenager, E., Koch-Henriksen, N., Brønnum-Hansen, H., Hyllested, K., Jensen, K., & Bille-Brahe, U. (1992). Suicide and multiple sclerosis: An epidemiological investigation. *Journal of Neurology, Neurosurgery & Psychiatry, 55*, 542–545.

Tate, R. L., Simpson, G. K., Flanagan, S., & Coffey, M. (1997). Completed suicide after traumatic brain injury. *Journal of Head Trauma Rehabilitation, 12*, 16–28.

US Department of Health and Human Services (USDHHS), Office of the Surgeon General, & National Action Alliance for Suicide Prevention. (2012, September). *2012 National strategy for suicide prevention: Goals and objectives for action*. Washington, DC: HHS.

Verrotti, A., Cicconetti, A., Scorrano, B., De Berardis, D., Cotellessa, C., Chiarelli, F., & Ferro, F. M. (2008). Epilepsy and suicide: Pathogenesis, risk factors, and prevention. *Neuropsychiatric Disease and Treatment, 4*, 365–370.

Voon, V., Krack, P., Lang, A. E., Lozano, A. M., Dujardin, K., Schüpbach, M., . . . Speelman, J. D. (2008). A multicentre study on suicide outcomes following subthalamic stimulation for Parkinson's disease. *Brain, 131*, 2720–2728.

Wasserman, L., Shaw, T., Vu, M., Ko, C., Bollegala, D., & Bhalerao, S. (2008). An overview of traumatic brain injury and suicide. *Brain Injury, 22*, 811–819.

Weisman, A. D., & Worden, J. W. (1972). Risk-rescue rating in suicide assessment. *Archives of General Psychiatry, 26*, 553–560.

Wortzel, H. S., Homaifar, B., Matarazzo, B., & Brenner, L. A. (2014). Therapeutic risk management of the suicidal patient: Stratifying risk in terms of severity and temporality. *Journal of Psychiatric Practice, 20*, 63–67.

Zung, W. W. K. (1974). Index of Potential Suicide (IPS): A rating scale for suicide prevention. In A. T, Beck, H. L. P Resnick, & D. J. Lettieri (Eds.), *The prediction of suicide* (pp. 221–249). Bowie, MD: Charles Press.

9 Evidence-Based Interventions

Introduction

Despite recent efforts, the evidence base for interventions (i.e., psychotherapeutic and psychopharmacologic) that are specifically focused on ameliorating suicidal thoughts and/or behaviors without a history of neurodisability is limited. In turn, even less work has been undertaken to develop and test suicide prevention interventions for those coping with symptoms associated with a history of neurodisability. In discussing suicide prevention for those with traumatic brain injury (TBI) and implications for general practice, Simpson and Tate (2007a) suggest several strategies, including providing existing frontline treatments and addressing comorbid psychiatric issues (e.g., substance abuse, depression) associated with self-directed violent thoughts and behaviors. In the absence of clinical trials in the field of neurodisability, "frontline treatments" refer to psychotherapeutic and psychopharmacologic interventions (as outlined in national clinical guidelines or evidence-based reviews) used to treat other (non–brain damaged) populations displaying suicidal thoughts and behaviors and that are extrapolated to the field of neurodisability.

The information provided in this chapter will focus on (1) the evidence-based treatments for suicide prevention among those without neurodisability; (2) the one existing evidence-based intervention for suicide prevention among those with a neurologic condition, Window to Hope; and (3) evidence-based treatments to decrease one of the most common psychiatric condition among individuals with neurodisability, depression, which is also a risk factor for suicidal thoughts and behaviors. In conclusion, strategies for engaging individuals with impairments (cognitive, hearing, physical, and visual) in treatment will also be discussed. These will elaborate on the initial strategies outlined in Chapter 8.

Suicide Prevention Interventions for Those Without Neurodegenerative Disease

O'Neil and colleagues (2012) conducted a systematic review of suicide prevention interventions. Although their primary key question was "What is the effectiveness of specific interventions to reduce rates of suicidal [self-directed violence] SDV in military and/or veteran populations?" (p. 16), the lack of any randomized controlled trials in the population of interest resulted in the review being focused on Key Question 1: "What lessons can be learned from SDV violence prevention intervention research conducted outside of military settings that can be applied to veteran and/or military populations?" Findings were grouped based on the type of intervention (i.e., pharmacotherapy versus psychotherapy).

PSYCHOPHARMACOTHERAPY

In terms of medical treatments, it was determined that existing evidence was low or insufficient to make strong conclusions regarding the effectiveness of antidepressants in reducing suicidal behavior. The authors (O'Neil et al., 2012) noted that low strength of the evidence was in part associated with methodological concerns (e.g., short duration of studies and small sample sizes). Despite black box warnings, observational studies show a correlation between increasing prescription rates for antidepressants and decreasing suicidal behavior. Similar findings were reported regarding antipsychotic and mood stabilizers medications, including lithium (O'Neil et al., 2012).

PSYCHOTHERAPY

Finding existing research to be heterogeneous in terms of psychotherapeutic interventions, durations of treatment, and populations studied, O'Neil and colleagues (2012) grouped trials by populations (those with borderline personality disorder, recent suicide attempts/prevention of suicide deaths, psychotic spectrum disorders, or depression/dysthymia). Therapies tested among those with borderline personality disorder included dialectic behavioral therapy (Linehan et al., 2006), mentalization-based treatment (Bateman & Fonagy, 2009), structured clinical management, systems training for emotional predictability and problem-solving (STEPPS; Bateman & Fonagy, 2009), and cognitive-behavioral therapy (CBT) specific to Cluster B personality disorders (Davidson et al., 2006; Davidson, Tyrer, Norrie, Palmer, & Tyrer, 2010) (see Table 9.1).

Despite the overall low strength of the evidence (in part because of the limited number of suicides that occurred during the trial), dialectic behavioral therapy and mentalization-based treatment were identified as having an evidence base. In terms of psychotherapies specifically designed to prevent suicide, existing studies were generally underpowered, and design flaws contributed to potential bias (O'Neil et al., 2012). Per O'Neil and colleagues (2012) the "strongest evidence" for an intervention for those with a recent suicide attempt is problem-solving treatment (PST; Hatcher, Sharon, Parag, & Collins, 2009). Similar weaknesses were identified regarding existing research for suicide prevention interventions among those with psychotic spectrum and depressive disorders.

PST-oriented interventions (D'Zurilla & Goldfried, 1971) have been successfully implemented among those with a history of neurodisability (Tsaosides & Gordon, 2009; Fong & Howid, 2009) as well as among those with a previous history of suicide (Hatcher et al., 2009). Rath and colleagues (2003) conducted a randomized controlled trial (RCT) of 60 individuals with mild to severe TBI (novel PST-oriented treatment or conventional group therapy) and found that those who received the PST intervention showed significant improvements in problem-solving. Results were maintained at 6 months. Fong and Howie (2009) investigated the effects of problem-solving training among 33 outpatients with moderate acquired brain injury using a metacomponential approach and found that those in the novel program demonstrated better outcomes regarding problem representation. As noted earlier, Hatcher et al. (2011) explored whether PST would improve outcomes (e.g., presenting again with self-harm) among adults presenting to a hospital after an SDV event (PST plus usual care vs. usual care alone). The outpatient PST intervention—up to nine, 1-hour sessions—focused on problem orientation, problem listing and definition, brainstorming, devising an action plan, and reviewing the plan. There was also a specific focus on the person's previous suicide attempt. Although the intervention was found to have little effect on the overall rate of repetition, among the 38% of people who presented with a repeat episode of SDV, those randomized to PST had a 39% lower risk of a further presentation after a year. At 3 months and 1 year, those in the PST group also showed significantly greater improvements on measures of hopelessness, suicidal

TABLE 9.1

Promising psychotherapeutic interventions for those without a history of neurodisability

Treatment	Population	Citation
Cognitive Behavioral Therapy (CBT) for Suicide Prevention	Individuals with a history of a suicide attempt; Adults	Brown, G. K., Ten Have, T., Henriques, G. R., Xie, S. X., Hollander, J. E., & Beck, A. T. (2005). Cognitive therapy for the prevention of suicide attempts: a randomized controlled trial. *JAMA, 294*, 563–570.
Dialectic Behavioral Therapy (DBT)	Individuals with Borderline Personality Disorder; Adults	Linehan, M. M., Comtois, K. A., Murray, A. M., Brown, M. Z., Gallop, R. J., Heard, H. L., . . . & Lindenboim, N. (2006). Two-year randomized controlled trial and follow-up of dialectical behavior therapy vs therapy by experts for suicidal behaviors and borderline personality disorder. *Archives of General Psychiatry, 63*, 757–766.
Mentalization-Based Treatment (MBT)	Individuals with Borderline Personality Disorder; Adults	Bateman, A., & Fonagy, P (2009). Randomized controlled trial of outpatient mentalization-based treatment versus structured clinical management for borderline personality disorder. *American Journal of Psychiatry, 166*, 1355–1364.
Problem-Solving Therapy (PST)	Individuals with a history of a suicide attempt; Adults	Hatcher, S., Sharon, C., Parag, V., & Collins, N. (2011). Problem-solving therapy for people who present to hospital with self-harm: Zelen randomised controlled trial. *British Journal of Psychiatry, 199*, 310–316.

From O'Neil et al. (2012).

thinking, problem-solving, anxiety, and depression. Also of note, Hatcher and colleagues (2009) suggested that PST may be an especially useful suicide prevention intervention for those with poor problem-solving skills (e.g., those with cognitive impairment). These findings suggest that PST is a promising candidate and a potential stand-alone effective intervention for those with neurodegenerative conditions and a history of suicidal thought and behaviors.

Moreover, to specifically address challenges in problem-solving hypothesized to increase risk among those with moderate to severe TBI Brenner and colleagues (2015) developed and tested the acceptability and feasibility of an intervention titled Problem-Solving Therapy for Suicide Prevention (PST-SP) (see also Barnes et al., 2017). Conducted in a group setting, problem-solving training (e.g., D'Zurilla & Goldfried, 1971) is paired with safety planning (Stanley & Brown, 2008) to facilitate suicide prevention among veterans with hopelessness and moderate-to-severe TBI. Quantitative and qualitative results suggested that PST-SP was an acceptable and feasible intervention for veterans at risk of suicide due to a history of moderate to severe TBI and clinically significant hopelessness. For example, one veteran participant stated, "It opened my eyes to the bad way in which I deal with problems. I did not even recognize them, and now I have the ability to define a problem that is confronting me . . . [and] understand that all problems can be worked through" (p. 604). Findings also supported readiness for Phase II randomized controlled trial to evaluate the efficacy of PST-SP.

Based on previous research that suggests that individuals with neurodisability can benefit from cognitive behavioral interventions (Stalder-Lüthy et al., 2013; Waldron, Casserly, & O'Sullivan, 2013), the authors would like to highlight cognitive therapy for the prevention of suicide attempts (Brown et al., 2005). Unfortunately, Brown et al.'s (2005) seminal publication regarding this intervention in the *Journal of the American Medical Association* seems to have fallen between O'Neil et al.'s (2012) recent review and previous reviews by Mann and colleagues (2005) and Gaynes et al. (2004). CBT for suicide prevention (Brown et al., 2005) is an individual psychotherapy for those with previous suicidal SDV. The "central feature of the intervention" is the "identification of proximal thoughts, images, and core beliefs" activated prior to the suicide attempt and the use of cognitive behavioral strategies to help the client develop adaptive coping strategies. One hundred and twenty adults with a recent suicide attempt were randomized to the CBT 10-week intervention or enhanced care as usual with tracking and referral services. From baseline to the 18-month follow-up assessment, 13 participants in CBT (24.1%) versus 23 (41.6%) made at least one subsequent suicide attempt ($p = .049$). Those in the CBT group also noted significantly less hopelessness ($p = .045$).

Since the review, additional data in support of CBT have emerged. Rudd and colleagues (2015) evaluated the effectiveness of a brief CBT intervention with the goal of preventing suicide attempts among military personnel. Active duty soldiers who had attempted suicide or reported suicidal ideation were randomized to treatment as usual or treatment as usual plus the brief CBT intervention. During the follow-up period, soldiers in the latter group were approximately 60% less likely to make a suicide attempt than those who received only treatment as usual.

LETHAL MEANS SAFETY AND COUNSELING

Reducing the lethality of the environment has proved to be one of the most effective interventions in reducing suicide (Mann et al., 2005). Historically, an early example of the efficacy of this approach was observed in the phasing out of the domestic use of coal gas in the United Kingdom (Kreitman, 1976). More recently, evidence from the United Kingdom and Australia suggests that legislation requiring changes in medication packaging has led to reductions in the total number of tablets taken in overdose and to subsequent decreases in morbidity and mortality (Buckley, Newby, Dawson, & Whyte, 1995; Hawton, 2002; Hawton et al., 2004; Hawton et al., 2001; Prince, Thomas, James, & Hudson, 2000; Robinson, Smith, & Johnston, 2000; Turvill, Burroughs, & Moore, 2000).

This, along with other research and clinical efforts, has increased focus on lethal means safety as a method of suicide prevention. *Lethal means* are objects, such as medications, firearms, and sharp objects, that can be used to engage in suicidal behavior. Counseling regarding lethal means safety is relevant to both inpatient and outpatient settings. In the inpatient settings, issues such as hanging points, open windows, and the hoarding of medication need to be carefully managed. In outpatient settings, the range of items that could be discussed includes firearms, medication, or other means that are part of an articulated suicide plan. Clinicians are encouraged to work with clients and family members to facilitate means safety during periods of crisis. This may include temporarily removing guns or bullets from the home or safely discarding medications that may be lethal but are no longer being taken by the individual. Reducing access to firearms during periods of crisis has particular applicability in the United States (Betz, Barber, & Miller, 2011; Miller, Barber, Azrael, Hemenway, & Molnar, 2009) where gun-related means of suicide are elevated compared to most other Western countries, both among the general population and within neurodisability (see Chapter 11). Efforts aimed at training clinicians to conduct lethal means counseling are under way in both civilian and veteran settings (for additional resources, see https://www.hsph.harvard.edu/means-matter/lethal-means-counseling/ and https://www.mirecc.va.gov/lethalmeanssafety/index.asp).

Suicide Specific Prevention Interventions for Those with Neurodisability

As noted earlier, research in this area has been sparse. In a recent systematic review regarding suicide and TBI, Bahraini and colleagues (2013) identified three studies in which suicidal ideation was an outcome. Only one (Window to Hope; Simpson, Tate, Whiting, & Cotter, 2011) had a low risk of bias. Nonetheless, this is an improvement from a similar previous review conducted by Simpson and Tate (2007b) which found that no treatments or clinical management approaches for people with TBI had been tested. To the best of our knowledge, no suicide prevention–specific interventions had been tested across the other seven neurologic conditions covered in this book. That being said, Window to Hope sets the stage for what is possible when interventions are designed and implemented for those with neurodisability more broadly.

This intervention, a 20-hour manualized group CBT program for those with moderate to severe TBI, is structured around four therapeutic strategies: behavioral activation, cognitive restructuring, problem-solving, and relapse prevention. As research suggests that hopelessness is both a risk factor for suicide and highly prevalent among those with TBI, it is specifically targeted both across the four sections of the program and in the primary treatment outcome. Therapeutic strategies aimed at compensating for cognitive impairment are woven into the intervention (e.g., small group size [2–3 participants]; handouts and worksheets containing limited amounts of text in large-sized font). To evaluate the efficacy of the intervention, Simpson et al. (2011) conducted a pilot RCT (treatment, $n = 8$; waitlist, $n = 9$) and identified a significant group-by-time interaction on the Beck Hopelessness Scale (Beck & Steer, 1988) in the treatment group ($F_{1,\ 15} = 13.20$; $P = .002$). More recently, the intervention has been culturally adapted for US military veterans, and a Phase II RCT was conducted among members of this population with moderate to severe TBI (Matarazzo et al., 2014; Brenner et al., 2017). Results from the RCT supported the efficacy of Window to Hope as a psychotherapeutic suicide-prevention intervention for veterans with a history of moderate to severe TBI. In specific, those who participated in the intervention reported significantly lower scores on the Beck Hopelessness Scale (Beck & Steer, 1988) than those who were initially allocated to the waitlist group. Also of note, to the best of our knowledge, this replication is a first among psychological interventions for psychological distress in those with moderate to severe TBI (Brenner et al., 2017).

Evidence-Based Treatments for Those with Neurodisability and Depression

As previously noted, depression is both highly prevalent among those with neurodisability and a significant risk factor for suicide. Although treatment of depressive symptoms alone is not a sufficient suicide prevention strategy, assessment and implementation of interventions aimed at ameliorating depression is warranted. Two recent reviews provide support for the use of CBT among those with acquired brain injury (Waldron et al., 2013; Stalder-Lüthy et al., 2013). Despite this support, Waldron et al. (2013) noted that CBT was not effective for all participants. Dose effects and poor generalization (e.g., CBT to target anger did not significantly impact symptoms of depression) were also discussed (Waldron et al., 2013). Fann, Hart, and Schomer (2009) conducted an earlier systematic review to evaluate the evidence regarding interventions for TBI and noted that, at that time, the largest pharmacological intervention to date had enrolled 54 patients. Despite the "paucity" of RCTs for depression following TBI, the "best" preliminary evidence seemed to support serotonergic antidepressants and cognitive-behavioral interventions. Unfortunately, a paucity of evidence also exists in terms of effective treatment of depression among other populations with neurodisability.

In a 2005 review regarding depression and multiple sclerosis (MS), Siegert and Abernethy (2005) noted that "there is a small body of controlled studies indicating that depression in people with MS respond well to two treatments—psychotherapy that emphasizes the development of active coping skills (such as CBT) and antidepressant medication" (p. 473). They also noted a previously conducted review/meta-analysis by Mohr and Goodkin (1999) that included five studies and provided support for psychotherapy or antidepressants. Seven years after this review was published, Mohr, Hart, Fonreva, and Tasch (2006) published a study regarding the adequacy of antidepressant pharmacotherapy in a sample of patients with MS being treated by neurologists. Although 25% ($n = 67$) of the 260 patients met criteria for major depressive disorder, 65.6% received no antidepressant medication, 4.7% received subthreshold doses from their neurologists, 26.6% received doses at threshold, and 3.1% received doses exceeding threshold (Mohr et al., 2006).

Modifying Treatment Strategies

As articulated in the discussion regarding Window to Hope, strategies can be employed to assist those with neurodegenerative conditions and associated impairments to participate in and benefit from interventions. In a recent systematic review, Gallagher, McLeod, and McMillan (2016) identified modifications for CBT for cognitive impairment across the domains of attention/concentration/alertness, communication, memory, executive functioning, and therapeutic education in relation to CBT (Table 9.2). In addition to cognitive impairments, Signoracci, Matarazzo, and Bahraini (2012) and Williams and Abeles (2004) have identified strategies to manage auditory, physical, and visual impairments. Although further research is required to provide an evidence-base for the presented suggestions, it is

TABLE 9.2

Intervention strategies to compensate for common cognitive and sensory impairments after neurodisability

Impairment	Strategies
Cognitive	• Shorter sessions
	• Increase frequency of sessions
	• Slower pace of conversation and presentation of information
	• Taking breaks mid-session
	• Presentation of less material during each session and on handouts
	• Limit use of lengthy, open-ended, or multiple questions
	• Use of clear structured questions
	• Place emphasis on behavioral techniques (such as behavioral activation)
	• Summarize and repeat salient points at frequent intervals during the session
	• Visual and verbal cues and mnemonics
	• Written, phone, text, and web-based reminders regarding session content, homework, and upcoming sessions
	• Employment of external supports (e.g., smartphones, support persons, family members) either in the session or in supporting homework tasks to enhance generalization
	• Use summarizing, verbal redirection or some cue to alert clients when they have become tangential
	• Focus on concrete examples and aid clients to generate alternative solutions (in such cases, it is then important for the client to decide whether or not they would like to adapt a proffered option/alternative)
	• Therapist takes a directive and structured approach if needed
	• Model between-session task completion
	• If doing group-based therapy, small group size (2–4 participants)
Auditory	• Openness to communication options (including sign language, writing, and other forms of verbal and visual communication)
	• Scheduling by mail, fax, or email
Physical	• Home or community-based treatment
	• Tele-interventions
Visual	• Use of multiple modalities to present materials

From Signoracci et al. (2012); Williams and Abeles (2004); Gallagher et al. (2016).

believed that such strategies will improve outcomes in both research and practice settings.

Conclusion

Although work in this area has been limited, existing research suggests that those with a history of neurological disabilities can benefit from therapeutic interventions aimed at directly reducing suicide risk (lethal means safety), as well as those that address secondary drivers of suicide (e.g., depression). Further work is needed to identify interventions aimed at meeting the specific needs of those living with neurodisabilities and their caregivers.

Implications for Clinicians

1. Individuals living with neurodisability can benefit from strategies aimed at reducing suicide risk, including pharmacologic, environmental (lethal means safety), and psychotherapeutic interventions.
2. Reducing the lethality of the environment should be a core therapeutic consideration.
3. Limited modifications can be made to evidence-based psychotherapies developed for those without a history of disability to increase the feasibility of implementation among those with cognitive impairments related to neurodisability.
4. In the case of chronic hopelessness after TBI, Window to Hope should be considered as a frontline therapeutic treatment option.
5. The delivery of psychotherapeutic interventions should be adapted to compensate for the cognitive, behavioral, and motor-sensory impairments faced by people with neurodisability, while maintaining intervention fidelity.

References

Bahraini, N., Simpson, G. K., Brenner, L., Hoffberg, A., & Schneider, A. L. (2013). Suicidal ideation and behaviours after traumatic brain injury: A systematic review. *Brain Impairment, 14*, 92–112.

Barnes, S. M., Monteith, L. L., Gerard, G. R., Hoffberg, A. S., Homaifar, B. Y., & Brenner, L. A. (2017). Problem-solving therapy for suicide prevention in veterans with moderate-to-severe traumatic brain injury. *Rehabilitation Psychology, 62*, 600–608.

Bateman, A., & Fonagy, P. (2009). Randomized controlled trial of outpatient mentalization-based treatment versus structured clinical management for borderline personality disorder. *American Journal of Psychiatry, 166*, 1355–1364.

Beck, A. T., & Steer, R. A. (1988). *Manual for the Beck Hopelessness Scale*. San Antonio, TX: Psychological Corp.

Betz, M. E., Barber, C., & Miller, M. (2011). Suicidal behavior and firearm access: Results from the second injury control and risk survey. *Suicide and Life Threatening Behavior, 41*, 384–391.

Brenner, L. A., Bahraini, N., Homaifar, B. Y., Monteith, L. L., Nagamoto, H., Dorsey-Holliman, B., & Forster, J. E. (2015). Executive functioning and suicidal behavior among veterans with and without a history of traumatic brain injury. *Archives of Physical Medicine and Rehabilitation, 96*, 1411–1418. http://dx.doi.org/10.1016/j.apmr.2015.04.010

Brenner, L. A., Forster, J. E., Hoffberg, A. S., Matarazzo, B. B., Hostetter, T. A., Signoracci, G., & Simpson, G. K. (2017). Window to hope: A randomized controlled trial of a psychological intervention for the treatment of hopelessness among veterans with moderate to severe TBI. *Journal of Head Trauma Rehabilitation*. doi: 10.1097/HTR.0000000000000351

Brown, G. K., Ten Have, T., Henriques, G. R., Xie, S. X., Hollander, J. E., & Beck, A. T. (2005). Cognitive therapy for the prevention of suicide attempts: A randomized controlled trial. *Journal of the American Medical Association, 294*, 563–570.

Buckley, N. A., Newby, D. A., Dawson, A. H., & Whyte, I. M. (1995). The effect of the introduction of safety packaging for carbamazepine on toxicity in overdose in adults. *Pharmacoepidemiology and Drug Safety, 4*(6), 351–354. doi:10.1002/pds.2630040606

Davidson, K., Norrie, J., Tyrer, P., Gumley, A., Tata, P., Murray, H., & Palmer, S. (2006). The effectiveness of cognitive behavior therapy for borderline personality disorder: Results from the borderline personality disorder study of cognitive therapy (BOSCOT) trial. *Journal of Personality Disorders, 20*, 450–465.

Davidson, K. M., Tyrer, P., Norrie, J., Palmer, S. J., & Tyrer, H. (2010). Cognitive therapy v. usual treatment for borderline personality disorder: Prospective 6-year follow-up. *British Journal of Psychiatry, 197*, 456–462.

Department of Veterans Affairs. (2017). *Lethal Means Safety & Suicide Prevention—MIRECC/CoE*. Retrieved from https://www.mirecc.va.gov/lethalmeanssafety/index.asp.

D'Zurilla, T. J. & Goldfried, M. R. (1971). Problem solving and behavior modification. *Journal of Abnormal Psychology, 78*, 271–281.

Fann, J. R., Hart, T., & Schomer, K. G. (2009). Treatment for depression after traumatic brain injury: A systematic review *Journal of Neurotrauma, 26*(12), 2383–2402. doi: 10.1089/neu.2009.1091

Fong, K., & Howid, D. (2009). Effects of an explicit problem-solving skills training program using a metacomponential approach for outpatients with acquired brain injury. *American Journal of Occupational Therapy, 63*, 525–534.

Gallagher, M., McLeod, H. J., & McMillan, T. M. (2016). A systematic review of recommended modifications of CBT for people with cognitive impairments following brain injury. *Neuropsychological Rehabilitation*, doi.org./10.1080/09602011.2016.1258367

Gaynes, B. N., West, S. L., Ford, C. A., Frame, P., Klein, J., & Lohr, K. N. (2004). Screening for suicide risk in adults: A summary of the evidence for the US Preventive Services Task Force. *Annals of Internal Medicine, 140*, 822–835.

Harvard School of Public Health. (2017, December 5). *Lethal means counseling.* Retrieved from https://www.hsph.harvard.edu/means-matter/lethal-means-counseling/

Hatcher, S., Sharon, C., Parag, V., & Collins, N. (2011). Problem-solving therapy for people who present to hospital with self-harm: Zelen randomised controlled trial. *British Journal of Psychiatry, 199,* 310–316.

Hawton, K. (2002). United Kingdom legislation on pack sizes of analgesics: Background, rationale, and effects on suicide and deliberate self-harm. *Suicide and Life Threatening Behavior, 32*(3), 223–229. doi:10.1521/suli.32.3.223.22169

Hawton, K., Simkin, S., Deeks, J., Copper, J., Johnston, A., Waters, K., . . .Simpson, K. (2004). UK legislation on analgesic packs: Before and after study of long term effect on poisonings. *British Medical Journal, 329*(7474), 1076. doi:10.1136/bmj.38253.527581.7C

Hawton, K., Townsend, E., Deeks, J., Appleby, L., Gunnell, D., Bennewith, O., & Cooper, J. (2001). Effects of legislation restricting pack sizes of paracetamol and salicylate on self poisoning in the United Kingdom: Before and after study. *British Medical Journal, 322*(7296), 1203–1207.

Kreitman, N. (1976). The coal gas story. United Kingdom suicide rates, 1960–71. *Journal of Epidemiology & Community Health, 30,* 86–93.

Linehan, M. M., Comtois, K. A., Murray, A. M., Brown, M. Z., Gallop, R. J., Heard, H. L., . . . Lindenboim, N. (2006). Two-year randomized controlled trial and follow-up of dialectical behavior therapy vs therapy by experts for suicidal behaviors and borderline personality disorder. *Archives of General Psychiatry, 63,* 757–766.

Mann, J. J., Apter, A., Bertolote, J., Beautrais, A., Currier, D., Haas, A., . . . Hendin, H. (2005). Suicide prevention strategies: A systematic review. *Journal of the American Medical Association, 294,* 2064–2074.

Matarazzo, B. B., Hoffberg, A. S., Clemans, T. A., Signoracci, G. M., Simpson, G. K., & Brenner, L. A. (2014). Cross-cultural adaptation of the Window to Hope: A psychological intervention to reduce hopelessness among US veterans with traumatic brain injury. *Brain Injury, 28,* 1238–1247.

Miller, M., Barber, C., Azrael, D., Hemenway, D., & Molnar, B. E. (2009). Recent psychopathology, suicidal thoughts and suicide attempts in households with and without firearms: Findings from the National Comorbidity Study Replication. *Injury Prevention, 15,* 183–187.

Mohr, D. C., & Goodkin, D. E. (1999). Treatment of depression in multiple sclerosis: Review and meta-analysis. *Clinical Psychology: Science and Practice, 6,* 1–9.

Mohr, D. C., Hart, S. L., Fonareva, I., & Tasch, E. S. (2006) Treatment of depression for patients with multiple sclerosis in neurology clinics. *Multiple Sclerosis,12,* 204–208.

O'Neil, M. E., Peterson, K., Low, A., Carson, S., Denneson, L. M., Haney, E., . . . Kansagara, D. (2012). *Suicide prevention interventions and referral/follow-up services: A systematic review.* VA-ESP Project 05-225.

Prince, M. I., Thomas, S. H., & James, O. F., & Hudson, M. (2000). Reduction in incidence of severe paracetamol poisoning. *Lancet, 355*(9220), 2047–2048. doi:10.1016/S0140-6736(00)02354-0

Rath, J., Simon, D., Langenbahn, D., Sherr, R., & Diller, L. (2003). Group treatment of problem-solving deficits in outpatients with traumatic brain injury: A randomized outcome study. *Neuropsychological Rehabilitation, 13,* 461–468

Robinson, D., Smith, A. M., & Johnston, G. D. (2000). Severity of overdose after restriction of paracetamol availability: A retrospective study. *British Medical Journal, 321,* 926–927.

Rudd, M. D., Bryan, C. J., Wertenberger, E. G., Peterson, A. L., Young-McCaughan, S., Mintz, J., ... Wilkinson, E. (2015). Brief cognitive-behavioral therapy effects on post-treatment suicide attempts in a military sample: Results of a randomized clinical trial with 2-year follow-up. *American Journal of Psychiatry, 172*, 441–449.

Siegert, R. J., & Abernethy, D. A. (2005). Depression in multiple sclerosis: A review. *Journal of Neurology, Neurosurgery and Psychiatry, 76*, 469–475. doi: 10.1136/jnnp.2004.054635

Signoracci, G. M., Matarazzo, B. B., & Bahraini, N. H. (2012) Traumatic brain injury and suicide: Contributing factors, risk assessment, and safety planning. In J. Lavigne (Ed.), *Frontiers in suicide prevention and risk research* (pp. 95–114). Hauppauge, NY: Nova Science.

Simpson, G. K., & Tate, R. L. (2007a). Preventing suicide after traumatic brain injury: Implications for general practice. *Medical Journal of Australia, 187*, 229–232.

Simpson, G., & Tate, R. (2007b). Suicidality in people surviving a traumatic brain injury: Prevalence, risk factors and implications for clinical management. *Brain Injury, 21*, 1335–1351.

Simpson, G. K., Tate, R. L., Whiting, D. L., & Cotter, R. E. (2011). Suicide prevention after traumatic brain injury: A randomized controlled trial of a program for the psychological treatment of hopelessness. *Journal of Head Trauma Rehabilitation, 26*, 290–300.

Stalder-Lüthy, F., Messerli-Bürgy, N., Hofer, H., Frischknecht, E., Znoj, H., & Barth, J. (2013). Effect of psychological interventions on depressive symptoms in long-term rehabilitation after an acquired brain injury: A systematic review and meta-analysis. *Archives of Physical Medicine and Rehabilitation, 94*, 1386–1397.

Stanley, B., & Brown, G. K. (2008). *Safety plan treatment manual to reduce suicide risk: Veteran version.* Washington, DC: United States Department of Veterans Affairs.

Tsaousides, T., & Gordon, W. A. (2009). Cognitive rehabilitation following traumatic brain injury: Assessment to treatment. *Mount Sinai Journal of Medicine: A Journal of Translational and Personalized Medicine, 76*, 173–181.

Turvill, J. L., Burroughs, A. K., & Moore, K. P. (2000). Change in occurrence of paracetamol overdose in UK after introduction of blister packs. *Lancet, 355*, 2048–2049.

Waldron, B., Casserly, L. M., & O'Sullivan, C. (2013). Cognitive behavioural therapy for depression and anxiety in adults with acquired brain injury. What works for whom? *Neuropsychological Rehabilitation, 23*, 64–101.

Williams, C. R., & Abeles, N. (2004). Issues and implications of deaf culture in therapy. *Professional Psychology: Research and Practice, 35*, 643–648.

10 Clinical Practice Approaches

Introduction

As outlined in Chapter 9, evidence-based methods to address suicide prevention for people with neurodisability are sparse. Therefore, current best practice involves a combination of limited evidence-based interventions (both interventions designed specifically for neurodisability and generic evidence-based approaches extrapolated from broader practice) integrated with rational clinical approaches (Department of Veterans Affairs/Department of Defense, 2013). The first half of this chapter will focus on these rational clinical approaches that can be combined with evidence-based approaches to formulate suicide prevention responses tailored to level of risk. Following this, the remaining half of the chapter will address postvention. *Postvention* can be defined as "those activities developed by, with, or for suicide survivors, in order to facilitate recovery after suicide, and to prevent adverse outcomes including suicidal behavior" (Andriessen, 2009, p. 43).

Treatment Approaches in Response to Assessed Level of Risk

The concept of tailoring interventions to levels of risk is widespread in suicidology (e.g., Bongar, 2002; Berman, 2006). In Chapter 8, key elements that make up a decision-making matrix that can structure the clinicians' conclusions about the degree of suicide risk after neurodisability were introduced. The matrix comprises three degrees of severity (high, intermediate, low) delineated across two time dimensions (acute, chronic). In this chapter, this matrix is fleshed out, detailing treatment approaches associated with the varied levels of risk (Table 10.1). In considering the

TABLE 10.1

Risk-related treatment approaches

	Acute	Chronic
High	Inpatient admission Direct observation Intensive treatment Environment limited access to lethal means Coordinated discharge plan between mental health and neurodisability services	Regular mental health follow-up Regular reassessment of suicide risk/Monitoring for warning signs Well-articulated safety plan Means restriction as part of safety plan Develop coping skills/protective factors Increase treatment intensity during crisis periods Increase supports
Intermediate	Treat as outpatient if meet sufficient criteria Intensive treatment Regular reassessment of suicide risk/monitoring for warning signs Well-articulated safety plan Increase supports	Routine mental health care Increase coping skills/protective factors Well-articulated safety plan
Low	Increase coping strategies/protective factors Well-articulated safety plan Monitoring for warning signs	

Adapted from Wortzel, Hofmaifar, Matarazzo, and Brenner (2014); Simpson (2001).

matrix, it is important to recognize that these categories are not static but can be dynamic, with a person moving from an intermediate to a high risk and, similarly, a lessening of risk intensity occurring with time and appropriate treatment.

Each category employs a multifaceted set of treatment approaches tailored to the level of risk. Some of these approaches have already been introduced in earlier chapters (suicide risk assessment/monitoring for warning signs in Chapter 8, and lethal means safety and psychological therapies in Chapter 9). The focus of this section will be on flagging the principles underpinning the treatment approach overall, followed by a description of additional treatment elements not previously outlined.

PRINCIPLES

The options detailed in Table 10.1 range from the minimally to highly restrictive (i.e., restricting an individual's freedom through an inpatient admission), and therefore it is important from the outset to be aware of three principles that can inform the selection of treatment decisions. First, it is important to provide treatment and support in the least restrictive environment (Objective 8, US Department of Health and Human Services [USDHHS], 2012). Not everyone who is suicidal requires inpatient treatment (Berman, 2006). This principle supports the notion that an inpatient admission should be the last option considered. Second, the individual's self-determination, operationalizing the principle of autonomy (DVA/DoD, 2013), should not be overridden without careful consideration. Weight needs to be given to the distressed individual's wishes as to how and where they should be treated or receive support during a suicidal crisis. The final principle is the staff's duty of care. In this context, staff need to balance the previous principles against their own responsibility (i.e., duty of care) to minimize the harm that could occur to a distressed individual. This takes on additional significance in the context of clients with significant cognitive impairment. In such cases, the balance of client autonomy and duty of care requires very careful consideration.

CRITERIA FOR INPATIENT VERSUS OUTPATIENT TREATMENT

A central application of these principles is in making a decision whether the person displaying suicidal thoughts and behaviors requires an inpatient admission or can be supported as an outpatient. Driving this decision is an assessment of whether the person is able to maintain his or her own safety; that is, to use a safety plan and get help and support if risk increases.

In the case of high acute suicide risk (see Table 10.1), there is broad consensus that an inpatient admission is usually warranted (e.g., Berman, 2006; Bongar, 2002).

People at acute intermediate risk need very careful review before making a decision about inpatient versus outpatient admission (Maltsberger & Stoklosa, 2012). The clinical features listed in Box 10.1 can help guide clinician decision-making around these decisions, although there are no "gold standard" criteria.

BOX 10.1
CRITERIA FOR INPATIENT VERSUS OUTPATIENT MANAGEMENT

Outpatient Treatment

If a suicidal person is assessed as being able to maintain his or her own safety (i.e., to use a safety plan and get help and support if risk increases), then outpatient management is a reasonable option. Criteria include:

- Able to keep self from self-harm
- Able to engage with counsellors and co-operate with treatment
- Is known to the people treating, and they have confidence in the person
- Has a clear diagnosis
- Has other protective factors including support of family and/or friends able to provide ongoing support
- Has service support networks in case of a further crisis or breakdown in family support systems

Inpatient Treatment

Inpatient treatment is reserved for people at greatest risk, and it is always important for staff to balance the least restrictive option with person's right of autonomy. Factors that may suggest that an inpatient admission is necessary apply to individual who are having difficulty managing their own safety due to:

- High levels of distress, agitation, or hopelessness
- Need for ongoing observation, monitoring, and support not available in the community
- History of a recent suicide attempt
- Intoxicated to a level that means it is not possible to conduct full assessment
- Suicidal and also experiencing severe depressive or psychotic problems
- Absence of viable support (family, friends, services)
- Need for admission to commence treatment (e.g., medication)

From Berman (2006); New South Wales Health (1999).

INPATIENT ADMISSIONS

An inpatient admission can keep individuals safe until they are able to keep themselves safe in a less restrictive environment. Such hospitalization can be voluntary, but in cases in which the client refuses, an involuntary admission to a secure ward may need to be arranged. The legalities surrounding who can approve and execute such admissions, the premises to which a person may be admitted, the length of time for which a person can be detained, and the processes of review for such admissions vary from jurisdiction to jurisdiction. It is crucial for staff who play a role in managing suicidal thoughts and behaviors among clients with neurodisability to familiarize themselves with the local context.

DIRECT OBSERVATION

Direct observation (see Table 10.1) within the context of such admissions aims to monitor the person for agitation or distress. Furthermore, direct observation helps limit the person's access to lethal means of suicide, such as hoarding medication or seeking hanging points within such an environment. The issue of direct observation also has applicability to voluntary residential environments (e.g., nursing homes, group homes, neurorehabilitation centers). While undertaking observation may seem like common sense, there has been limited research into its efficacy (Manna, 2010), and a number of factors need to be considered in its implementation.

Observation can only work if it is delivered effectively and safely (Janofsky, 2009). The level of observation is an important consideration (Janofsky, 2009). It should be commensurate with the degree of assessed risk; for example, continual observation versus close (or intermittent) observation, which might involve checking every 15 minutes (Konrad et al., 2007; Meehan et al., 2006). For example, if the assessment is that a suicide attempt might be imminent, it is important to remember that it only takes 5–7 minutes for a lethal hanging to occur (Konrad et al., 2007). Suicide by hanging is one of the potential means of death after neurodisability, having been reported among people with traumatic brain injury (TBI; Achte, Lonnqvist, & Hillbom, 1971), epilepsy (Nilsson, Ahlbom, Farahmand, Åsberg, & Tomson, 2002), Huntington's disease (Baliko, Csala, & Czopf, 2004), and multiple sclerosis (Stenager, Koch-Henriksen, & Stenager, 1996).

However, continuous observation is difficult to implement and staff may have different understandings of whether direct observation means line of sight at arms' length or some other distance, whether it means observation of the patient in bathroom, and what sort of breaks in observation are allowable. Patients may also resent this continuous monitoring (Fletcher, 1999). Furthermore, some staff perceive observation as a low-level task with limited clinical utility (Doughty, 2002). Janofsky (2009) presents a useful observation workflow model developed for nurses-physicians in the context of shift-based episodes of care that addresses many of the implementation problems identified in the literature.

INTENSIVE TREATMENT

Intensive treatment is important for inpatients with high acute risk, outpatients with intermediate acute risk, or outpatients with chronic risk who are experiencing a crisis period (e.g., Jones et al., 2003; Soden et al., 2000; see Table 10.1). Overall, the goal is to "reduce the hurt and/or widen the vision and/or pull back from action and/or lighten the pressure—even a little bit" (Shneidman, 1989). Intensity can refer to either the number of treatment modalities that comprise the intervention or the frequency with which a single modality is provided. In the context of tailoring interventions to the level of suicide risk, mental health treatments can be intensive (i.e., daily), regular (i.e., weekly), or routine (less than weekly) (see Table 10.1).

Treatment of mental health disorders constitutes a traditional frontline approach in suicide prevention generally, and it is assumed that it will be of equal importance in managing suicide risk among individuals with neurodisability (e.g., Wasserman et al., 2008). Treatment approaches principally comprise pharmacotherapy or psychological interventions. The importance of referral to a mental health professional who has experience with suicide prevention–focused intervention, as well as familiarity with evidence-based treatments for mental health conditions, has been stressed by authors in the field (e.g., Jones et al., 2003; Simpson & Tate, 2007). One of the challenges in achieving this goal is the low rates of mental health treatment accessed by people with neurodisability, and this has been highlighted across several types of neurodisability (e.g., Fann et al., 2011; Simpson, Sabaz, Daher, Gordon, & Strettles, 2014).

Where mental health treatment can be accessed, the types of psychotherapeutic interventions that could be delivered were detailed in Chapter 9. This included Dialectic Behavior Therapy (Linehan et al., 2006), Mentalization-Based Treatment (Bateman & Fonagy, 2009), and Problem-Solving Treatment (Hatcher, Sharon, Parag, & Collins, 2011) among others.

However, based on the reality that not all individuals with suicidal thoughts have psychiatric conditions, as well as the fact that some treatments (e.g., medication for depression) take time to work, providing individuals with strategies to cope with suicidal thoughts and urges is vital. Examples of such suicide prevention interventions include cognitive behavioral therapy (CBT) for suicide prevention and brief CBT for the prevention of suicide attempts (Brown et al., 2005; Rudd et al., 2015). Moreover, there is evidence for PST as an efficacious prevention strategy for both risk factors for suicide (depression) and suicidal thoughts and behaviors (https://www.sprc.org/resources-programs/problem-solving-therapy-pst; https://nrepp.samhsa.gov/ProgramProfile.aspx?id=108#hide1), as well as initial data about PST as a feasible approach among those with moderate to severe TBI (see Chapter 9).

Potentially equally important is the treatment of other health-related factors that are common among those with neurodisabilities and that might be exacerbating the suicide risk. For example, chronic pain (Archibald et al., 1994; Fishbain, 1999; Halbauer, Lew, & Yesavage, 2009; Ruan, & Luo, 2017) and/or poor sleep (Bernert, & Joiner, 2007; Matthews, Signoracci, Stearns-Yoder, & Brenner, 2016) are known suicide risk factors.

COORDINATED DISCHARGE PLAN

Although an acute inpatient admission may reduce the intensity of a high acute crisis, it does not guarantee longer term safety. One general risk factor for suicide among all clinical groups is a postcrisis discharge from an inpatient psychiatric unit (Wasserman et al., 2012), with one element being poorer continuity of care (Desai, Dausey, & Rosenheck, 2005). Cases of suicide following discharge from inpatient psychiatric units have been documented after neurodisability (e.g., Tate, Simpson, Flanagan, & Coffey, 1997; Achte et al., 1971).

If the admission to an acute inpatient unit took place while the client was under active management by a neurodisability agency and/or sole practitioner and that agency and/or practitioner is planning to resume services once the individual is discharged back into the community, then seeking to coordinate with the mental health service around the transition out of the inpatient unit is very important. Collaboration between agencies is recommended as part of best practice (Wasserman et al., 2012). However, clinical experience suggests that mental health services can discharge clients without any notification to treating neurodisability agencies. Furthermore, people with neurodisability often have difficulties accessing mainstream community mental health services (Simpson et al., 2014), and this may not be part of the discharge plan. Therefore it is important to be proactive in contacting and seeking to coordinate with mental health services, the person's family, and the individual herself to ensure appropriate follow-up is provided in a timely manner.

SAFETY PLANNING

For patients at risk for suicide, a safety plan should be considered an important evidence-based element of treatment (see Table 10.1). Stanley and Brown (2012) identified the need for such an intervention based on clinical experiences in which individuals were evaluated for care and given a date for a follow-up appointment but were not provided with help to identify strategies to maintain safety in the interim. The need for this type of intervention is further highlighted by the fact that many individuals do not return for follow-up care. In response, Stanley and Brown (2012) introduced a brief intervention for use among veteran health administration (VHA) clinicians (http://www.mentalhealth.va.gov/docs/va_safety_planning_manual.pdf) (Figure 10.1).

Due to the brief nature of this intervention, it can be implemented in a wide range of settings (e.g., emergency department, psychiatric inpatient unit; Stanley et al., 2016; 2018). The structured intervention, which usually takes between 20 and 45 minutes to complete, facilitates a collaborative process by which the patient and the provider work together to develop a personalized plan for safety that the patient can reference and use during future periods of distress. During the safety planning process, the dyad works together to identify (1) warning signs (thoughts, feelings, and behaviors that contribute to suicidal behavior); (2) personal coping strategies; (3) family members, friends, and safe places that can serve as distractors; (4) family and friends who can assist during a suicidal crisis; (5) health professionals to be contacted during a crisis; and (6) strategies to restrict access to lethal means. Materials regarding safety planning, as well as documents that can be used to facilitate the process, can be found at http://www.suicidesafetyplan.com/ or http://www.mentalhealth.va.gov/docs/va_safety_planning_manual.pdf. In addition, several mobile applications have been developed (e.g., http://www.my3app.org/safety-planning/). Such applications may be particularly useful for individuals with cognitive impairment. Coupled with the timer on a mobile phone, an individual could be cued to look at and implement steps of his safety plan throughout the day or during stressful events.

INCREASE SUPPORT

In the general suicide prevention literature, the involvement of an individual's family and broader social network is recommended as an important treatment element (Wasserman et al., 2012). In particular, education of families in relation to risk and protective factors, available treatments for addressing elevated suicidal thoughts or behaviors, the need for treatment adherence, and the need to restrict access to lethal means within the environment have been highlighted (Wasserman et al., 2012). The

SAFETY PLAN: VA VERSION

Step 1: Warning signs:

1. _____
2. _____
3. _____

Step 2: Internal coping strategies - Things I can do to take my mind off my problems without contacting another person:

1. _____
2. _____
3. _____

Step 3: People and social settings that provide distraction:

1. Name _____ Phone_____
2. Name _____ Phone_____
3. Place _____ Place_____

Step 4: People whom I can ask for help:

1. Name_____ Phone_____
2. Name_____ Phone_____
3. Name_____ Phone_____

Step 5:Professionals or agencies I can contact during a crisis:

1. Clinician Name_____Phone_____
   Clinician Pager or Emergency Contact #_____
2. Clinician Name_____Phone_____
   Clinician Pager or Emergency Contact_____
3. Local Urgent Care Services_____
   Urgent Care Services Address_____
   Urgent Care Services Phone_____
4. VA Suicide Prevention Resource Coordinator Name_____
   VA Suicide Prevention Resource Coordinator Phone_____
5. VA Suicide Prevention Resource Coordinator Phone_____
   VA Suicide Prevention Hotline Phone: 1-800-273-TALK (8255), push 1 to reach a VA mental health clinician_____

Step 6: Making the environment safe:

1. _____
2. _____

Safety Plan Treatment Manual to Reduce Suicide Risk: Veteran Version (Stanley & Brown, 2008).

FIGURE 10.1 Safety plan.

importance of mobilizing family and/or broader social networks has been flagged in the neurodisability literature (Wasserman et al., 2008). Specifically, authors have highlighted the importance of preserving the family structure as a protective factor (Hartkopp, Brønnum-Hansen, Seidenschnur, & Biering-Sørensen, 1998; Long & Miller, 1991) and that patients and families should be warned of the potential for suicidal thoughts or behaviors (Voon et al., 2008).

Our clinical experience suggests that family and friends can play four important roles in the context of a suicidal crisis. First, they can act as a source of support to the person who is suicidal. In doing this, they can reduce perturbation and provide the person with emotional support during the crisis. Second, they can act as an early warning system if some new crisis or problem arises, allowing for intervention at the earliest possible time. Third, they can monitor the person who is suicidal, assist in observing and preventing them from taking steps to harm themselves or from becoming intoxicated, which might then lead to a suicide attempt being made. However, in some cases such observation in untenable, and as such a higher level of care (e.g., inpatient) may be indicated. For example, maintaining 24 hour observation in light of immenent intent is not recommended. Finally, families and friends can also act as a conduit of care, helping people to get to necessary appointments, ensuring the person is taking prescribed medication, and reinforcing themes and messages that are part of the counseling process. Finally, staff without formal mental health qualifications (e.g., allied health, rehabilitation nursing, attendant carers) can also play similar support roles (Simpson, Franke, & Gillett, 2007). This may be in the absence of family support or to complement family support. It should also be noted, however, that in some cases familial/friends can be drivers of suicidal thoughts and behaviors.

COPING STRATEGIES/PROTECTIVE FACTORS

Building active coping strategies and a positive lifestyle can act as important protective factors (Wasserman et al., 2012). In addition to the coping that can be acquired from current CBT approaches, new programs drawing on the "third wave" of behavior therapy, such as acceptance and commitment therapy, can promote psychological flexibility after neurodisability (Whiting, Deane, Simpson, Ciarrochi, & McLeod, 2017; Whiting, Deane, Simpson, McLeod, & Ciarrochi, 2017). Furthermore, precepts drawn from positive psychology are starting to be applied to conceptualizing the process of psychological adjustment to neurodisability (Evans, 2011). Early interventions based on these precepts have been tested (e.g., Cullen et al., 2018) and, with further evidence, may be useful ways to build psychological resilience to the challenges of living with a neurodisability.

Psychological interventions can be complemented by broader social programs. In the context of spinal cord injury (SCI) suggested approaches include providing meaningful activities to improve quality of life (Hartkopp et al., 1998) and improving community reintegration (Ahoniemi, Pohjolainen, & Kautiainen, 2011). In respect to this last suggestion, the possible benefit of linking clients into disability-specific support groups to increase access to emotional support and social connection has also been canvassed (Wasserman et al., 2008).

CONCLUSION

Suicide prevention involves ensuring that the person expressing suicidal thoughts and/or behaviors receives the appropriate level of treatment. There is a growing range of psychological and psychosocial interventions that can complement frontline pharmacotherapy. However, the evidence base underpinning these approaches is still very weak, and further research is urgently needed to strengthen this evidence base.

Postvention

Clinicians working in the field of neurodisability for any length of time are likely to encounter the suicide of a patient or client within their agencies' caseload, if not within their own caseload. In an early account, the impact of two client suicides on the treating team in a specialist neuropsychological treatment center for clients with TBI has been detailed (Klonoff & Lage, 1995, see Box 10.2). The authors raised a question about whether the impact of the suicides may have been greater for reha-bilitation professionals given the relative lack of exposure to training on suicide as part of their formal training. However, mainstream mental health professionals such as psychiatrists also report little if any training about suicide postvention, and the personal impact seems to be just as challenging (Balon, 2007).

The term "postvention" was coined by Shneidman (1969), and his dictum that "postvention is prevention" (Shneidman, 1981) is still relevant today (Aguirre & Slater, 2010). Therapists or agencies working with a client who dies by suicide need to know what to do in response to the death. Furthermore, the personal impact on staff and their ongoing needs must be considered (Balon, 2007; Klonoff & Lage, 1995, Wurst et al., 2010). In addition, activities are required at an organizational level to improve knowledge of and interventions for the next suicidal client, to en-sure that care was conducted at a suitable standard (both at a clinical level and in terms of service systems), and to examine whether any risk management issues can be identified (Stelovich, 1999).

There has been a lack of research into postvention relative to prevention, and this imbalance is also true in the case of neurodisability. Historically, the lack of any focus on postvention was a shortcoming of national and state suicide prevention

BOX 10.2

IMPACT OF TWO CLIENT SUICIDES ON A TEAM PROVIDING A
NEUROPSYCHOLOGICAL TREATMENT PROGRAM FOR CLIENTS WITH TBI

In reflecting on the impact of the deaths, salient points about the staff experiences were
highlighted:

- Initial reactions of shock, disbelief, and profound sadness
- Feelings of anger toward the patient (among some staff)
- Anger was linked to questions about
  - Why the client could not see the impact that the suicide would have on other
    patients, staff, and family members
  - Why the client did not more clearly communicate his intentions and thereby allow
    for the staff to intervene and prevent the death
- Self-questioning about why their best efforts to provide treatment had failed
- Feeling helpless and discouraged because the client's behavior had not been better
  anticipated in order for the death to have been prevented
- Although the two clients had been depressed, the lack of warning about the immi-
  nence of the suicides
- Clinicians reminded of their limitations in the face of the insurmountable suffering
  and loss that some clients experience as a result of TBI, despite the best efforts of the
  clinicians
- The value of a psychological autopsy in reviewing the clients' pre- and postinjury history, treatment course, and the staff's personal reactions to the death
- Renewed determination to provide a treatment milieu that promoted hope, effectiveness, and self-worth for clients

From Klonoff & Lage (1995).

plans (Aguirre & Slater). However, Objective 10 of the current US National Suicide
Prevention Plan (USDHHS, 2012) clearly addresses postvention.

THE NEED FOR POSTVENTION

Postvention is important because of the far-reaching consequences and impact of
a suicide. Recent work by Cerel et al. (2018) suggests that each suicide results in
135 individuals who knew the person being impacted by the death. The recovery of
survivors is still hampered by the societal taboos that surround suicide (Dyregrov,
2011). Up to 50% of survivors will report depression and guilt (Andriesson, 2009).

They may have a distorted sense of responsibility for the death ("Could I have prevented it? Did I drive the person to do it?"; Cerel & Campbell, 2008; Saarinen, Viinamäki, Hintikka, Lehtonen, & Lönnqvist, 1991) and experience feelings of shame and rejection (Andriesson, 2009; Van Dongen, 1993). They may encounter pejorative judgments of the decedent from others (e.g., "How selfish the person was . . . "; Aguirre & Slater, 2010) or about their own role ("You drove the person to it"; Silverman, Range, & Overholser, 1995). Survivors may develop posttraumatic stress disorder (PTSD; Jordan, 2001), particularly if they discovered or were exposed to the body. Complicated bereavement reactions also arise (Aguirre & Slater, 2010), with some survivors reporting a prolonged and intense search for meaning about the suicide (Wagner & Colhoun, 1992). Fueling the dictum that postvention is prevention, there is also the concern that, without support, suicide survivors may be at greater risk of future suicide themselves. Despite the unique features of bereavement following suicide, there still may be more similarities than differences to other forms of bereavement (Andriessen, 2009).

Postvention seeks to address the needs and concerns of suicide survivors. In considering intervention or support, a distinction can be made between the broader group of people who are exposed to a suicide but not substantively affected and the smaller group who experience a negative impact arising from the death (Jordan & McMenamy, 2004). Among this group that experiences a negative impact, studies have found that approximately one-third feel that they are able to cope without help (Provini, Everett, & Pfeffer, 2000). Despite the needs of the other two-thirds for assistance, surveys in the United States have found that only 25% of survivors received formal or informal help (Dyregrov, 2011; Jordan & McMenamy, 2004; Provini et al., 2000). Families with young children indicated significantly more concerns compared to families without young children (Jordan & McMenamy, 2004). In the European context, higher levels of contact with professionals (85%) are reported by survivors (Dyregrov, 2011); however, the support is generally of short duration, with 67% reporting that the support lasted less than 6 months (Dyregrov, 2011). One caution about the differences in these levels of support are the differences in timeframes, with the US data collected 5 months after the death compared to 15 months in the Norwegian study.

INTERVENTIONS FOR SUICIDE SURVIVORS

Sources of support and intervention include general practitioners, specialist therapists, survivor or bereavement self-help groups, and specialized reading material and Internet sites (Hawton & Simkin, 2003). Although a number of specialized suicide bereavement programs have been described (particularly school-based postvention programs), there are a lack of evaluated specialist programs (Jordan & McMenamy, 2004). In a systematic review, McDaid, Trowman, Golder, Hawton, and Sowden (2008) found only a handful of evaluated programs. Three programs were identified that provided modest benefits compared to no treatment (an 8-week group-based program provided by a mental health professional and volunteer; a 10-session psychologist-led bereavement group for children; a 4-session cognitive behavior family program delivered by a psychiatric nurse); however, all but one of the studies had major methodological shortcomings, and, when two active treatments were compared, less benefit was observed (McDaid et al., 2008).

In clinical practice, bereavement support groups are a common option. A significant proportion of people who are bereaved by suicide are interested in meeting others who have had the same experience, but this is not universal (Dyregrov, 2011; Feigelman, Gorman, Beal Chastain, & Jordan, 2008). A detailed consideration of support groups is provided by Cerel, Padgett, Cornwell, and Reed (2009). While the benefits are commonly reported, the possibility has been raised that some people might experience harm from taking part in self-help groups, either through retraumatization arising from group participants recounting their experiences of violent deaths, or that people with avoidant styles of coping may not respond well to self-disclosure or sharing of feelings among group participants (Jordan & McMenamy, 2004).

The research suggests that proactive contact from services and social supports is also important (not just providing survivors with a contact number). When left to their own devices, some studies have found that it takes years before a survivor will contact services or help (e.g., 4.5 years, Aguirre & Slater, 2010). Survivors have also identified information needs, particularly around helping bereaved children and how to communicate within the family (Dyregrov, 2011). Survivors also nominated the importance of longer term contact and support (i.e., extending beyond the first year) in comparison to current experience that services are typically available for the first few weeks.

STAFF AND ORGANIZATION-RELATED CONSIDERATIONS

Although neurodisability staff are not first responders (i.e., police, firemen, paramedics), they may inadvertently be the first person to discover a body. More commonly, however, staff in neurodisability agencies will be notified about the death of a patient or client. Whatever the circumstances, the impact on staff can be profound (Balon, 2007; Klonoff & Lage, 1995; Wurst et al., 2010). Staff may lose confidence and question their professional competence (Balon, 2007; Klonoff & Lage, 1995)—even their suitability for their chosen career (Balon, 2007). They also may experience concerns about professional liability (see Chapter 13).

There is little if any training for staff about postvention, in particular how to respond to the emotional impact of having a client die by suicide (Balon, 2007). A common practice is for senior management or supervisors to conduct a psychological autopsy with staff who worked with the patient or client (Balon, 2007; Shneidman, 1969; Shneidman & Ross, 1971; Klonoff & Lage, 1995). The emotional impact of the experience can also be substantial, and senior management or supervisors need to directly provide support to staff (Balon, 2007) or ensure that such support is available.

At an organizational level, an agency audit is an important step to take after a suicide (Jenkins & Singh, 2000). In other fields, agency audits have found that a low weight was placed on the mental illness of clients or on the problem of compliance with treatment (Jenkins & Singh, 2000). Stelovich (1999) describes in some detail the importance of and procedures for conducting such an audit.

From a clinical and organizational perspective, postvention activities are time-dependent. The workplace postvention taskforces of the American Association of Suicidology and the National Action Alliance for Suicide Prevention have produced a guide for managers addressing suicide postvention in the workplace. The guide addresses workplace responses that need to occur immediately, within 24 hours, and within 1 week.

Conclusion

The clinical management of people with an identified suicide risk is still both a science and an art. This involves taking the best of current evidence about suicide prevention and extrapolating it to the person with neurodisability and combining this with rational clinical approaches. Over time, a greater number of treatments will be validated for treating mental health conditions among people with neurodisability, and this will add greatly to the options available to clinicians. However, any such interventions will need to be combined with broader psychosocial support approaches to ensure a comprehensive approach. Developing a safety plan provides one structured approach to achieve this. Monitoring for warning signs can be a useful component or adjunct to such a plan. If a death by suicide does occur, there is still much work to do to respond to the psychosocial and emotional impact felt by the survivors, focusing not only on the family of the decedent, but also on the clinical staff who worked with the person.

Implications for Clinicians

1. Provide treatment and support in the least restrictive environment commensurate with the degree of suicide risk and level of cognitive ability, balancing the principle of autonomy with duty of care.
2. In deciding the level of treatment, determine the degree to which the person is able to maintain his or her own safety; that is, to use a safety plan and get help and support if risk increases.
3. Consider the combination of appropriate psychological treatments in combination with other clinical support strategies.
4. Mobilizing social support systems can complement clinical interventions.
5. Postvention is needed to address the far-reaching consequences and impact of a suicide.

References

Achte, K. A., Lonnqvist, J., & Hillbom, E. (1971). Suicides following war brain-injuries. *Acta Psychiatrica Scandinavica,* Suppl, 1–94.

Aguirre, R. T. P., & Slater, H. (2010). Suicide postvention as prevention: Improvement and expansion in the United States. *Death Studies, 34,* 529–540.

Ahoniemi, E., Pohjolainen, T., & Kautiainen, H. (2011). Survival after spinal cord injury in Finland. *Journal of Rehabilitation Medicine, 43,* 481–485.

Andriessen, K. (2009). Can postvention be prevention? *Crisis: The Journal of Crisis Intervention and Suicide Prevention, 30,* 43–47.

Archibald, C. J., McGrath, P. J., Ritvo, P. G., Fisk, J. D., Bhan, V., Maxner, C. E., & Murray, T. J. (1994). Pain prevalence, severity and impact in a clinic sample of multiple sclerosis patients. *Pain, 58,* 89–93

Baliko, L., Csala, B., & Czopf, J. (2004). Suicide in Hungarian Huntington's disease patients. *Neuroepidemiology, 23,* 258–260.

Balon, R. (2007). Encountering patient suicides: The need for guidelines. *Academic Psychiatry, 31,* 336–337.

Bateman, A., & Fonagy, P. (2009). Randomized controlled trial of outpatient mentalization-based treatment versus structured clinical management for borderline personality disorder. *American Journal of Psychiatry, 166,* 1355–1364.

Berman, A. L. (2006). Risk management with suicidal patients. *Journal of Clinical Psychology: In Session, 62,* 171–184.

Bernert, R. A., & Joiner, T. E. (2007). Sleep disturbances and suicide risk: A review of the literature. *Neuropsychiatric Disease and Treatment, 3,* 735–743.

Bongar, B. (2002). *The suicidal patient: Clinical and legal standards of care* (2nd ed.) Washington, DC: American Psychological Association.

Brown, G. K., Have, T. T., Henriques, G. R., Xie, S. X., Hollander, J. E., & Beck, A. T. (2005). Cognitive therapy for the prevention of suicide attempts: A randomized controlled trial. *Journal of the American Medical Association, 294*, 563–570.

Cerel, J., Brown, M. M., Maple, M., Singleton, M., van de Venne, J., Moore, M., & Flaherty, C. (2018). How many people are exposed to suicide? Not six. https://onlinelibrary.wiley.com/doi/epdf/10.1111/sltb.12450

Cerel, J., & Campbell, F. R. (2008). Suicide survivors seeking mental health services: A preliminary examination of the role of an active postvention model. *Suicide and Life Threatening Behavior, 38*, 30–34.

Cerel, J., Padgett, J. H., Conwell, Y., & Reed, G. A. Jr. (2009). A call for research: The need to better understand the impact of support groups for suicide survivors. *Suicide and Life Threatening Behavior, 39*, 269–281.

Cullen, B., Pownall, J., Cummings, J., Baylan, S., Broomfield, N., Haig, C., . . . Evans, J. J. (2018). Positive PsychoTherapy in ABI Rehab (PoPsTAR): A pilot randomised controlled trial. *Neuropsychological Rehabilitation, 28*, 17–33.

Department of Veterans Affairs/Department of Defense (DVA/DoD). (2013). *VA/DoD Clinical Practice Guideline for assessment and management of patients at risk for suicide. Version 1.0.* The Office of Quality, Safety and Value, VA, Washington, DC & Office of Evidence Based Practice, U.S. Army Medical Command. Retrieved from http://www.guideline.gov/content.aspxid=47023

Desai, R. A., Dausey, D. J., & Rosenheck, R. A. (2005). Mental health service delivery and suicide risk: The role of individual patient and facility factors. *American Journal of Psychiatry, 162*, 311–318.

Doughty, C. (2002). Suicide prevention topic 9: What evidence is there about the use of seclusion or containment for patients presenting with suicidal behaviours at emergency departments, tertiary mental health services or inpatient units? NZHTA Report 2002. Retrieved from http://nzhta.chmeds.ac.nz/publications/topic9.pdf

Dyregrov, K. (2002). Assistance from local authorities versus survivors' needs for support after suicide. *Death Studies, 26*(8), 647–668.

Dyregrov, K. (2011).What do we know about needs for help after suicide in different parts of the world: A phenomenological perspective. *Crisis: The Journal of Crisis Intervention and Suicide Prevention, 32*, 310–318.

Evans, J. J. (2011). Positive psychology and brain injury rehabilitation. *Brain Impairment, 12*, 117–127.

Fann, J. R., Bombardier, C. H., Richards, J. S., Tate, D. G., Wilson, C. S., & Temkin, N. (2011). Depression after spinal cord injury: Comorbidities, mental health service use, and adequacy of treatment. *Archives of Physical Medicine and Rehabilitation, 92*, 352–360.

Feigelman, W., Gorman, B. S., Beal Chastain, K., & Jordan, J. R. (2008). Internet support groups for suicide survivors: A new mode for gaining bereavement assistance. *Omega, 57*, 217–243.

Fishbain, D. A. (1999). The association of chronic pain and suicide. *Seminars in Clinical Neuropsychiatry, 4*, 221–227.

Fletcher, R. F. (1999). The process of constant observation: Perspectives of staff and suicidal patients. *Journal of Psychiatric and Mental Health Nursing, 6*, 9–14.

Halbauer, J. D., Lew, H. L., & Yesavage, J. A. (2009). Neuropsychiatric diagnosis and management of chronic sequelae of war-related mild to moderate traumatic brain injury. *Journal of Rehabilitation Research and Development, 46*, 757.

Hartkopp, A., Brønnum-Hansen, H., Seidenschnur, A.-M., & Biering-Sørensen, F. (1998). Suicide in a spinal cord injured population: Its relation to functional status. *Archives of Physical Medicine and Rehabilitation, 79*, 1356–1361.

Hatcher, S., Sharon, C., Parag, V., & Collins, N. (2011). Problem-solving therapy for people who present to hospital with self-harm: Zelen randomised controlled trial. *British Journal of Psychiatry, 199*, 310–316.

Hawton, K., & Simkin, S. (2003). Helping people bereaved by suicide: Their needs may require special attention. *Bereavement Care, 22*, 41–42.

Janofsky, J. S. (2009). Reducing inpatient suicide risk: Using human factors analysis to improve observation practices. *Journal of the American Academy of Psychiatry and the Law Online, 37*, 15–24.

Jenkins, R., & Singh, B. (2000). Policy and practice in suicide prevention. *The British Journal of Forensic Practice, 2*, 3–11.1`

Jones, J. E., Hermann, B. P., Barry, J. J., Gilliam, F. G., Kanner, A. M., & Meador, K. J. (2003). Rates and risk factors for suicide, suicidal ideation and suicide attempts in chronic epilepsy. *Epilepsy and Behavior, 4*, S31–S38.

Jordan, J. R. (2001). Is suicide bereavement different? A reassessment of the literature. *Suicide and Life-Threatening Behavior, 31*, 91–102.

Jordan, J. R., & McMenamy, J. (2004). Interventions for suicide survivors: A review of the literature. *Suicide and Life-Threatening Behavior, 34*, 337–349.

Klonoff, P. S., & Lage, G. A. (1995). Suicide in patients with traumatic brain injury: Risk and prevention. *Journal of Head Trauma Rehabilitation, 10*, 16–24.

Konrad, N., Daigle, M. S., Daniel, A. E., Dear, G. E., Frottier, P., Hayes, L. M., . . . Sarchiapone, M. (2007). Preventing suicide in prisons, Part I: Recommendations from the International Association for Suicide Prevention task force on suicide in prisons. *Crisis: The Journal of Crisis Intervention and Suicide Prevention, 28*, 113.

Linehan, M. M., Comtois, K. A., Murray, A. M., Brown, M. Z., Gallop, R. J., Heard, H. L., . . . Lindenboim, N. (2006). Two-year randomized controlled trial and follow-up of dialectical behavior therapy vs therapy by experts for suicidal behaviors and borderline personality disorder. *Archives of General Psychiatry, 63*, 757–766.

Long, D. D., & Miller, B. J. (1991). Suicidal tendency and multiple sclerosis. *Health and Social Work, 16*, 104–109.

Manna, M. (2010). Effectiveness of formal observation in inpatient psychiatry in preventing adverse outcomes: The state of the science. *Journal of Psychiatric and Mental Health Nursing, 17*, 268–273.

Maltsberger, J. T., & Stoklosa, J. B. (2012). Outpatient treatment. In R. I. Simons & R. E Hales (Eds.), *The American Psychiatric Publishing textbook of suicide assessment and management* (2nd ed., pp. 303–314). Arlington, VA: American Psychiatric Publishing.

Matthews, E. E., Signoracci, G. M., Stearns-Yoder, K., & Brenner, L. A. (2016). A qualitative study of sleep–wake disturbance among Veterans with post–acute moderate to severe traumatic brain injury. *The Journal of Head Trauma Rehabilitation, 31*(2), 126–135.

McDaid, C., Trowman, R., Golder, S., Hawton, K., & Sowden, A. (2008). Interventions for people bereaved through suicide: Systematic review. *British Journal of Psychiatry, 193*, 438–443.

Meehan, J., Kapur, N., Hunt, I. M., Turnbull, P., Robinson, J., Bickley, H., . . . Shaw, J. (2006). Suicide in mental health in-patients and within 3 months of discharge. *British Journal of Psychiatry, 188*, 129–134.

Nilsson, L., Ahlbom, A., Farahmand, B. Y., Åsberg, M., & Tomson, T. (2002). Risk factors for suicide in epilepsy: A case control study. *Epilepsia, 43*, 644–651.

New South Wales Health. (1999). *Suicide risk assessment and management: Training manual.* Sydney, NSW: Author.

Provini, C., Everett, J. R., & Pfeffer, C. R. (2000). Adults mourning suicide: Self-reported concerns about bereavement, needs for assistance, and help-seeking behavior. *Death Studies, 24*, 1–19.

Ruan, X., & Luo, J. J. (2017). Suicide before and after spinal cord injury. *The Journal of Spinal Cord Medicine, 40*, 280–281.

Rudd, M. D., Bryan, C. J., Wertenberger, E. G., Peterson, A. L., Young-McCaughan, S., Mintz, J., . . . Wilkinson, E. (2015). Brief cognitive-behavioral therapy effects on post-treatment suicide attempts in a military sample: Results of a randomized clinical trial with 2-year follow-up. *American Journal of Psychiatry, 172*(5), 441–449.

Saarinen, P., Viinamäki, H., Hintikka, J., Lehtonen, J., & Lönnqvist, J. (1999). Psychological symptoms of close relatives of suicide victims. *European Journal of Psychiatry, 13*, 33–39.

Schneidman, E. S. (1969). Prologue: Fifty-eight years. In E. S. Shneidman (Ed.), *On the nature of suicide* (pp. 1–30). San Francisco: Jossey-Bass.

Schneidman, E. S. (1981). Postvention: The care of the bereaved. *Suicide and Life Threatening Behavior, 11*, 349–359.

Shneidman, E. S. (1989). Overview: A multidimensional approach to suicide. In D. Jacobs & H. Brown (Eds.), *Suicide: Understanding and responding* (pp. 1–30). Madison, CT: International Universities Press.

Shneidman, E. S., & Ross, E. B. (1971). Prevention, intervention and postvention. *Annals of Internal Medicine, 75*, 441–458.

Silverman, E., Range, L., & Overholser, J. (1995). Bereavement from suicide as compared to other forms of bereavement. *Omega, 30*, 41–51.

Simpson, G. (2001). Suicide prevention after traumatic brain injury: A resource manual. Sydney, Australia: South Western Sydney Area Health Service, Brain Injury Rehabilitation Unit.

Simpson, G. K., Franke, B., & Gillett, L. (2007). Suicide prevention training outside the mental health service system: Evaluation of a state-wide program in Australia for rehabilitation and disability staff in the field of traumatic brain injury. *Crisis: The Journal of Crisis Intervention and Suicide Prevention, 28*, 35–43.

Simpson, G. K., & Tate, R. L. (2007). Suicidality in people surviving a traumatic brain injury: Prevalence, risk factors and implications for clinical management. *Brain Injury, 21*, 1335–1351.

Simpson, G. K., Sabaz, M., Daher, M., Gordon, R., & Strettles, B. (2014). Service utilisation and service access among community-dwelling clients with challenging behaviours after severe traumatic brain injury: A multicentre study. *Brain Impairment, 15*, 28–42.

Soden, R. J., Walsh, J., Middleton, J. W., Craven, M. L., Rutkowski, S. B., & Yeo, J. D. (2000). Causes of death after spinal cord injury. *Spinal Cord, 38*, 604–610.

Stanley, B., & Brown, G. K. (2012). Safety planning intervention: A brief intervention to mitigate suicide risk. *Cognitive and Behavioral Practice, 19*, 256–264.

Stanley, B., Brown, G. K., Brenner, L. A., . . . Green, K. L. (2018). Comparison of the safety planning intervention with follow-up vs usual care of suicidal patients treated in the emergency department. *JAMA Psychiatry, 75*(9), 894–900.

Stanley, B., Chaudhury, S. R., Chesin, M., Pontoski, K., Bush, A. M., Knox, K. L., & Brown, G. K. (2016). An emergency department intervention and follow-up to reduce suicide risk in the VA: Acceptability and effectiveness. *Psychiatric Services, 67*, 680–683.

Stelovich, S. (1999). Guidelines for conducting a suicide review. In D. G. Jacobs (Ed.), *The Harvard Medical School guide to suicide assessment and intervention* (pp. 482–490) San Francisco: Jossey-Bass.

Stenager, E. N., Koch-Henriksen, N., & Stenager, E. (1996). Risk factors for suicide in multiple sclerosis. *Psychotherapy and Psychosomatics, 65*, 86–90.

Tate, R. L., Simpson, G. K., Flanagan, S., & Coffey, M. (1997). Completed suicide after traumatic brain injury. *Journal of Head Trauma Rehabilitation, 12*, 16–28.

US Department of Health and Human Services (HHS), Office of the Surgeon General, & National Action Alliance for Suicide Prevention. (2012). *2012 National strategy for suicide prevention: Goals and objectives for action.* Washington, DC: HHS.

Van Dongen, C. J. (1993). Social contexts of postsuicide bereavement. *Death Studies, 17*, 125–141.

Voon, V., Krack, P., Lang, A. E., Lozano, A. M., Dujardin, K., Schüpbach, M., . . . Speelman, J. D. (2008). A multicentre study on suicide outcomes following subthalamic stimulation for Parkinson's disease. *Brain, 131*, 2720–2728.

Wagner, K. G., & Calhoun, L. G. (1992). Perceptions of social support by suicide survivors and their social networks. *Omega, 24*, 61–73.

Wasserman, D., Rihmer, Z., Rujescu, D., Sarchiapone, M., Sokolowski, M., Titelman, D., . . . Carli, V. (2012). The European Psychiatric Association (EPA) guidance on suicide treatment and prevention. *European Psychiatry, 27*, 129–141.

Wasserman, L., Shaw, T., Vu, M., Ko, C., Bollegala, D., & Bhalerao, S. (2008). An overview of traumatic brain injury and suicide. *Brain Injury, 22*, 811–819.

Whiting, D. L., Deane, F. P., Simpson, G. K., Ciarrochi, J., & McLeod, H. J. (2017). The feasibility of using acceptance and commitment therapy to address psychological distress after severe traumatic brain injury: Two case studies. *Clinical Psychology*. doi: 10.1111/cp.12118

Whiting, D. L., Deane, F. P., Simpson, G. K., McLeod, H. J., & Ciarrochi, J. (2017). Cognitive and psychological flexibility after a traumatic brain injury and the implications for treatment: A conceptual review. *Neuropsychological Rehabilitation, 27*, 263–299.

Wortzel, H. S., Homaifar, B., Matarazzo, B., & Brenner, L. A. (2014). Therapeutic risk management of the suicidal patient: Stratifying risk in terms of severity and temporality. *Journal of Psychiatric Practice, 20*, 63–67.

Wurst, F. M., Mueller, S., Petitjean, S., Euler, S., Thon, N., Wiesbeck, G., & Wolfersdorf, M. (2010). Patient suicide: A survey of therapist's reactions. *Suicide and Life Threatening Behavior, 40*, 328–336.

11 Cross-Cultural Practice in Suicide Prevention

Introduction

Adopting a cultural perspective provides an important lens through which to develop a deeper, more nuanced understanding of the relationship between suicide and neurodisability. Elevated levels of risk are not simply the product of neurodisability, but also reflect an interaction between neurodisability and the cultural context (differences between countries and differences within countries). Around the world, the degree of internal cultural difference widely varies, from countries that are predominantly monocultural, with a high degree of racial and cultural homogeneity, to countries that are bicultural or multicultural, having significant variability in terms of racial/ethnic diversity.

After defining key terms, some background on inter- and intranational differences in suicide rates will be provided. Within this context, the following links between culture and suicide after neurodisability will be explored: Is there an invariant increase in the level of suicide risk associated with neurodisability across different countries? How do neurodisability and racial/ethnic minority status interact in association with suicidal behavior within countries? How can we increase cultural sensitivity in the assessment and management of suicidality among people with neurodisability?

Culture, Race, and Ethnicity

"Culture," "race," and "ethnicity" are overlapping terms and are often mistakenly used interchangeably and without consistency. The term "culture" refers to the world-view, ideas, customs, and social behavior of a defined group or society (Leenaars, 2008). "Race" refers to a group of persons related by common descent or heredity. People of the same race do not necessarily share the same culture (Tseng & Streltzer, 1997). "Ethnicity" then refers to groups that have racial, religious, linguistic, and other cultural traits in common (Leenaars, 2008).

Applying these definitions to the United States, there are certain cultural characteristics that define the American population as a whole. However, the United States is a highly multicultural society, comprising a mixture of different racial groups (e.g., white/Caucasian, black, Asian). Within these racial groups, further ethnic subgroups exist (e.g., white is further divided into Hispanic and non-Hispanic), many with distinct linguistic, cultural, and/or religious traditions. Racial and ethnic groups other than white (non-Hispanic) are commonly termed "minority groups."

Cross-National Differences in Suicidal Behavior

CROSS-NATIONAL DIFFERENCES IN SUICIDE AT THE GENERAL POPULATION LEVEL

As outlined in this book's Introduction, there is considerable cross-national variation in the rates of suicide. National differences in the ascertainment and reporting of suicide deaths account for some of the heterogeneity (Lester, 2008a; Wendler, Matthews, & Morelli, 2012). For example, ascertainment is influenced by the degree of cultural attitudes to the acceptability of suicide as well as the bureaucratic procedures employed to manage accidental deaths (Windfuhr & Karpur, 2011).

Differences in national rates also reflect underlying variations in the levels of comorbidities such as mental illness, substance abuse, and self-directed violence, as well as societal factors such as the availability of mental health services, the level of poverty, the degree of religiosity, divorce rates, significant political change, and the presence of social deprivation/fragmentation (Wendler et al., 2012; Windfur & Kapur, 2011). Furthermore, it has been argued that diversity in the underlying genetic structure and/or physiology of national populations may result in some populations having a higher vulnerability, for example, due to greater susceptibility to depressive disorders (Wendler et al., 2012; Lester, 2008a, 2008b). Similarly, national populations differ in their demographic profiles (e.g., age and sex composition) and therefore in the proportion of people at risk of suicide. For example, countries with higher proportions of known at-risk groups such as elderly males may have higher rates of suicide (Lester, 2008a, 2008b).

CROSS-NATIONAL STUDIES OF SUICIDAL BEHAVIOR
AFTER NEURODISABILITY

Studies involving cross-national comparisons of suicide in neurodisability are almost unknown. However, a small number of studies have highlighted different aspects of the links among culture, neurodisability, and suicide. The findings illustrate how suicidal behavior after neurodisability reflects the social characteristics of the country within which it occurs.

Voon et al. (2008) reported on the postoperative rate of suicide in the first 4 years after neurosurgical intervention (subthalamic nucleus deep brain stimulation) for the treatment of advanced Parkinson's disease (PD) across centers in North American, Europe, South America, and Asia. The incidence of deaths from centers in countries with high suicide rates was compared to the incidence of deaths from centers in countries with moderate suicide rates, based on World Health Organization (WHO, 2013) age-matched data. The percentage of suicides (0.59%, 12/2037) in countries with a high baseline rate of suicide (>13/100,000/yr) was greater than the percentage (0.37%, 12/3274) for countries with moderate baseline rates (6–13/100,000/yr). Although the raw data provided an indication that the increase of suicide after neurodisability varies in relation to underlying national rates, correlational analysis found the difference was nonsignificant.

In addition to the degree of suicide risk, national culture also potentially influences the means of suicidal behavior. Date from two studies conducted in the United States were aggregated (DeVivo, Black, Richards, & Stover, 1991; Charlifue & Gerhart, 1991) and compared to combined data from Australia (Soden et al., 2000) and Sweden (Hartkopp, Bronnum-Hansen, Seidenschnur, & Biering-Sorensen, 1998), respectively. The results are contained in Figure 11.1.

As displayed on the chart, more than half of the deaths in the United States were caused by gunshot, with 78% of the 87 deaths employing violent means. In contrast, overdoses, drowning, and hanging were more common in the two non-US countries, with 57% of the 37 deaths occurring through violent means. The methods of suicide after spinal cord injury (SCI) in the United States versus Sweden and Australia differed significantly, reflecting the influence of national characteristics in the choices and access to means for suicide.

A similar pattern is found in multiple sclerosis (MS). In the United States, the methods of suicide among 22 people with MS (identified through MS chapters)

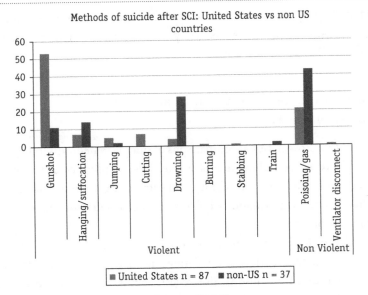

FIGURE 11.1 Cross-national comparison of means of suicide.

US data from DeVivo et al. (1991); Charlifue & Gerhart (1991); non-US data from Soden et al. (2000); Hartkopp et al. (1998).

were gunshot (46%), overdose and/or gas (44%), and other (jump 4%, cutting 4%) (Berman & Samuel, 1993). Stenager, Koch-Henriksen, and Stenager (1996) reviewed 50 suicides that occurred over 35 years in Denmark. Poisoning (38%) and hanging (30%) were the two most common methods across all deaths, with only one death by gunshot recorded.

In making this type of cross-national comparison, the additional check that needs to be made is whether the pattern of means used by people with neurodisability is the same pattern as for the underlying population. In one neurodisability group (traumatic brain injury [TBI]), two independent studies found that the means of suicide employed by people with TBI were significantly different from the pattern for the national population (Achte, Lonnqvist, & Hillbom, 1971; Maino et al., 2007).

Intranational Differences in Suicide

INTRANATIONAL DIFFERENCES IN SUICIDE ASSOCIATED WITH RACE/ETHNICITY AMONG THE GENERAL POPULATION

The previous section addressed the differences in suicide rates and behaviors between countries. This section addresses the differences in rates of suicidal thoughts and behaviors within countries among people from various racial and/or ethnic groups. For example, within the United States, white American males have much higher rates of suicide compared to African American males, all Hispanics, all Native Americans, and all Asian/Pacific Islanders (American Association of Suicidology, 2014; 2016). Similarly, lifetime estimated rates of suicide attempts vary by ethnic group (Oquendo, Lizardi, Greenwald, Weissman, & Mann, 2004). These racially and ethnically based discrepancies in suicide rates are also found in other countries with indigenous populations and/or large immigrant groups (e.g., Raleigh, 1996; McKenzie, Serfaty, & Crawford, 2003; Wendler et al., 2012).

A MODEL OF THE RELATIONSHIP BETWEEN RACE/ETHNICITY, NEURODISABILITY, AND SUICIDE

Before addressing findings from studies in neurodisability that have tested the relationship between race/ethnicity and suicidal behaviors, broader contextual information about factors that could underpin differences in the level of risk need to be outlined. Understanding suicide after neurodisability from a cultural perspective involves three interrelated factors (Figure 11.2). The first factor is the national suicide rate and behaviors, as discussed in the preceding sections. The available evidence suggested that rates of suicide after neurodisability are generally influenced by underlying national patterns. The link between the national suicide rate and suicide after neurodisability is then mediated by two additional factors. First is the generic risk and protective factors for suicide associated with being part of a racial/ethnic

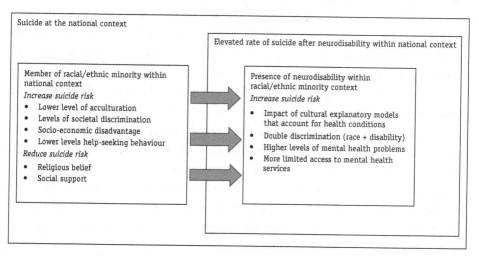

FIGURE 11.2 Suicide after brain injury in the cross-cultural context.

minority. Second, the experience of neurodisability within specific racial/ethnic contexts can also give rise to particular risk and protective factors.

MEMBERSHIP OF A RACIAL/ETHNIC MINORITY

Several dimensions of the racial/ethnic minority experience are associated with elevated suicide risk. These include the degree and process of acculturation, levels of racism/discrimination, broader socioeconomic disadvantage, and differences in help-seeking behavior (Table 11.1). Acculturation can apply both to the process of settlement arising from immigration as well as to the relationship between indigenous populations and the dominant colonizing culture. There is a complex relationship between each of these different sets of circumstances and suicide (see Table 11.1).

The complexities of the relationship between race and suicide extends to settled minority groups within dominant cultures. Although the relationship between socioeconomic disadvantage and suicide risk has been frequently documented, it may be overly simplistic to postulate a linear relationship between decreasing socioeconomic status, race/ethnicity, and increasing suicide. Not every study has found a relationship between racially based economic disparities and suicide (Burr, Hartman, & Matteson, 1999). For example, in the United States, African Americans who are in the middle class have been reported as having a higher suicide rate than those in lower socioeconomic classes (Burr et al., 1999) despite putatively experiencing less acculturation-related stress. One possible reason for this finding is suggested by Walker, Utsey, Bolden, and Williams (2005), who found that the relationship between acculturation and suicidal thoughts and behaviors was moderated by religion. Based on their study, the authors suggested that the degree of religiosity may be a stronger predictor of levels of suicidal distress among African Americans than the level of acculturation.

This leads to the consideration of protective factors that have been demonstrated as offsetting the challenges arising from acculturation, racism/discrimination, socioeconomic disadvantage, and differences in help-seeking behavior. The two key protective factors are religious belief and social support (Table 11.2). However, once again, although the importance of these factors has been frequently documented, the protective benefit is not universal. For example, religion can also be a source of strain when it is associated with dynamics such as guilt and punishment (Ismail, Wright, Rhodes, & Small, 2005, p. 26). Similarly, access to extensive family support is not universal among racial/ethnic minorities. Migration can lead to the break up of extended families across countries, and differing levels of acculturation between the first and succeeding generations of a family often provide a sources of intergenerational misunderstanding, conflict, and division (McKenzie et al., 2003; Diego, Yamamoto, Nguyen, & Hifumi, 1994, Simpson, Mohr, & Redman, 2000).

TABLE 11.1

Risk factors Race/ethnicity	Risk for suicide thoughts and behaviors
Degree of acculturation— new immigrants	Some studies have found that recent arrivals had suicide rates characteristic of their country of origin for the first generation (Lester, 2008b). The means of suicide was also more in keeping with their country of origin (Burvill et al., 1983). However, other studies have found that the rate of suicide among newly arrived migrants were higher than both the national rates of their adopted country and their country of origin (Hjern, 2002; Johansson et al., 1997).
Degree of acculturation— indigenous population	Being part of an indigenous group within a larger culture is a cause of stress for members of the less dominant cultural groups across several countries (Lester, 2008b). The strains associated with acculturation can give rise to mental health problems and elevated suicide risk. The degree of acculturation can be associated with suicide risk, with those reporting lower levels of acculturation having higher suicide rates (e.g., Van Winkle & May, 1986).
Degree of racism/ discrimination	Chronic exposure to racism, including discrimination across minority groups in the United States, leads to increased mental health problems such as depression or stress which mediate levels of suicidality (Utsey et al., 2008; Takahashi, 1989).
	One possible mechanism is that dealing with daily racial stresses and associated microaggression places strain on existing coping resources, with an associated vulnerability to psychological distress (Constantine & Sue, 2007; Pieterse & Carter, 2007).
Broader socioeconomic disadvantage as a source of suicide risk	People from racial and/or ethnic minorities often have poorer education levels, lower occupational profiles, lower income, poorer physical health, greater levels of unemployment, and limited access to health services with related higher levels of poverty, substance abuse, and mental health problems. These factors, individually or in combination, can increase the risk of suicide (Rehkopf & Buka, 2006; Canino & Roberts, 2001).

(continued)

TABLE 11.1 CONTINUED

Race/ethnicity	Risk for suicide thoughts and behaviors
Differences in help-seeking behavior	Barriers reduce the likelihood of people from racial/ethnic minorities accessing needed mental health services at times of elevated suicidality, including language, unequal power relationship implicit in seeking help from professionals within the dominant culture, the individualistic focus of Western mental health practices, problems among some cultures for male clients seeing female therapists, differing cultural expectations about the role of the therapist (e.g., collaborator vs. learned teacher and authority figure), and lack of culturally appropriate assistance available from Western-based service providers (Wendler et al, 2012; Akutsu & Chu, 2006).

Acculturation refers to the process of sociocultural changes arising from contact dynamics between two identifiable groups (Cuellar, Harris, & Jasso, 1980).

CULTURALLY MEDIATED IMPACT OF NEURODISABILITY

The culturally mediated impact of neurodisability may also contribute to suicide risk. These impacts of culture, race, and ethnicity are multilayered and include the

TABLE 11.2

Protective factors Race/ethnicity	Protective factors to reduce suicide thoughts and behaviors
Religious belief	Religious belief is a well-known protective factor for suicide, and is particularly strong in some racial/ethnic minority groups. Different dimensions of religion have been identified as playing potential protective role; namely, a source of comfort and reduction of emotional distress, a source of social connection through membership, and containing strong prohibitions about suicide (Utsey et al., 2007).
Extended family	Provides a social buffer and support against many of the other sources of stress already outlined. For example, African American woman have much denser social networks than African American men, and this is one explanatory factor accounting for their low rate of suicide (Utsey et al., 2007).

cultural differences in explanatory models that account for the onset, characteristics, and outcome of neurodisability; a double disadvantage in socioeconomic status; and higher levels of mental health problems and more limited access to mental health services when compared to their racial group in general.

There are differences in the explanatory models (Kleinman, Eisnberg, & Good, 1978; Kleinman, 1980) that cultures use that shape understanding about health problems. The explanatory model provides the basis for the culturally mediated interpretation of the causes, signs, and symptoms of the different types of neurodisability. In some cultures, greater weight may be given to understanding neurodisability as linked to madness, witchcraft, demon possession, or psycho-pathology rather than disease processes or injury (e.g., Wexler, 2010; Jacoby, Snape, & Baker, 2005; Simpson et al., 2000). While most commonly associated with the "folk beliefs" of ethnic cultures, it should be noted that mainstream Western scientific and biomedical culture has not been immune from making such misattributions (Wexler, 2010). The associated level of stigma fosters a sense of shame a individual, family and societal levels (e.g., Burneo et al., 2009; Wexler, 2010). Linked to this, social groups may shun or actively discriminate against individuals so afflicted, thus leading to feelings of alienation from one's racial/ethnic group, an important source of individual identity and social connection.

People with neurodisability may also be doubly disadvantaged in key areas of social integration such as workforce participation. For example, people with neurodisability have poor rates of return to work as a whole. However, people with neurodisability from minority groups often have even lower levels of return to work than comparable members of their racial group (Saltipidas & Ponsford, 2007; Buchanan et al., 2010) as part of a broader pattern of minority disadvantage, thereby increasing the risk of suicidal thoughts and behaviors.

In addition, people with neurodisability from racial/ethnic minorities can have higher rates of depression or mental health problems compared to people from white (non-Hispanic) backgrounds (e.g., Krause, Saladin, & Adkins, 2009; Buchanan et al., 2010). These problems may be compounded by stronger social sanctions applied to people with mental health conditions among some minority groups (Cultural Competence in Mental Health, www.upennrrtc.org). Any heightened level of mental health problems increases the suicide risk. Despite this concern, not all studies have reported such findings. Jia et al. (2010) found that people from black and other racial groups had lower levels of self-reported depression after stroke than non-Hispanic whites, with the authors speculating whether this reflected a racial/ethnic effect of underreporting of symptoms or poor symptom recognition by service providers.

Exacerbating these problems, people from racial/ethnic minorities often have more limited access to needed mental health services than their non-Hispanic white counterparts (US Department of Health and Human Services [USDHH], 2001). These problems can be compounded in the case of people with neurodisability. People with neurodisability from racial/ethnic minorities have poorer access to needed health, rehabilitation, and mental health care than do non-Hispanic whites (Mitch, 2011; Buchanan et al., 2010; Burneo et al., 2009). The lack of access to services for treatable mental health problems may contribute to the problem of elevated suicidal thoughts and behaviors (Feinstein, 2002).

As outlined in various sections of the book, many of the factors already listed are associated with suicide risk. Despite this, most of these hypothesized relationships of the elevated risk arising from an interaction between neurodisability and racial/ethnic background are untested. However, the absence of evidence should not be interpreted as evidence of absence. Many of these factors are important considerations when seeking to undertake assessment and intervention to manage suicide risk among racial/ethnic minority groups.

RACE AS A MEDIATING FACTOR FOR SUICIDAL THOUGHTS AND BEHAVIORS IN NEURODISABILITY

Although only two studies undertook cross-national comparisons of neurodisability and suicide, eight within-country studies of neurodisability and suicidal thoughts or behavior included race as a variable. All eight reports were situated in North America, with seven from the United States and one from Canada. The studies included race-related variables in a broader examination of risk factors for suicide or suicide ideation.

The two studies that examined race as a possible risk factor for suicide among people with SCI and PD, respectively, came to different conclusions. In an early study, DeVivo et al. (1991) found that racial background was associated with different levels of suicide risk among people with SCI. In the study, whites with any type of SCI were significantly more likely to die by suicide (standard mortality ratio [SMR] 5.4, 95% CI 3.8–7.0) compared to non-whites (SMR 2.6, 0.3–4.9) when compared to the general population. In contrast, although elevated, the SMR for non-whites was nonsignificant, albeit calculated on only 5 deaths. In contrast, Myslobodsky, Lalonde, and Hicks (2001) found a lower rate of suicide among people with PD compared to the general population. In their study, the variable of race (Caucasian, African American, other) was non-significant, acting as neither a risk factor nor a protective factor.

Six studies that investigated suicide ideation included race as a potential sociodemographic risk factor. In a Canadian population-based study into depression and suicide ideation among people with cerebrovascular accident (CVA;

Fuller-Thomson, Tulipano, & Song, 2012), people identified as white were twice as likely to report suicide ideation compared to non-whites (odds ratio [OR] 1.95, 95% CI 1.07, 3.57). The authors speculated that the difference may be due to protective factors among non-white groups (e.g., greater religious affiliation, social support), but could also reflect a greater openness among people from white backgrounds to report such symptoms. The remaining studies found no significant race-based differences in the frequency of suicide ideation after CVA (Kishi, Koiser, & Robinson, 1996a; Kishi, Robinson, & Koiser, 1996b); TBI (Tsaousides, Cantor, & Gordon, 2011), MS (Turner, Williams, Bowen, Kivlahan, & Hasselkorn, 2006), and PD (Nazem et al, 2008), respectively. In each study, people from the white (Caucasian) racial group were compared to an aggregated category of all other racial groups.

In reflecting on these limited findings, the elevated level of suicide risk associated with being white is consistent with the broader population data over the past two decades. However, in most studies, the US data were generally inconclusive, and this reflects at least three problems. First, the proportion of non-white participants in the samples was generally very low, resulting in a lack of power to detect any significant differences if they did exist. Furthermore, as a direct consequence of the small numbers of non-white participants, various minority groups were often aggregated into a "non-white" category, thus further reducing any chance of identifying significant patterns of association given the diversity among non-White racial groups. Finally, these problems were compounded by the different sets of nomenclature used to classify racial groups within the United States, including the terms white (or non-Hispanic white), African American (or black or non-Hispanic black), Hispanic, Asian, Asian American or Pacific Islander, North American Indian, and Alaskan Native.

With the establishment of core data elements for the reporting of findings among various diagnostic groups within neurology, the future will hopefully see greater consistency in the reporting of race and ethnicity data (e.g., Maas et al., 2010). Furthermore, seeking to oversample non-white participants in studies interested in investigating cultural differences will help alleviate some of the difficulties just outlined. Finally, increasing numbers of studies have been published that investigate outcomes for specific non-white racial/ethnic groups, and this avenue could be broadened to include suicide.

Assessment and Intervention

As outlined, the evidence base relating to cultural impact on the prevalence, risk factors, and treatment of suicidal thoughts and behaviors after neurodisability is too limited to draw any substantive conclusions. In the majority of studies, the findings relating to suicide were incidental to the primary purpose of the research. Only one or two studies have been conducted with the primary purpose of investigating the mediating impact of cultural issues on suicidal thoughts and/or behavior within any neurodisability group. In the absence of such data, the recommended clinical approach is to marry best practice in culturally sensitive approaches to suicide assessment and intervention for the general population with best practice in the culturally informed approaches to the assessment and treatment of neurodisability-related impairments and mental health issues.

The assessment and treatment of suicide build on broader cultural competencies for mental health (Stuart, 2004). Some key clinical starting points for addressing cross-cultural issues in the assessment and management of suicide after neurodisability are displayed in Box 11.1. The practice options outlined in this section build on content from previous chapters on suicide risk assessment and management.

BOX 11.1

CLINICAL APPROACH TO MANAGING SUICIDAL THOUGHTS AND
BEHAVIORS AMONG PEOPLE WITH NEURODISABILITY FROM CULTURALLY
AND LINGUISTICALLY DIVERSE BACKGROUNDS

1. Develop general cultural competence in mental health evaluation.
2. Develop knowledge of the epidemiological data regarding minority groups (e.g., American Association of Suicide Prevention Fact Sheets).
3. Ensure that representatives from different cultural groups have input into the development of suicide prevention assessment and management tools and approaches.
4. Identify whether mental health staff from same ethnic/racial background are available (if desired by client).
5. Pay careful attention to cultural issues when assessing and treating suicidal thoughts and behaviors, including sensitivity to

> Avoiding projecting one's own value system onto the patient and recognizing that stressors may be of great cultural import
>
> The fact that people from various racial/ethnic groups may be less likely to disclose suicide thoughts or behaviors
>
> The cultural context of help-seeking behavior and the varying expectation of patients from different racial/ethnic minorities toward the clinician.

Adapted from Westefeld et al. (2008, p. 230) and Wendler et al. (2012, p. 85).

ASSESSMENT

One approach to informing suicide risk assessment among different minority groups has been to develop specific profiles for each group (e.g., for African Americans, Hispanics, etc.). However, it is difficult to apply this approach to every racial/ethnic minority that might be encountered in the service setting, particularly in communities with high rates of racial/ethnic diversity. To circumvent this problem, Westefeld, Range, Greenfeld, and Kettman (2008) proposed modifying the Multicultural Assessment Procedure (MAP; Ridley, Li, & Hill, 1998, p. 244), a generic approach to multicultural assessment, to the assessment of suicide risk among ethnic minorities. The MAP can be further adapted to inform assessment of people with neurodisability who need suicide risk assessment. The MAP has four phases: (1) identifying, (2) interpreting, (3) incorporating cultural data, and then (4) arriving at a sound assessment decision based on steps 1–3.

IDENTIFYING CULTURAL DATA

The authors emphasize collecting data about the client's cultural background alongside the other standard elements of a biopsychosocial assessment. In collecting data about cultural background, the clinical interview is identified as the central tool in the assessment process. This centrality of the clinical interview is consistent with the assessment approach outlined for a standard suicide risk assessment in Chapter 8. Information should come from clients themselves, as well as from multiple other sources (e.g., family, health professionals from the same cultural background, key community informants). In applying the model to suicide assessment, Westefeld et al. (2008) stress the importance of drawing on cultural information to help interpret the degree of risk associated with various degrees of depression, hopelessness, and other key suicide risk factors. In extending the scope of any such assessment to also include neurodisability, it is also important to also focus on cultural factors associated with acquiring neurodisability and whether any such factors are exacerbating the suicide risk.

Cultural background can also shape beliefs about suicide. These can include beliefs that suicide is a sign of weakness, that suicide is a sin or immoral, that suicide is a taboo topic that cannot be discussed, or that thinking about suicide means that a person is "going crazy" (Westefeld et al., 2008). Gathering information about the presence of such belief systems within the cultural background of a client is important as it may influence the extent to which the person is willing to communicate about his or her levels of suicidal distress (Wendler et al., 2012).

In terms of standardized assessments that complement the clinical interview, a growing number of cognitive, behavioral, and affect-related measures have standardized translations in other languages. Books addressing the conduct of cross-cultural neuropsychological assessments (Uzzell, Ponton, & Ardila, 2007) assist in the culturally sensitive assessment of cognitive and behavioral functioning after neurodisability. However, there are still limited suicide assessment instruments validated for non–English speaking cultures. One option, however, is that some depression scales (e.g., Hamilton, the Beck Depression Inventory) that have been widely translated and validated contain items measuring suicide ideation, and these can provide a source of data to assist in making a risk assessment.

INTERPRETING CULTURAL DATA

Clients may display normative (i.e., behavior consistent with the culture) and idiosyncratic (i.e., unique to the client, not necessarily culturally expected behavior) behaviors in their presentation. According to Ridley et al. (1998), the first step to interpreting cultural data involves understanding the clients' idiosyncratic experience of his or her culture to see how it coincides or differs from the cultural norm. Second, the authors suggest that "base rates about particular psychological disorders, co-morbid conditions, medical conditions that present as psychological symptom patterns and suicide rates in various populations" (p. 875) form crucial contextual information within which to understand the condition of an individual client. As outlined earlier, although there is limited information about suicide risk after neurodisability, there are some initial data about variations in depression and/or psychological distress across different racial/ethnic minorities that provide some guidance. The authors finally provide several guidelines to assist the clinician in formulating a working hypothesis about the nature of their client's distress.

INCORPORATE CULTURAL DATA

The cultural data that have been collected are then integrated with the broader biopsychosocial assessment data to assist in refining assessment conclusions. The authors stress the importance of ruling out any medical condition that might be contributing to the psychological symptoms, drawing on the results of psychological assessments (preferably culturally sensitive ones) and comparing the data to criteria in the *Diagnostic and Statistical Manual of Mental Disorders* (DSM), albeit with appropriate caution, given the problems in cross-cultural application of the DSM nosology. This latter challenge is exacerbated in the case of neurodisability. To give one example, there has been wide documentation of the confounding effect of symptoms arising from the neuropathology of most types of neurodisability (particularly somatic symptoms) complicating the assessment of depression and potentially creating a number of false-positive diagnoses. Therefore, establishing the presence of defined mental health conditions is doubly complicated due to the influence of culture and neurodisability. Clinicians will need to draw on their knowledge of these complexities in order to modulate decisions in determining the severity of suicide risk.

ARRIVE AT ASSESSMENT DECISION

The final phase involves drawing on the data from the previous three steps. As summarized by Westefeld et al. (2008), this comprises "combining cultural variables/ history, the base rates, the direct assessment data and the clinical interview in order to determine risk" (p. 245). The synthesis of these data forms the basis for arriving at an assessment decision.

SUICIDE PREVENTION

The brief discussion on intervention in this section builds on the detailed suicide prevention guidelines for neurodisability detailed in earlier chapters. In considering the international application of suicide prevention guidelines, Mishara (2006, p. 259) observed that "there are more commonalities in suicide prevention activities around the world than diversity" (p. 1).

At the universal level (targeting all people with neurodisability), the first step is to ensure that all people with neurodisability, regardless of racial/ethnic background, are able to access the appropriate treatment for and management of their neurodisability. This includes neurorehabilitation, as well as appropriate neurological and/or neuropsychiatric care supported by appropriate functional and psychosocial interventions. Furthermore, the physicians and therapists delivering care should ensure that they have the appropriate cross-cultural competencies in mental health (Stuart, 2004). In relation to psychological distress, it is also important to balance the sensitivity toward possible diversity issues while not assuming that between-group differences are greater than within-group cultural differences (Sue & Sue, 2012; Choi, Rogers, & Werth, 2009).

At the level of indicated interventions (targeting people with neurodisability who have displayed suicidal thoughts or behaviors), the American Association of Suicide Prevention information resources (as referred to earlier) also provide useful culturally specific data about US suicide rates and rates of suicide attempts. Similarly, the World Health Organization provides international data (www.who.int/mental_ health/prevention/suicide/suicideprevent/en/) about the rates of suicide for approximately 100 countries. The limited evidence from the neurodisability literature highlights the importance of tailoring means restriction to reflect the local cultural conditions within different countries. Finally, mobilizing family support and/or reinforcing religious beliefs/connections may play important protective roles in reducing suicidal distress and the likelihood of future suicidal thoughts or behavior.

Conclusion

There is extremely limited data available about the impact of culture in mediating suicide risk after neurodisability. However, it does appear that the nature of suicidal thoughts and behavior after neurodisability is significantly shaped by the national cultural context. Suicide risk in neurodisability appears to be elevated from the national baseline. Similarly, the means of suicide may be influenced by national context, although the pattern of means for suicide and suicide attempts after neurodisability can differ from national norms. Furthermore, there is the possibility that people with neurodisability within racial/ethnic minorities experience double disadvantage, which may increase their suicide risk, although much more research needs to be done to confirm such a possibility.

Based on such approximations of risk, clinicians will then need to tailor suicide prevention responses to people with neurodisability from diverse cultural and linguistic backgrounds by drawing on broader cultural competencies, particularly cultural competencies developed within mental health. The illustration of how one tool, the MAP, could be adapted to assist with the assessment of suicide risk after neurodisability provides an example of how this challenging task might be accomplished.

Implications for Clinicians

1. Although the degree of elevated risk for suicidal thoughts and behaviors seems to be similar across Western developed countries, the actual types of behaviors (e.g., means of death) will reflect local cultures.
2. People with neurodisability from minority groups can face additional stressors because of a "double disadvantage" (disability + minority status) in seeking social goals such as employment and accommodation. They also report higher levels of depression and mental illness and may face greater challenges in accessing treatment.
3. As current evidence regarding neurodisability, diversity, and suicide is so limited, the MAP provides a model for assessing suicidal thoughts and behaviors in a culturally appropriate manner.

4. A growing number of measures of cognitive, behavioral, or affect-related functioning have validated translations for a range of different languages and can assist clinical practice.

5. Culturally or nationally specific suicide information resources from organizations including the American Association of Suicide Prevention and the World Health Organization can help inform the clinical management of people with neurodisability from diverse cultural, racial, or ethnic backgrounds.

References

Achte K. A., Lonnqvist J., & Hillbom E. (1971). Suicides following war brain-injuries. *Acta Psychiatrica Scandinavica: Supplementum, 225*, 1–94.

Akutsu, P. D., & Chu, J. P. (2006). Clinical problems that initiate professional help-seeking behaviors from Asian Americans. *Professional Psychology: Research and Practice, 37*, 407–415.

American Association of Suicidology. (2016). *African Americans and suicide*. Retrieved from https://www.suicidology.org/Portals/14/Re-Formatted%20African%20American%20 Suicide%20Fact%20Sheet%202016.pdf?ver=2016-11-16-105239-947

American Association of Suicidology. (2014). *American Indian and Alaska Natives*. Retrieved from https://www.suicidology.org/Portals/14/docs/Resources/FactSheets/2011/AI-AN2011.pdf

American Association of Suicidology. (2014). *Hispanic suicide*. Retrieved from https://www.suicidology.org/Portals/14/docs/Resources/FactSheets/Hispanic2012.pdf

American Association of Suicidology. (2016). *Suicide in the US*. Retrieved 14 from from https://www.suicidology.org/Portals/14/Re-Formatted%20Suicide%20in%20the%20United%20 States%202016%20Fact%20Sheet.pdf?ver=2016-11-16-105533-437

Berman, A. L., & Samuel, L. (1993). Suicide among people with multiple sclerosis. *Journal of NeuroRehabilitation, 7*, 53–62.

Buchanan, R. J., Zuniga, M. A., Carrillo-Zuniga, G., Chakravorty, B. J., Tyry, T., Moreau, R. L.,... Vollmer, T. (2010). Comparison of Latinos, African Americans, and Caucasians with multiple sclerosis. *Ethnicity and Disease, 20*(4), 451–457.

Burneo, J. G., Jette, N., Theodore, W., Begley, C., Parko, K., Thurman, D. J., & Weibe, S. (2009). Disparities in epilepsy: Report of a systematic review by the North American Commission of the International League Against Epilepsy. *Epilepsia, 50*(10), 2285–2295.

Burr, J. A., Hartman, J. T., & Matteson, D. W. (1999). Black suicide in U.S. metropolitan areas: An examination of the racial inequality and social integration-regulation hypotheses. *Social Forces, 77*, 1049–1080.

Burvill, P., McCall, M., Woodings, T., & Stenhouse, N. (1983). Comparison of suicide rates and methods in English, Scots and Irish immigrants in Australia. *Social Science and Medicine, 17*, 705–708.

Canino, G., & Roberts, R. E. (2001). Suicidal behavior among Latino youth. *Suicide and Life-Threatening Behavior, 31*, 66–78.

Charlifue, S. W., & Gerhart, K. A. (1991). Behavioral and demographic predictors of suicide after traumatic spinal cord injury. *Archives of Physical Medicine and Rehabilitation, 72*, 488–492.

Choi, J. L., Rogers, J. R., & Werth, J. L. Jr. (2009). Suicide risk assessment with Asian American college students: A culturally informed perspective. *The Counseling Psychologist, 37*, 186–218.

Constantine, M. G., & Sue, D. W. (2007). Perceptions of racial microaggressions among Black supervisees in cross-racial dyads. *Journal of Counseling Psychology, 54*, 142–153.

Cuellar, I., Harris, L., Jasso, R. (1980). An acculturation scale for Mexican American normal and clinical populations. *Hispanic Journal of Behavioral Sciences, 2*(3), 199–217.

DeVivo, M. J., Black, K. J., Richards, J. S., & Stover, S. L. (1991). Suicide following spinal cord injury. *Paraplegia, 29*, 620–627.

Diego, A. T., Yamamoto, J., Nguyen, L. H., & Hifumi, S. S. (1994). Suicide in the elderly: Profiles of Asians and Whites. *Asian American and Pacific Islander Journal of Health, 2*, 49–57.

Feinstein, A. (2002). An examination of suicidal intent in patients with multiple sclerosis. *Neurology, 59*, 674–678.

Fuller-Thomson, E., Tulipano, M. J., & Song, M (2012). The association between depression, suicidal ideation and stroke in a population-based sample. *International Journal of Stroke, 7*, 188–194.

Hartkopp, A., Brønnum-Hansen, H., Seidenschnur, A., & Biering-Sørensen, F. (1998). Suicide in a spinal cord injured population: Its relation to functional status. *Archives of Physical Medicine and Rehabilitation, 79*(11), 1356–1361.

Hjern, A. (2002). Suicide in first and second generation immigrants in Sweden: A comparative study. *Social Psychiatry and Psychiatric Epidemiology, 37*, 423–429.

Ismail, H., Wright, J., Rhodes, P., & Small, N. (2005). Religious beliefs about causes and treatment of epilepsy. *British Journal of General Practice, 55*, 26–31.

Jacoby, A., Snape, D., & Baker, G. A. (2005). Epilepsy and social identity: The stigma of a chronic neurological disorder. *Lancet Neurology, 4*, 171–178.

Jia, H., Chumbler, N. R., Wang, X., Chuang H. C., Damush, T. M., Cameon, R., & William, L. S. (2010). Racial and ethnic disparities in post-stroke depression detection. *International Journal of Geriatric Psychiatry, 25*, 298–304.

Johansson, L. M., Johansson, S. E., Bergman, B., & Sundquist, J. (1997). Suicide, ethnicity and psychiatric in-patient care: A case control study. *Archives of Suicide Research, 3*, 257–269.

Kishi, Y., Kosier, J. T., & Robinson, R. G. (1996a). Suicidal plans in patients with acute stroke. *The Journal of Nervous and Mental Disease, 184*, 274–280.

Kishi, Y., Robinson, R. G., & Kosier, J. T. (1996b). Suicidal plans in patients with stroke: Comparison between acute-onset and delayed-onset suicidal plans. *International Psychogeriatrics, 8*, 623–634.

Kleinman, A. (1980). *Patients and healers in the context of culture.* Berkeley, CA: University of California Press.

Kleinman, A., Eisnberg, L., & Good, B. (1978). Culture, illness and care: Clinical lessons from cross-cultural research. *Annals of Internal Medicine, 88*, 251–258.

Krause, J. S., Saladin, L. K., & Adkins, R. H. (2009). Disparities in subjective well-being, participation, and health after spinal cord injury: A 6-year longitudinal study. *NeuroRehabilitation, 24*(1), 47–56.

Leenars, A. A. (2008). Suicide: A cross-cultural theory. In F. T. L. Leong & M. M. Leach (Eds.), *Suicide among racial and ethnic minority groups: Theory, research and practice* (pp. 13–38). New York: Taylor & Francis.

Lester, D. (2008a). Theories of suicide. In F. T. L. Leong & M. M. Leach (Eds.), *Suicide among racial and ethnic minority groups: Theory, research and practice* (pp. 39–53). New York: Taylor & Francis.

Lester, D. (2008b). Suicide and culture. *World Cultural Psychiatry Research Review, 3,* 51–68.

Maas, A. I., Harrison-Felix, C., Menon, D., Adelson, P. D., Balkin, T., Bullock, R., . . . Schwab, K. (2010). Common data elements for traumatic brain injury: Recommendations from the interagency working group on demographics and clinical assessment. *Archives of Physical Medicine and Rehabilitation, 91*(11), 1641–1649.

Maino, A., Kyllönen, T., Viilo, K., Hakko, H., Säkioja, T., & Räsänen, P. (2007). Traumatic brain injury, psychiatric disorders and suicide: A population-based study of suicide victims during the years 1988-2004 in Northern Finland. *Brain Injury, 21,* 851–855.

McKenzie, K., Serfaty, M., & Crawford, M. (2003). Suicide in ethnic minority groups. *British Journal of Psychiatry, 183,* 100–101.

Mishara, B. (2006). Cultural specificity and the universality of suicide. *Crisis, 27,* 1–3.

Mitch, V. (2011). Acquired Brain Injury Rehabilitation Service Delivery Project: Developing a model of care for rural and remote NSW. Sydney, NSW: Agency for Clinical Innovation.

Myslobodsky, M., Lalonde, F. M., & Hicks, L. (2001). Are patients with Parkinson's Disease suicidal? *Journal of Geriatric Psychiatry and Neurology, 14,* 120–124.

Nazem, S., Siderowf, A. D., Duda, J. E., Brown, G. K., Have, T. T., Stern, M. B., & Weintraub, D. (2008). Suicidal and death ideation in Parkinson's disease. *Movement Disorders, 23*(11), 1573–1579.

Oquendo, M. A., Lizardi, D., Greenwald, S., Weissman, M. M., & Mann, J. J. (2004). Rates of lifetime suicide attempt and rates of lifetime major depression in different ethnic groups in the United States. *Acta Psychiatrica Scandinavica, 110,* 446–451.

Pieterse, A. L., & Carter, R. J. (2007). An examination of the relationship between general life stress, racism-related stress, and psychological health among Black men. *Journal of Counseling Psychology, 54,* 101–109.

Raleigh, V. S. (1996). Suicide patterns and trends in people of Indian subcontinent and Caribbean origin in England and Wales. *Ethnicity and Disease, 1,* 55–64.

Rehkopf, D. H., & Buka, S. L. (2006). The association between suicide and the socio-economic characteristics of geographical areas: A systematic review. *Psychological Medicine, 36,* 145–157.

Ridley, C. R., Li, L. C., & Hill, C. L. (1998). Multicultural assessment: Reexamination, reconceptualization, and practical application. *The Counseling Psychologist 26,* 827–910.

Saltipidas, H., & Ponsford, J. (2007). The influence of cultural background on motivation for and participation in rehabilitation and outcome following traumatic brain injury. *Journal of Head Trauma Rehabilitation, 22,* 132–139.

Simpson, G. K., Mohr, R., & Redman, A. (2000). Cultural variations in the understanding of brain injury and brain injury rehabilitation. *Brain Injury, 14,* 125–140.

Soden, R. J., Walsh, J., Middleton, J. W., Craven, M. L., Rutkowski, S. B., & Yeo, J. D. (2000). Causes of death after spinal cord injury. *Spinal Cord, 38,* 604–610.

Stenager, E. N., Koch-Henriksen, N., & Stenager, E. (1996). Risk factors for suicide in multiple sclerosis. *Psychotherapy and Psychosomatics, 65,* 86–90.

Stuart, R. B. (2004). Twelve practical suggestions for achieving multicultural competence. *Professional Psychology: Research and Practice, 35*, 3–9.

Sue, D. W., & Sue, D. (2003).*Counseling the culturally diverse: Theory and practice* (6th ed.). New York: Wiley.

Takahashi, Y. (1989). Suicidal Asian patients: Recommendations for treatment. *Suicide and Life-Threatening Behavior, 19*, 305–313.

Tsaousides, T., Cantor, J. B., & Gordon, W. A. (2011). Suicidal ideation following traumatic brain injury: Prevalence rates and correlates in adults living in the community. *Journal of Head Trauma Rehabilitation, 26*, 265–275.

Tseng, W. S., & Streltzer, J. (Eds.). (1997). *Culture and psychopathology.* New York: Bruner/Mazel.

Turner, A. P., Williams, R. M., Bowen, J. D., Kivlahan, D. R., & Hasselkorn, J. K. (2006). Suicidal ideation in multiple sclerosis. *Archives of Physical and Medical Rehabilitation, 87*, 1073–1078.

US Department of Health and Human Services (USDHH). (2001). *Mental health: Culture, race, and ethnicity.* Rockville, MD: US Department of Health and Human Services, Public Health Service, Office of the Surgeon General. Retrieved from http://www.mentalhealth.samhsa.gov/cre/toc.asp

Utsey, S. O., Stanard, P., & Hook, J. N. (2008). Understanding the role of cultural factors in relation to suicide among African Americans. In F. T. L. Leong & M. M. Leach (Eds.), *Suicide among racial and ethnic minority groups: Theory, research and practice* (pp. 57–79). New York: Taylor & Francis.

Uzzell, B. P., Ponton, M., & Ardila, A. (Eds.). (2007). *International handbook of cross-cultural neuropsychology.* Mahwah, NJ: Lawrence Erlbaum.

Van Winkle, N. W., & May, P. A. (1986). Native American suicide in New Mexico, 1959–1979. *Human Organization, 45*, 296–309.

Voon, V., Krack, P., Lang, A. E., Lozano, A. M., Dujardin, K., Schüpbach, M., . . . Moro, E. (2008). A multicentre study on suicide outcomes following subthalamic stimulation for Parkinson's disease. *Brain, 131*(10), 2720–2728.

Walker, R. L., Utsey, S. O., Bolden, M. A., & Williams, O. III (2005). Do sociocultural factors predict suicidality among persons of African descent living in the US? *Archives of Suicide Research, 9*, 203–217.

Wendler, S., Matthews, D., & Morelli, P. T. (2012). Cultural competence in suicide risk assessment. In R. I. Simon & R. E. Hales (Eds.), *The American Psychiatric Publishing textbook of suicide assessment* (pp. 75–88). Washington, DC: American Psychiatric Publishing.

Westefeld, J. S., Range, L., Greenfeld, J. M., & Kettman, J. J. (2008). Testing and assessment. In F. T. L. Leong & M. M. Leach (Eds.), *Suicide among racial and ethnic minority groups: Theory, research and practice* (pp. 229–253). New York: Taylor & Francis.

Wexler, A. (2010). The art of medicine: Stigma, history, and Huntington's disease. *Lancet, 376*, 18–19.

Windfuhr, K., & Karpur, N. (2011). International perspectives on the epidemiology and aetiology of suicide and self-harm. In R. C. O'Connor, S. Platt, & J. Gordon (Eds.), *International handbook of suicide prevention: Research, policy and practice* (pp. 27–57). West Sussex, UK: Wiley-Blackwell.

World Health Organization. (2013). *World Health Organization Suicide prevention (SUPRE).* Retrieved from www.who.int/mental_health/prevention/suicide/suicideprevent/en/

12 Public Health and Organizational Approaches

Introduction

The concept of preventing diseases or illness has had a long history in Western medicine. In the second half of the twentieth century, models originally developed for broader prevention of disease or illness were adapted to suicide prevention. These include the primary/secondary/tertiary triad and the universal/selective/indicated models (Gordon, 1983). Such models provide a framework of conceptually and/or empirically based intervention strategies for suicide prevention (Metha, Weber, & Webb, 1998). Although these models had their origins in public health-oriented approaches to disease management, in their application to suicide prevention they have commonly combined elements of public health and individual approaches (Pitman & Caine, 2012).

Public health strategies target groups or whole populations (Wasserman & Durkee, 2009). For example, within this context, people with a neurodisability could be seen as an indicated population (i.e., an at-risk group). Common public health activities include surveillance (identifying the epidemiology and risks for diseases or disorders), public education campaigns, screening to identify undetected cases, and introduction of legislation. In contrast, individual-oriented strategies are characterized as "healthcare approaches" to suicide prevention (Wasserman & Durkee, 2009). Such individual approaches have been the primary focus of the previous four chapters (i.e., approaches to suicide risk assessment, evidence-informed interventions, clinical management strategies, and cross-cultural applications).

Therefore, this chapter starts by focusing on public health strategies. The first section of the chapter addresses the underlying rationale and also highlights some examples of public health approaches to suicide prevention. The relevance of such public health initiatives for people with neurodisability will be emphasized.

The next section of the chapter then outlines two models of suicide prevention (primary/secondary/tertiary and universal/selective/indicated), which are informed by multimodal approaches (i.e., include both public health and individual approaches). Results from two well-known international examples of the coordinated application of multimodal suicide prevention approaches in large human service organizations (i.e., the UK mental health sector; the US Air Force) are then briefly outlined. Following this, an example is given of a model (based on the universal/selective/indicated model) applied to the field of neurodisability, providing ideas about how sole practitioners, small-scale agencies, and larger scale organizations can create "stepped care" models of suicide prevention. The last section of the chapter addresses suicide prevention training, with a discussion of application to staff working in the field of neurodisability.

Rationale and Public Health Approaches to Suicide Prevention

RATIONALE

The rationale for public health approaches to suicide prevention has been persuasively advanced by Lewis, Hawton, and Jones (1997). The authors suggested that health-based approaches that focus on high-risk groups only would have limited impact on national suicide rates (Pitman & Caine, 2012; Yip, 2005). Such approaches needed to be complemented by upstream public health-based approaches that addressed larger social and ecological forces (e.g., unemployment) and that aim to reduce suicide rates "by shifting modal behaviors and improving mental well-being across society as a whole" (Pitman & Caine, 2012, p. 175).

COMMON PUBLIC HEALTH APPROACHES

Among members of the general population, initiatives have focused on a range of areas. The importance of reducing the lethality of the environment (means safety) as applied to neurodisability was addressed in Chapter 9. Additional population-level efforts that contribute to suicide prevention have involved establishing voluntary media guidelines for the reporting of suicides (e.g., not glamorizing the deaths or portraying them as "heroic"; not providing details about the actual means of dying; providing information about suicide helplines with any reporting on suicides). Evidence suggests that media adherence to such guidelines has helped limit the risk of contagion, as outlined in Chapter 4. Other common approaches have included conducting mental health awareness campaigns and implementing gatekeeper or staff training (Mann et al., 2005; Hawton & Williams, 2002; Dumesnil & Verger, 2009; Matthieu, Cross, Batres, Flora, & Knox, 2008; Jenkins & Singh, 2000).

RELEVANCE OF PUBLIC HEALTH APPROACHES TO NEURODISABILITY

Worldwide, those with neurodisability are rarely highlighted as a priority "at-risk" group. Rather, neurodisability is usually aggregated with other health conditions such as cancer and HIV/AIDS into a "medical" risk factor group (e.g., US Department of Health and Human Services [USDHHS], 2012). In keeping with the population focus, public health measures have rarely targeted neurodisability. One exception is the contested US Food and Drug Administration alert on the association between antiepileptic drugs and suicidal thoughts and behavior (Hesdorffer, Berg, & Kanner, 2010; Wen et al., 2010; Fountoulakis et al., 2012). However, people with neurodisability benefit indirectly, as part of the general population, from public health initiatives that contribute to suicide prevention more broadly.

Despite the promise of such public health initiatives, Jenkins and Singh (2000) have reaffirmed the point that, in terms of suicide prevention, "general population approaches need to be complemented by specific interventions with groups that appear to be at high risk" (p. 8). In the context of neurodisability, however, little work has been undertaken in devising effective suicide prevention strategies in response to the findings about elevated suicidality. With few exceptions, the extent of consideration has comprised piecemeal clinical suggestions (i.e., falling within the healthcare approach) with no discussion of how these suggestions could be combined to produce a coherent and coordinated approach. The next section introduces two broader models of suicide prevention that have been influential in national suicide prevention policy frameworks and then explores how one of these models could be adapted to provide a systematic model for neurodisability.

Models of Suicide Prevention

A model of suicide prevention provides a framework that incorporates both clinical management approaches and the application of public health initiatives into the field. Such models highlight the multistranded approach needed in thinking about effective suicide prevention (Wasserman & Durkee, 2009), and they can provide a basis for the needed coordination of strategies for suicide prevention (Caine, 2013). To provide clarity regarding intervention-related terms (National Research Council, 2009), definitions for the key elements of the two models outlined here are provided in Table 12.1 (for a discussion of definitional issues, see National Research Council and Institute of Medicine, 2009).

PRIMARY/SECONDARY/TERTIARY MODEL

In the Primary/Secondary/Tertiary model, the *primary prevention* component focuses on prophylaxis through reducing risk factors and strengthening protective

TABLE 12.1

Key terms with definitions and examples

Key term	Definition
Prevention	Interventions that occur prior to the onset of a disorder that are intended to prevent or reduce risk for the disorder (National Research Council and Institute of Medicine, 2009)
Mental Health Promotion Interventions	Interventions that aim to enhance the ability to achieve developmentally appropriate tasks (developmental competencies) and a positive sense of self-esteem, mastery, well-being, and social inclusion and to strengthen the ability to cope with adversity (National Research Council and Institute of Medicine, 2009)
Primary	Primary component focuses on prophylaxis, reducing risk factors, and strengthening protective factors
Secondary	Reduce the prevalence of already existing disorders by treatment, early detection of unknown cases, and their appropriate treatment
Tertiary	Reduce the incidence of relapses through rehabilitation among people who have experienced the disorder to prevent supplementary deterioration
Universal	Interventions that target the general public or a whole population group that have not been identified on the basis of individual risk (National Research Council and Institute of Medicine, 2009)
Selective	Interventions that target individuals or subgroups whose risk of developing mental disorders is significantly higher than average (National Research Council and Institute of Medicine, 2009)
Indicated	Interventions that target individuals who are identified as having signs, symptoms, or genetic markers related to mental disorders, but who do not yet meet diagnostic criteria (National Research Council and Institute of Medicine, 2009)

factors (Hadlaczky, Wasserman, Hoven, Mandell, & Wasserman, 2011). De Leo and Meneghal (2001) describe this as being proactive in working among people not currently suicidal to reduce the likelihood of later suicide risk.

Secondary prevention focuses on reducing risk among people with the existing targeted condition, in particular through identifying the target condition in its earliest stages. As applied to suicide prevention, this can include targeting mental disorders, providing mental health treatment, conducting screening to facilitate early detection, undertaking gatekeeper training, and conducting interventions to treat suicidal behaviors (Wasserman & Durkee, 2009). *Tertiary prevention* refers to reducing the incidence of relapse through rehabilitation after having suffered from diseases or disorder. As applied to suicide prevention, this might mean treating people who have made repeated suicide attempts or who have had a previous history of suicide ideation (Andersson & Jenkins, 2006).

UNIVERSAL/SELECTED/INDICATED MODEL

The original adaptation of the Universal/Selected/Indicated (USI) model to suicide prevention was contained in a report produced by the Institute of Medicine (Mrazek & Haggerty, 1994). At the universal level, the whole population of concern is targeted (e.g., all adults). Selected strategies focus on groups at risk of developing the target condition (e.g., among adults, those with mental health problems), and the indicated level is aimed at people who already have condition (i.e., adults displaying suicidal thoughts or other behaviors) (see also Table 12.1). The USI model has been used as part of the conceptualization of suicide prevention in US national policy documents (Goldsmith, Pellmar, Kleinman, & Bunney, 2002; USDHHS, 2012).

In discussing the USI model, Yip (2005) suggests that examples of universal-level interventions include public programs that highlight the dangers of substance abuse. Examples of selective-level interventions include programs for children of parents with manic depressive illness or for victims of physical or sexual abuse. Examples of indicated-level interventions include programs for people who already have had suicidal ideation or attempts (Yip, 2005).

The USI devotes more attention to proactively treating presuicidal individuals than does the Primary/Secondary/Tertiary model, with both universal and selected interventions targeting people who may have never contemplated or displayed suicidal behavior. In contrast, the Primary/Secondary/Tertiary model's tertiary level has a tail (treating relapse), an area in which no real provision is made within the USI model. While the treatment of people who continue to actively self-harm can reduce suicidal behaviors and suicide (e.g., Hawton et al., 1998), this is counterbalanced by the fact that the majority of people who do die by suicide do so on their first attempt.

The application of the USI model to suicide prevention after neurodisability is further discussed later.

ORGANIZATION-BASED SUICIDE PREVENTION APPROACHES

The potential efficacy for coordinated multilayered suicide prevention approaches (as suggested by the Primary/Secondary/Tertiary and USI models) in reducing suicide in bounded, managed, large-scale organizations has been illustrated in both the United Kingdom and the United States.

In the United Kingdom, the improved take-up of nine mental health service recommendations by psychiatric hospitals at a national level across England and Wales resulted in significantly reduced suicide rates among patients (While et al., 2012). The nine recommendations are outlined in Box 12.1. The provision of 24-hour crisis care was the one recommendation most strongly associated with a decline in suicide rates (While et al., 2012).

The second example of a sector-based approach is the successful US Air Force Suicide Prevention Program (Knox, Litts, Talcott, Feig, & Caine, 2003). This servicewide program comprised 11 initiatives and had a broader focus that also included other forms of violence, including homicide, accidental death, and severe

---

BOX 12.1
SUICIDE PREVENTION STRATEGIES TO BE ADOPTED BY ALL PSYCHIATRIC
HOSPITALS IN THE UNITED KINGDOM

1. Providing 24-hour crisis teams
2. Removing ligature points (physical points in a ward that could be used for hanging)
3. Conducting follow-up with patients within 7 days of discharge
4. Conducting assertive community outreach, including providing intensive support for people with severe mental illness
5. Providing regular training to frontline clinical staff on the management of suicide risk
6. Managing patients with co-occurring disorders (mental and substance use disorder)
7. Responding to patients who are not complying with treatment
8. Sharing information with criminal justice agencies
9. Conducting multidisciplinary reviews and sharing information with families after a suicide

---

From While et al. (2012); Department of Health (2012).

family violence (Knox et al., 2003). The initiatives focused on reducing modifiable risk factors and strengthening protective factors, including strengthening social supports, building effective coping skills, and reducing stigma that acted as barriers to help-seeking behavior (Knox et al., 2003).

Both these examples highlight the important contribution that organizational policies and programs can make to suicide prevention in addition to the efforts of individual staff members. This integrative focus is reflected in the model of suicide prevention for neurodisability outlined in the following section.

A Model of Suicide Prevention for Neurodisability

There are three reasons for considering the adoption of a model of suicide prevention after neurodisability rather than simply shunting this off as an issue for mental health services. First, people with neurodisability have indicated that neurorehabilitation services would be a preferred source for accessing support during suicidal crises (Brenner, Homaifar, Adler, Wolfman, & Kemp, 2009; Kuipers & Lancaster, 2000). Furthermore, data about the idiosyncratic factors that increase risk within specific neurodisability groups, as outlined in Chapter 6, are not well known across generic mental health and suicide prevention agencies. Finally, frontline management approaches applied with other clinical groups may need adapting to ensure effective delivery to people with neurodisability (e.g., the SAD-PERSONS example from Chapter 7).

Despite this, as mentioned earlier in the chapter, discussion of suicide prevention approaches among other neurodisability groups has been relatively fragmented. The most detailed discussions have been produced in the field of epilepsy (Blumer et al., 2002; Blumer, 2008; Robertson, 1997). Robertson (1997) outlined several strands of suicide prevention under the heading of "prophylaxis and management of suicide attempters," invoking the language of the Primary/Secondary/Tertiary model although not explicitly referring to that model. In contrast, Blumer (2008) has outlined a specific clinically oriented approach to suicide prevention after epilepsy involving the early assessment and treatment of comorbid psychiatric conditions in tandem with the management of epilepsy. The clinical model has been developed at the Epi-Center for Epilepsy in the United States and is predicated on a single mechanism that Blumer asserts accounts for all suicides after epilepsy (Blumer et al., 2002; Blumer, 2008).

To the best of our knowledge, no systematic discussion of suicide prevention has been undertaken in the fields of stroke (with the exception of any early paper by Garden, Garrison, & Jain, 1990), spinal cord injury (SCI), amyotrophic lateral sclerosis (ALS), or Huntington's disease (HD) (the major focus for the limited discussion that has taken place has been on responses to the crisis period associated with people undergoing predictive testing rather than approaches to managing suicide prevention across the whole course of HD), multiple sclerosis (MS), or Parkinson's disease (PD).

However, work on the application of suicide prevention models or neurodisability has received initial attention in the field of traumatic brain injury (TBI). Simpson and Tate (2007a) employed the USI model as a framework to organize knowledge about suicide risk and prevention after TBI. The model was originally proposed to address the civilian context but was subsequently adapted to provide suicide prevention guidelines for general practitioners in the primary healthcare network who have patients with TBI (Simpson & Tate, 2007b) and in the context of veterans with TBI (Simpson & Tate, 2009). The model was elaborated further by Wasserman et al. (2008) with the inclusion of additional psychiatric management approaches.

The USI model that has been applied to TBI can also be broadened to the field of neurodisability (Table 12.2). Within the model, the universal level refers to the population of people with neurodisability, the selected level to at-risk groups within neurodisability (e.g., people with comorbid psychiatric conditions, comorbid substance abuse), and the indicated level to individuals with neurodisability for whom suicide is an identified issue (e.g., suicidal thoughts or behaviors have been reported or observed). Although it can be argued that. people with neurodisability, as an "at-risk" group, should fit at the selective level of the USI model, there are interventions that can be considered at the universal, selective, and indicated levels in promoting suicide prevention, and, therefore, employing a more expansive application of the model is warranted.

Elements of the model are applicable to a wide range of organizational settings. These can range from sole practitioners (e.g., individual therapists in private practice), to small independent agencies (e.g., a community epilepsy support service) or units that are part of larger service systems (e.g., a brain injury outpatient clinic in a health service), to larger organizations (e.g., free-standing rehabilitation hospitals). One caveat is that most strategies included in the model are clinically generated or extrapolated from research in other clinical or population settings rather than arising from a validated evidence base of research in the field of neurodisability.

UNIVERSAL LEVEL

The clinical management strategy most commonly referred to by authors across all types of neurodisability at the universal level is proactive screening or monitoring for warning signs of suicide risk. The targets of any such screening could include depression, hopelessness, suicide ideation, or broader risk factors. However, any such initiative needs to be tempered by the logistic challenges highlighted in Chapter 7. Awareness of heightened times of suicide risk during the course of the various types of neurodisability may also assist in identifying subgroups who could be the focus

TABLE 12.2

A working model of suicide prevention for neurodisability

Level	Clinical management	Organizational strategies
Universal	Conduct screening for depression, hopelessness or suicide ideation	Broader public education campaigns to dispel stigma and ignorance about neurodisability (e.g., epilepsy)
	Monitor for warning signs that increase risk level	Ensure appropriate intervention to treat neurodisability is provided
	Recognize that time periods of elevated suicide risk may vary among neurodisability groups	Treatment to include focus on (i) building social supports and decreasing social isolation, (ii) build participation and meaning
	Make provision for the availability of long-term support for neurodisability groups for whom there is evidence that suicide is a chronic or late complication	Consider programs health and wellness programs
		Ensure staff trained in suicide prevention
		Introduce agency-based suicide prevention policy and procedures
		Educate primary care network about potential suicide risk
		Educate family and friends about possible suicide risk (as appropriate)
Selected	If unable to screen at universal level, target at-risk groups	Identify programs/professionals that clients can access for treatment of psychiatric conditions (either within the service or externally)
	Monitor people injured as the result of a suicide attempt (SCI, TBI)	Primary care network have access information about evidence-base treatment guidelines for the assessment and treatment of depression after neurodisability
	Positive finding from screening or warning signs trigger suicide risk assessment	
	Pay careful attention to treatments for which there is evidence that they exacerbate suicidal thoughts or behaviors	Identify an agreed-on procedure for a suicide risk assessment
	Provide evidence-based treatments for psychiatric disorders (e.g., CBT, IPT for depression; SSRIs for depression, aggression; treatment for substance abuse problems)	

(continued)

TABLE 12.2 CONTINUED

Level	Clinical management	Organizational strategies
Indicated	Reduce the lethality of the environment	Agency conducts an audit of the potential lethality of physical environment
	Provide frontline treatments (pharmacotherapy, psychotherapy)	Agency framework for how staff record suicide assessment in files
	Keep individual safe (e.g., provide "emergency contact card" with crisis contacts, develop safety plan)	Agency protocols for dealing with a suicidal crisis
	Increase formal and informal supports (e.g., more clinician hours, family involvement)	
	Conduct careful history taking and collect data from other sources as compatible with privacy legislation	
	If assess that suicide attempt is imminent, contact suicide crisis service—take to psychiatric emergency service	
	In managing someone with a history of attempts, plan for the possibility that people may use more than one method	
	Provide support/monitor for at least 12 months after a suicide attempt	
	Closely monitor in the months after discharge from a psychiatric hospital	

of strategies at the selected level. Furthermore, support should be tailored to ensure that it is available over the long term for groups at chronic risk of suicidality (e.g., those with TBI).

However, early detection of risk is not the only strategy to be considered at the universal level. Caine (2013) asserts that prevention-related priorities must be shifted to include "distal preventive interventions" focused on interpersonal factors and social contexts aimed at altering the "trajectories of people before they become suicidal." Applying this principle to the field of neurodisability, public health strategies would highlight the importance of people with neurodisability accessing appropriate treatment for their condition. In providing treatment, special attention could be provided for building social supports and reducing social isolation (e.g., career training programs in cerebrovascular accident (CVA) patients; Ostwald et al.,

2014), building participation (e.g., providing effective interventions to increase employment options for people with SCI; Ottomanelli et al., 2012), and promoting health and wellness among people with neurodisability (e.g., the intervention titled *Promoting Wellness for Women with MS*; Stuifbergen, Becker, Blozis, Timmerman, & Kullberg, 2003). Broader public education campaigns to dispel stigma and ignorance about neurodisability have also been recommended (Robertson, 1997), as well as ensuring that staff have access to suicide prevention training, that appropriate policies and procedures for suicide prevention are introduced, and that outreach to the primary care network is provided (Caine & Schwid, 2002; Robertson, 1997; Simpson & Tate, 2007b).

SELECTED LEVEL

If universal screening is not viable, an alternative is to screen for suicidal thoughts and behaviors among at-risk groups (see Chapter 7) or individuals who have multiple suicide risk factors. For example, research has shown that people who sustained their TBI or SCI as the results of a suicide attempt are at higher risk of post-injury suicide (see Chapter 6) and therefore require additional monitoring. Any positive findings from screening or warning signs should trigger a suicide risk assessment. Timely treatment of comorbid psychiatric disorders is also important (e.g., Blumer et al., 2002; Wasserman et al., 2008; National Stroke Foundation, 2010) although the evidence base for effective pharmacotherapy or psychotherapy in treating such disorders is still extremely limited across several of the neurodisability groups. Careful attention needs to be paid to medical treatments (e.g., surgery, pharmacotherapy) that might exacerbate suicidal thoughts and behaviors (Robertson, 1997; Blumer, 2008; Voon et al., 2008) to ensure that appropriate assessment, monitoring, and intervention is provided. Finally, it is essential to ensure that a clinical pathway to needed treatment has been devised, that general practitioners have access to the latest research and/or evidence-based clinical guidelines for the assessment and treatment of depression after neurodisability, and that there is an agreed on protocol for the assessment of suicide risk.

INDICATED LEVEL

In cases where suicidal thoughts and behaviors have been identified, the lethality of the immediate environment should be assessed, and there are a number of strategies to facilitate safe storage/disposal of firearms or medication (e.g., Adekoya & Majumder, 2004). As with selected interventions, the provision of frontline treatments for any psychiatric disorders or broader psychological distress is crucial.

Furthermore, increasing support, safety planning, and ensuring access to needed services in times of crisis (Jones et al., 2003; Stanley & Brown, 2008; Wasserman et al., 2008) can complement frontline treatments. Thorough history-taking (e.g., review of medical records) can identify previous suicidal behavior that may not be disclosed by the client (Simpson & Tate, 2007a). Monitoring of patients in the immediate postdischarge period of psychiatric inpatient crisis care is important (Simpson & Tate, 2007a). Finally, agencies should conduct an audit of the potential lethality of the environment. It is also important to ensure necessary and accurate documentation in service records of staff action in the assessment and management of a suicidal client (this point is further discussed in Chapter 13).

Training in Suicide Prevention

GENERAL APPROACHES TO SUICIDE PREVENTION TRAINING

The provision of staff training is a key plank in building capacity for suicide prevention (Metha et al., 1998; Krysinska et al., 2016). Training is one of the 13 goals making up the US National Suicide Prevention Strategy (USDHHS, 2012) and is a typical element in suicide prevention programs internationally (e.g., European Commission and World Health Organization, 2008). The activity of staff training is normally located within the primary (PST) or universal (USI) components of broader suicide prevention strategies.

The benefits of training can include the possibility of preventing suicidal behaviors through appropriate intervention, improving staff attitudes toward suicide, increasing clinical knowledge, reducing staff anxiety and increasing confidence, and training in early identification of suicide risk (Chagnon, Houle, Marcoux, & Renaud, 2007, Gask, Lever-Green, & Hays, 2008, Matthieu et al., 2008, Simpson et al., 2003, Tierney, 1994). Van der Feltz-Cornelis et al. (2011) propose that training addresses (1) theoretical aspects of depression and suicide, (2) practical elements (how to talk about suicidality, detect suicidality, handle an acute suicidal crisis), (3) what to do when treatment needs are encountered, (4) populations at risk of suicide, and (5) provide information materials to vulnerable populations for distribution.

A number of training programs exist to address the distinct needs of various groups (Suicide Prevention Resource Center and Suicide Prevention Action Network USA, 2010) including community groups (e.g., first responders, crisis line volunteers, individuals working in the justice system and/or in law enforcement) and health professionals (at undergraduate or graduate level). The National Suicide Plan also proposes that suicide prevention training should be included in recertification or licensing programs for professionals by certifying and/or accrediting agencies (USDHHS, 2012).

The World Health Organization (2006) asserts that suicide prevention is everybody's business. Reflecting this, the target audience for training is broad, given that people with neurodisability come into contact with a wide range of different staff (e.g., frontline nonclinical staff, volunteers, paraprofessionals, health professionals) from civilian and veteran medical, rehabilitation, mental health, and community-based disability service systems. The training needs across these groups are varied, reflecting differences in qualifications, experience, and the roles that staff play in suicide prevention. The suicide prevention training currently accessed is generic, with limited options available for curriculum tailored specifically to the neurodisability sector.

In evaluating the impact of training, intermediate outcomes are most typically measured (e.g., improvements in attitudes, knowledge, skills, and confidence pertaining to suicide prevention; Metha et al., 1998, Simpson, Franke, & Gillet, 2007) rather than reductions in suicidal behavior per se. Measurement of these intermediate outcomes has typically involved completing objective knowledge tests, pencil-and-paper self-reports (e.g., attitudes, confidence, knowledge), and, less frequently, observational ratings of trainee performance in a specific skill (Cross, Matthieu, Cerel, & Knox, 2007; Morriss, Gask, Battersby, Francheschini, & Robson, 1999; Neimeyer & Pfeiffer, 1994; Tierney, 1994).

SUICIDE PREVENTION TRAINING IN THE NEURODISABILITY FIELD

There have been calls to improve staff awareness and provide access to suicide prevention training within the field of neurodisability (Brenner et al., 2009; Kuipers & Lancaster, 2000), SCI (Ahoniemi et al., 2011; Hartkopp et al., 1997), and epilepsy (Robertson, 1997) as well as providing training to other sectors, such as the primary healthcare network (Simpson & Tate, 2007b). General practitioners often play an active role in managing people with neurological conditions living in the community, and the importance of providing training to general practitioners about the particular needs and suicide risks associated with specific neurodisability groups has been highlighted (Robertson, 1997; Simpson & Tate, 2007b). This is line with broader suicide prevention strategies within which general practitioners are identified as playing a pivotal role (Van der Feltz-Cornelis et al., 2011).

Some initial accounts of training devised specifically for staff within the neurodisability field have been published. Simpson and colleagues (2004, 2007) conducted a controlled trial of a 6-hour suicide prevention program delivered to 86 staff from rehabilitation and community disability organizations working in the field of TBI across the state of Victoria, Australia. Compared to a matched group of staff who did not attend the training, staff attending the program reported significant increases in knowledge and skills immediately post-workshop, and a number of these gains were maintained at the 6-month follow-up. Kuipers and Lancaster (2000) have also referred to conducting brain injury–specific suicide prevention training, but supplied no information about the curriculum, training delivery, or outcomes.

In addition to core topics proposed in the National Suicide Prevention Strategy (USDHHS, 2012) as part of a generic training program, curriculum for suicide prevention training targeting neurodisability could be enhanced by the inclusion of disability-specific content. This is in line with the contention of Clarke and Fawcett (1992) that clinical/diagnostic groups have unique patterns of suicide risk factors in comparison to the general community. Such a curriculum would cover information about the specific prevalence, risk factors, and protective factors for suicidality as well as the adjustment of screening, assessment, and management approaches to compensate for motor-sensory, cognitive, or emotional/behavioral impairments.

Despite the face validity of such an adapted curriculum, there is no evidence to date that such a curriculum leaves staff better prepared to manage suicide prevention than generic training. Simpson et al. (2007) found that staff rated their knowledge and skills about generic suicide prevention significantly more highly than they rated their knowledge and skills pertaining to a specific group (i.e., TBI) that was the focus of the training. However, the two scores were highly intercorrelated ($r = .87$), suggesting that the commonalities in the screening, assessment, and management of suicide across different clinical/diagnostic groups outweighed any idiosyncratic differences. In the absence of widespread access to training tailored to specific neurodisability groups, staff appear to extrapolate and adapt established generic suicide prevention training in undertaking the identification, assessment, and management of suicide risk after neurodisability.

Conclusion

A comprehensive approach to suicide prevention will incorporate both clinical management and adapted public health initiatives synthesized into a hybrid model of suicide prevention. Such initiatives can be implemented on an organizational basis (i.e., within service systems or in single agencies). The model outlined in this chapter is based on current best evidence in suicide prevention for neurodisability and can serve as a starting point. Further testing and evaluation of suicide prevention approaches across all types of neurodisability is still needed to better inform approaches to suicide prevention.

Implications for Clinicians

1. Suicide prevention involves the mobilization of organizations, not just individual clinicians.
2. Comprehensive models of suicide prevention typically incorporate a combination of public health–based and individually oriented strategies.
3. Seeking to build well-being at individual and societal levels for people with neurodisability is an important, albeit distal, component of a multilayered suicide prevention approach.
4. Initiatives for lethal means safety at a population level will also help to reduce the suicide risk for individuals with neurodisability.
5. Staff training helps to operationalize the principle that suicide prevention is everyone's business, but it also needs to clearly articulate the roles of staff relevant to their level of training, experience, and their normal work duties.

References

Adekoya, N., & Majumder, R. (2004). Fatal traumatic brain injury, West Virginia, 1989–1998. *Public Health Report, 119*(5), 486–492.

Ahoniemi, E., Pohjolainen, T., & Kautiainen, H. (2011). Survival after spinal cord injury in Finland. *Journal of Rehabilitation Medicine, 43*, 481–485.

Andersson, M., & Jenkins, R. (2006). The national suicide prevention strategy for England: The reality of a national strategy for the nursing profession. *Journal of Psychiatric and Mental Health Nursing, 13*, 641–650.

Blumer, D. (2008). Suicide: Incidence, psychopathology, pathogenesis, and prevention. In J. Engel & T. A. Pedley (Eds.), *Epilepsy: A comprehensive text book* (pp. 2196–2202). Philadelphia, PA: Lippincott Williams and Wilkins.

Blumer, D., Montouris, G., Davies, K., Wyler, A., Phillips, B., & Hermann, B. (2002). Suicide in epilepsy: Psychopathology, pathogenesis, and prevention. *Epilepsy and Behavior, 3*, 232–241.

Brenner, L. A., Homaifar, B. Y., Adler, L. E., Wolfman, J. H., & Kemp, J. (2009). Suicidality and veterans with a history of traumatic brain injury: Precipitating events, protective factors and prevention strategies. *Rehabilitation Psychology, 54*, 390–397.

Caine, E. D. (2013). Forging an agenda for suicide prevention in the United States. *American Journal of Public Health, 103*(5), 822–829.

Caine, E. D., & Schwid, S. R. (2002). Multiple sclerosis, depression, and the risk of suicide. *Neurology, 59*, 662–663.

Chagnon, F., Houle, J., Marcoux, I., & Renaud, J. (2007). Control-group study of an intervention training program for youth suicide prevention. *Suicide and Life-Threatening Behavior, 37*, 135–144.

Clarke, D. C., & Fawcett, J. (1992). Review of empirical risk factors for evaluation of the suicidal patient. In B. Bongar (Ed.), *Suicide: Guidelines for assessment, management, and treatment* (pp. 16–48). New York: Oxford University Press.

Cross, W., Matthieu, M. M., Cerel, J., & Knox, K. L. (2007). Proximate outcomes of gatekeeper training for suicide prevention in the workplace. *Suicide and Life-Threatening Behavior, 37*, 659–670.

De Leo, D., & Meneghal, G. (2001). The elderly and suicide. In D. Wasserman (Ed.), *Suicide: An unnecessary death* (pp. 195–207). London: Martin Dunitz.

Department of Health. (2012). *Preventing suicide in England: A cross-government outcomes strategy.* Retrieved from www.dh.gov.uk/publications

Dumesnil, H., & Verger, P. (2009). Public awareness campaigns about depression and suicide: A review. *Psychiatric Services, 60*, 1203–1213.

European Commission and World Health Organization. (2008, June 12–13). *European pact for mental health and well-being.* Presented at the EU High Level conference: Together for mental health and well-being, Brussels.

Fountoulakis, K. N., Gonda, X., Samara, M., Siapera, M., Karavelas, V., Ristic, D. I., & Iacovides, A. (2012). Antiepileptic drugs and suicidality. *Journal of Psychopharmacology, 26*, 1401–1407.

Garden, F. H., Garrison, S. J., & Jain, A. (1990). Assessing suicide risk in stroke patients: Review of two cases. *Archive of Physical Medicine & Rehabilitation, 71*, 1003–1005.

Gask, L., Lever-Green, G., & Hays, R. (2008). Dissemination and implementation of suicide prevention training in one Scottish region. *BMC Health Services Research, 8*, 246. doi:10.1186/1472-6963-8-246

Goldsmith, S., Pellmar, T., Kleinman, A., & Bunney, W. (Eds.). (2002). *Reducing suicide: A national imperative.* Washington, DC: Institute of Medicine, The National Academies Press.

Gordon, R. (1983). An operational classification of disease prevention. *Public Health Reports, 98*, 107–109.

Hadlaczky, G., Wasserman, D., Hoven, C. W., Mandell, D. J., & Wasserman, C. (2011). Suicide prevention strategies: Case studies from across the globe. In R. C. O'Connor, S. Platt, & J. Gordon (Eds.), *International handbook of suicide prevention: Research, policy and practice* (pp. 475–485). Chichester, UK: Wiley-Blackwell.

Hartkopp, A., Brønnum-Hansen, H., Seidenschnur, A.-M., & Biering-Sørensen, F. (1997). Survival and cause of death after traumatic spinal cord injury: A long-term epidemiological survey from Denmark. *Spinal Cord, 35*(2), 76–85.

Hawton, K., Arensmen, E., Townsend, E., Bremner, S., Feldman, E., Goldney, R., . . . Traskman-Bendz, L. (1998). Deliberate self harm: Systematic review of efficacy of psychosocial and pharmacological treatments in preventing repetition. *British Medical Journal, 317*, 441–447.

Hawton, K., & Williams, K. (2002). Influences of the media on suicide: Researchers, policy makers, and media personnel need to collaborate on guidelines. *British Medical Journal, 325*, 1374–1375.

Hesdorffer, D. C., Berg, A. T., & Kanner, A. M. (2010). An update on antiepileptic drugs and suicide: Are there definitive answers yet? *Epilepsy Currents, 10*(6), 137–145.

Jenkins, R., & Singh, B. (2000). Policy and practice in suicide prevention. *The British Journal of Forensic Practice, 2*, 3–11

Jones, J. E., Hermann, B. P., Barry, J. J., Gilliam, F. G., Kanner, A. M., & Meador, K. J. (2003). Rates and risk factors for suicide, suicidal ideation and suicide attempts in chronic epilepsy. *Epilepsy and Behavior, 4*, S31–S38.

Knox, K. L., Litts, D. A., Talcott, G. W., Feig, J. C., & Caine, E. D. (2003). Risk of suicide and related adverse outcomes after exposure to a suicide prevention programme in the US Air Force: Cohort study. *British Medical Journal, 327*, 1376.

Krysinska, K., Batterham, P. J., Tye, M., Shand, F., Calear, A. L., Cockayne, N., & Christensen, H. (2016). Best strategies for reducing the suicide rate in Australia. *Australian & New Zealand Journal of Psychiatry, 50*, 115–118.

Kuipers, P., & Lancaster, A. (2000). Developing a suicide prevention strategy based on the perspective of people with brain injuries. *Journal of Head Trauma Rehabilitation, 15*, 1275–1284.

Lewis, G., Hawton, K., & Jones, P. (1997). Strategies for preventing suicide. *British Journal of Psychiatry, 171*, 351–354.

Mann, J. J., Apter, A., Bertolote, J., Beautrais, A., Currier, D., Haas, A., . . . Hendin, H. (2005). Suicide prevention strategies: A systematic review. *Journal of the American Medical Association, 294*, 2064–2074.

Matthieu, M. M., Cross, W., Batres, A. R., Flora, C. M., & Knox, K. L. (2008). Evaluation of gatekeeper training for suicide prevention in Veterans. *Archives of Suicide Research, 12*, 148–154.

Metha, A., Weber, B., & Webb, L. D. (1998). Youth suicide prevention: A survey and analysis of policies and efforts in the 50 states. *Suicide and Life-Threatening Behavior, 28*, 150–164.

Morriss, R., Gask, L., Battersby, L., Francheschini, A., & Robson, M. (1999). Teaching frontline health and voluntary workers to assess and manage suicidal patients. *Journal of Affective Disorders, 39*, 77–83.

Mrazek, P. J., & Haggerty, R. J. (1994). *Reducing risks from mental disorders: Frontiers for preventive intervention research*. Washington DC: National Academies Press.

National Research Council and Institute of Medicine. (2009). *Preventing mental, emotional, & behavioral disorders among young people: Progress and possibilities*. Washington, DC: National Academies Press (US).

National Stroke Foundation. (2010). *Clinical guidelines for stroke management*. Melbourne, Australia: Author.

Neimeyer, R. A., & Pfeiffer, A. M. (1994). Evaluation of suicide intervention effectiveness. *Death Studies, 18*, 131–166.

Ostwald, S. K., Godwin, K. M., Cron, S. G., Kelley, C. P., Hersch, G., & Davis, S. (2014). Home-based psychoeducational and mailed information programs for stroke-caregiving dyads post-discharge: A randomized trial. *Disability and Rehabilitation, 36*, 55–62.

Ottomanelli, L., Goetz, L. L., Suris, A., McGeough, C., Sinnott, P. L., Toscano, R., . . . Thomas, F. P. (2012). Effectiveness of supported employment for veterans with spinal cord injuries: Results from a randomized multisite study. *Archives of Physical Medicine and Rehabilitation, 93*, 740–747.

Pitman, A., & Caine, E. (2012). The role of the high-risk approach in suicide prevention. *British Journal of Psychiatry, 201*, 175–177.

Robertson, M. M. (1997). Suicide, parasuicide and epilepsy. In J. Engel & T. A. Pedley (Eds.), *Epilepsy: A comprehensive textbook* (pp. 2141–2151). Philadelphia, PA: Lippincott-Raven Publishers.

Simpson, G. K., Franke, B., & Gillett, L. (2007). Suicide prevention training outside the mental health service system: Evaluation of a state-wide program in Australia for rehabilitation and disability staff in the field of traumatic brain injury. *Crisis: The Journal of Crisis Intervention and Suicide Prevention, 28*, 35–43.

Simpson, G. K., & Tate, R. L. (2007a). Suicidality in people surviving a traumatic brain injury: Prevalence, risk factors and implications for clinical management. *Brain Injury, 21*, 1335–1351.

Simpson, G. K., & Tate, R. L. (2007b). Preventing suicide after traumatic brain injury: Implications for general practice. *Medical Journal of Australia, 187*, 229–232.

Simpson, G. K., & Tate, R. L. (2009). Suicidality and suicide prevention among war veterans with traumatic brain injury. In L. Sher & A. Vilens (Eds.), *Suicide in the military* (pp. 161–182). New York: Nova Science.

Simpson, G. K., Winstanley, J., & Bertapelle, T. (2003). Evaluation of a suicide prevention training workshop for staff working in the field of traumatic brain injury. *Journal of Head Trauma Rehabilitation, 18*, 445–456.

Stanley, B., & Brown, G. (2008). *Safety plan treatment manual to reduce suicide risk: Veteran version.* Department of Veterans Affairs. Retrieved from http://www.mentalhealth.va.gov/docs/va_safety_planning_manual.pdf

Stuifbergen, A. K., Becker, H., Blozis, S., Timmerman, G., & Kullberg, V. (2003). A randomized clinical trial of wellness intervention for women with multiple sclerosis. *Archives of Physical Medicine and Rehabilitation, 84*, 467–476.

Suicide Prevention Resource Center (SPRC); Suicide Prevention Action Network USA (SPAN USA). (2010, August). *Charting the future of suicide prevention: A 2010 progress review of the National Strategy and recommendations for the decade ahead* (D. Litts, Ed.). Newton, MA: Education Development Center, Inc.

Tierney, R. J. (1994). Suicide intervention training evaluation: A preliminary report. *Crisis, 15*, 69–76.

United Nations. (1996). *Prevention of suicide: Guidelines for the formulation and implementation of national strategies.* New York: United Nations, Department for Policy Coordination and Sustainable Development.

US Department of Health and Human Services (USDHHS), Office of the Surgeon General, & National Action Alliance for Suicide Prevention. (2012). *2012 National strategy for suicide prevention: Goals and objectives for action.* Washington, DC: HHS.

Van der Feltz-Cornelis, C. M., Sarchiapone, M., Postuvan, V., Volker, D., Roskar, S., Grum, A. T., ... Hegerl, U. (2011). Best practice elements of multilevel suicide prevention strategies: A review of systematic reviews. *Crisis, 32*, 319–333.

Voon, V., Krack, P., Lang, A. E., Lozano, A. M., Dujardin, K., Schüpbach, M., ... Moro, E. (2008). A multicentre study on suicide outcomes following subthalamic stimulation for Parkinson's disease. *Brain, 131*, 2720–2728.

Wasserman, D., & Durkee, T. (2009). Strategies in suicide prevention. In D. Wasserman, & C. Wasserman (Eds.), *Oxford textbook of suicidology and suicide prevention: A global perspective* (pp. 381–384). New York: Oxford University Press.

Wasserman, L., Shaw, T., Vu, M., Ko, C., Bollegala, D., & Bhalerao, S. (2008). An overview of traumatic brain injury and suicide. *Brain Injury, 22*, 811–819.

Wen, X., Meador, K. J., Loring, D. W., Eisenschenk, S., Segal, R., & Hartzema, A. G. (2010). Is antiepileptic drug use related top depression and suicidal ideation among patients with epilepsy? *Epilepsy and Behavior, 19*, 494–500.

While, D., Bickley, H., Roscoe, A., Windfur, K., Rahman, S., Shaw, J., . . . Kapur, N. (2012). Implementation of mental health service recommendations in England and Wales and suicide rates, 1997–2006: A cross-sectional and before-and-after observational study. *Lancet, 379*, 1005–1012.

World Health Organization. (2006). *Suicide Prevention (SUPRE)*. Retrieved from www.who.int/mental_health/prevention/suicide/suicideprevent/en/. Accessed December 31, 2013.

Yip, P. S. F. (2005). A public health approach to suicide prevention. *Hong Kong Journal of Psychiatry, 15*, 29–31.

13 Legal and Ethical Issues

Introduction

The clinical and legal dimensions of healthcare are closely intertwined (Appelbaum & Gutheil, 2000). As such, working with patients to manage suicide risk gives rise to a range of "clinical-legal" issues (Simon & Shuman, 2009). In fact, Simon and Shuman observe that "the law derives its requirements from professional practice, [therefore] good clinical practice and good laws are often complementary" (p. 155). The information in this chapter aims to assist clinicians in finding an appropriate balance.

In the United States, the predominant legal issue associated with suicide is malpractice. Therefore, salient clinical management strategies aimed at minimizing the risk of litigation will be discussed. This focus is consistent with Objective 7.2 of the National Strategy for Suicide Prevention (US Department of Health and Human Services [USDHHS], 2012): "Equip practitioners with attitudes, knowledge, and skills to cope with sentinel events (unanticipated events resulting in death or serious physical or psychological injury), along with effective clinical preventive procedures to minimize risk of litigation" (p. 46).

Following this, issues associated with the wish to hasten death or end one's life will be addressed. As applied to neurodisability, the issue of physician-assisted suicide has been most frequently considered in relation to those living with amyotrophic lateral sclerosis (ALS) due to its aggressive degenerative course and the debilitating impairments associated with the end stages of the condition. Brief mention of the issue has also been raised in relation to multiple sclerosis (MS). However, as legislation continues to pass, questions regarding the right to die in relation to a wide range of diagnoses have come to the fore. Although psychologists do not play the central medical management role in end-of-life decision-making, their services may be called upon for assessment or counseling as part of the clinical evaluation process. Therefore, rehabilitation psychologists need to be aware of a range of issues associated with this complex area of health practice.

Legal Issue of Malpractice

Legal action can be brought against individual clinicians, organizations (e.g., hospitals, health management organizations), or both. In this chapter, our focus is on the legal responsibilities and exposure of the clinician. Compared to those in other areas of medical specialty, malpractice suits are less frequently brought against mental health professionals (Bongar, 2002). Suicide is a low base rate event, and, in the eventuality of a suicide, there are few cases that involve litigation. Cases that go to court have generally been settled in favor of the defendant, and therefore, in cases in which litigation is initiated, most are settled out of court (Bongar, 2002). However, this should not minimize the personal impact on mental health staff who do get caught up in such proceedings (Simon & Shuman, 2009), and concerns just about the possibility of litigation seem to have dissuaded some clinicians from working with individuals who are at high risk for suicide (Bongar, 2002).

In the field of psychiatry, Simon and Shuman (2009) report that between 1998 and 2008 17% of claims against psychiatrists were related to suicide/attempted suicide. Furthermore, a proportion of the largest category of claims (incorrect treatment, 38% of claims) were also related to a suicide/attempted suicide. One difficulty in interpreting the significance of these data is that the base number of claims on which the percentages were calculated was not reported.

Malpractice: The Most Common Form of Litigation

The most common form of litigation in cases of suicide is malpractice suits. In legal terms, malpractice is a *tort* or *civil wrong* (i.e., as distinct from a criminal or contract-related wrong) arising from the negligence of the practitioner. *Negligence* refers to a failure to have done something (a sin of omission or a sin of commission) that represents a breach of the practitioner's duty of care (Berman, 2006). The four elements that need to be established to uphold a case of malpractice are encapsulated in the 4D mnemonic "a Dereliction of a Duty that Directly Damages" (Sadoff, 1975). *Duty* refers to the duty of care; *dereliction* to the breach in that duty of care. A *direct* (proximate) relationship needs to be proved between any such dereliction and the adverse outcome (in this case, suicide), and, finally, there need to be *damages* arising from the outcome that can be compensated. Simon (1992) highlighted three areas on which claims for damages have focused. These are (1) inadequate assessment of the potential and severity of suicide risk, (2) failure to use reasonable treatment interventions and precautions, and (3) inadequate follow-through in the reasonable implementation of treatment. These areas of liability apply to inpatient and outpatient settings (Bongar, 2002).

THE EXISTENCE OF A THERAPEUTIC RELATIONSHIP

A clinician's duty of care comes into being once a therapeutic relationship exists between clinician and client. Simon (1988) has outlined a number of actions by clinicians that might create a clinician–patient relationship; namely, giving advice, making psychological interpretations, supervising treatment by another clinician, having a lengthy phone call with a prospective client, treating an unseen client by mail (e-mail or surface mail), giving a client an appointment, telling walk-in clients they will be seen, acting as a substitute clinician, and/or providing treatment during an evaluation. The treatment relationship with a client may also create duties to nonclient third parties (e.g., *Tarasoff* duty).

STANDARD OF CARE

In determining whether there has been a dereliction related to duty of care, it has to be determined whether the clinician provided a satisfactory standard of care. No universal agreement exists about the meaning of "standard of care," and its definition varies, as outlined in statute, across different states within the United States. That being said, national associations such as the American Psychological Association have ethical principles and codes of practice (http://www.apa.org/ethics/code/index.aspx) to facilitate clinical decision-making. At its heart, however, the standard of care provided by the clinician needs to be judged by experts as that of a *reasonable* and *prudent* practitioner (Peters, 2000); namely, consistent with approaches customarily employed by clinicians in similar circumstances and with similar training, experience, and skill (Simon, 2004). Berman (2006) refers to two key factors pertaining to suicide deaths that are the focus in evaluating the standard of care provided: Was the death *forseeable*? And, was *reasonable care* provided?

Foreseeability of risk should be distinguished from prediction of suicide, as there is broad understanding that current best practices do not allow for an individual suicide to be accurately predicted. For example, there is no "professional standard" of clinical practice for the prediction of suicide (Simon, 2012). Furthermore, as has been outlined in Chapters 7 and 8, there are no psychological tests or suicide risk checklists that can accurately predict which individual might die by suicide (Simon, 2012). Foreseeability also needs to be distinguished from *preventability*. Rather, foreseeability refers to the "reasonable evaluation of the potential for a suicidal act on the basis of an assessment of risk" (Berman, 2006, p. 172). The possibility of suicide risk should be recognized with all clients who display suicidal thoughts/behaviors or other warning signs, display moderate to severe levels of hopelessness, are diagnosed with any disorders listed in the *Diagnostic and Statistical Manual of Mental Disorders* (DSM-5), or in other ways display known risk factors for suicide (see Chapters 6, 7, and 8). According to Simon (2012), systematically evaluating an individual's suicidal thoughts (e.g., intensity and duration) and behaviors (e.g., past attempts, preparatory behavior), as well as risk and protective factors should meet any reasonable definition of adequate (Simon, 2012). To this could also be added the systematic monitoring for warning signs of imminent suicidal behavior. The clinician then arrives at a judgment about the imminence of suicide risk and documents this judgment (see Chapter 8). If a client does engage in lethal suicidal behavior, it does not automatically follow that this was due to some negligence on the clinician's part. If the clinicians' judgment was reasonably made based on the collected data, and reasonable attempts had been made to collect the data, then it is defensible to argue that the suicide had not been forseeable.

Reasonable care implies that the clinician has outlined and followed a systematic treatment approach that does not widely deviate from what other clinicians with similar skills and training would offer to a client with a similar presentation. Treatment plans should be a reasonable response to the specific problems the client is experiencing and include appropriate measures to deal with the level of suicide risk. For example, if a client was adjudged to be at a high level of suicide risk, then it would be reasonable to expect that the clinician would have taken appropriate steps to minimize the possibility of client self-directed violence (SDV) (e.g., reduce the lethality of the local environment, ensure appropriate levels of monitoring/support and of ability to maintain safety). If a client is not able or willing to comply with a treatment plan (e.g., safety plan), this should be documented, and a more intensive interventions may be required (e.g., hospitalization). Finally, an important element of reasonable care is *dependability*; namely, the responsibility of the clinician to ensure timely follow-through in the implementation of the treatment plan elements, whether delivered directly by the clinician or indirectly through other staff.

Part of the history of litigation around malpractice has been the recognition that, within psychology and psychiatry, there are multiple therapeutic methods available. Therefore, the concept of standard care has not been limited to those therapeutic modalities that would be considered "mainstream." It also encompasses a wider range of therapeutic modalities, on the basis that the modality is practiced by a *respectable minority* of clinicians. Applying this doctrine, standard care would suggest that the clinician needs to have made reasonable attempts to identify elevated risk for suicide. In cases where an elevated risk is detected, the clinician then needs to demonstrate that reasonable clinical management efforts have been made. However, more recently, this doctrine has been challenged by the growth of the evidence-based movement, which provides a separate set of criteria by which the validity of treatments can be evaluated, and the movement of professions to identify "best treatments" or best practices for various conditions (Bongar, 2002). One example of this is the VA/DOD Clinical Practice Guidelines for suicide prevention (https://www.guideline.gov/summaries/summary/47023/vadod-clinical-practice-guideline-for-assessment-and-management-of-patients-at-risk-for-suicide).

FAILURE OF DUTY OF CARE AS PROXIMATE CAUSE OF SUICIDE

If a failure to meet the standard of care occurred, then it needs to be established that this "dereliction of duty" was the proximate cause of the client's death. The standard for establishing proximate causation involves proving that, without the failure to uphold an acceptable standard of care, the client's suicide more likely than not could have been avoided (Bongar, 2002).

DAMAGES ARISING FROM MALPRACTICE SUITS

Plaintiffs need to be able to demonstrate that damages have been linked with the suicide. Family members and/or heirs may outline direct financial losses (e.g., loss of income that would have been earned by the decedent) or less tangible emotional injuries such as grief and suffering or the loss of the social dimensions of the relationship (e.g., companionship, comfort, etc.) (Gutheil,1999). In cases for which a breach of the standard of care has been causally linked to a client's death, two principle types of damages can be awarded. These are *compensatory damages* or *punitive damages* (Bongar, 2002; Robertson, 1988; Simon, 1988). Compensatory damages refer to compensation that 'is calculated to replace the loss or injury to the plaintiff' (Robertson, 1988, p.8). Punitive damages are awarded when the defendents behavior is judged to be 'wilful, wanton, malicious or reckless' (Simon, 1988, p. 4). Punitive damages are typically awarded in addition to a compensatory award (Simon, 1988).

Integrating Legal, Ethical, and Clinical Standards of Care

Integrating legal, ethical, and clinical standards of care involves the clinician displaying an appropriate attitudinal approach to the client, assessing clinical practice considerations, and understanding the extent and limits of client confidentiality in the case of suicide prevention.

ATTITUDINAL APPROACH TO CLIENT

Clinicians are expected to be proactive, positive, and life-affirming in their approach to suicidal patients (Berman, 2006). It is also important to adopt a nonjudgmental stance (i.e., not stereotyping the client as "weak" or "manipulative"). Clinicians need to monitor for any negative affect arising in their feelings toward the client (e.g., frustration, anger, hopelessness about the client's prospects) as this may be inadvertently communicated to the person and/or significant others. Within this context, clinical supervision and/or consultation is an important source of support, guidance, and oversight. It is equally important as a risk management strategy.

CLINICAL PRACTICE CONSIDERATIONS

Clinical practice needs to be rooted in the value of respect for patient autonomy and provision of the least restrictive care (see Chapter 10). The issue of autonomy is complicated in the context of potential suicidal behavior per se, in which considerations about autonomy need to be balanced with a concern for client safety. Additional complications arise in the case of cognitive impairment associated with neurodisability. The presence of such impairments may reduce decision-making capacity, but even in cases in which substitute decision-making may be required, seeking the assent of the client to proposed treatment options is important. Moreover, cognitive impairments associated with neurodisability should not be confused with one's ability to make medical preferences known or to challenge decisions pertaining to one's health. Clinicians are encouraged to work with such patients as well as family members and support persons to identify means of ascertaining individual preferences.

As outlined in Chapter 8, a suicide risk assessment needs to be multidimensional, gathering information from the client himself, as well as from the client's social network and other health professionals as appropriate (also see Simon, 2012). In gathering data, reviewing available medical records can also be of value. Simpson and Tate (2005) found that 15.5% (7/45) of clients did not disclose previous suicidal behavior in a research interview. Developing some form of structured or semi-structured assessment protocol is recommended as a means of ensuring thoroughness in assessment (Malone, Szanto, Corbitt, & Mann, 1995; Simon, 2012) and can also assist with documentation. The importance of documentation will be further discussed later.

Treatment ideally aims to reduce warning signs and modifiable risk factors contributing to the elevated suicidal risk and to strengthen protective factors, including supports. In terms of maximizing a risk management approach, consultation with colleagues and the review of treatment approaches in any previous crisis/crises are useful resources in informing the current treatment plan (Berman, 2006). Close collaboration is required between the prescribing physician and clinicians/other support staff, as well as the client's broader supports in managing medication. Appropriate risk management ensures that communication occurring as a part of this collaborative effort is also documented in medical charts. Close collaboration is also required when clients are discharged from inpatient mental health or hospital settings to ensure that adequate community supports and follow-up are in place (see Chapters 10 and 12). For example, the failure to make timely follow-up appointments and reasonable efforts to ensure attendance at such appointments by clinicians has been adjudged as failing to meet an acceptable standard of care (Berman, 2006). Clinicians need to ensure that clients and/or family members know who to contact if an emergency arises during the times that the clinician is not available (e.g., 24-hour crisis lines for an out-of-hours emergency). This information, as well as other strategies for coping, can be addressed in a personalized safety plan (see Chapter 10).

Contemporaneous documentation of the assessment and treatment of suicidal clients is a critical component (the "sine qua non," Berman, 2006, p. 173) of risk management (Simon, 2012; Gutheil, 1999). Despite this being widely known, reviews of mental health clinician notes in medical charts identified important gaps in documentation when compared to a full research review of available documentation (Malone et al., 1995). Furthermore, when documentation is completed, it is often telegraphic (Simon, 2012), too terse to capture important details of the client's presentation or the underlying clinical reasoning of the clinician. Although poor documentation is not linked to the suicide per se, it compounds the difficulty for clinicians in explaining and defending their decisions and actions. According to Jacobs and Brewer (2004), the clinician should "indicate the reason for the assessment and review of the factors that may contribute to increased risk"; document "the basis for the determination of risk, any changes made in the treatment plan, and the rationale for those changes [as well as] any treatment changes that were considered but rejected . . . along with reasons for rejection"; and note the "presence or absence of firearms . . . [and] any measures taken to limit access to or remove preferred means for engaging in suicidal behavior" (p. 378).

Finally, in the case of a death by suicide, offering outreach to members of the decedent's social network is important. This can serve several purposes. It addresses the need of responding therapeutically to the emotional reaction to the loss, it can allow for opportunity to clarify with family members the process and any challenges of treatment, and it can also aids in preserving the alliance between family members and the treating clinician or team (Gutheil, 1999).

CONFIDENTIALITY, DUTY TO INFORM, AND SUICIDE RISK

The 2012 National Strategy for Suicide Prevention (USDHHS, 2012) includes an objective to "Educate practitioners about how to exchange confidential patient information appropriately to promote collaborative care while safeguarding patient rights" (p. 46). The need to waive confidentiality may arise in situations of acute risk of self-harm in which the clinician needs to communicate with relatives or close others (Simon, 2012; Berman, 2006). Berman (2006) recommends that clients should be informed by clinicians at the beginning of the therapeutic relationship that the clinician will break confidentiality in order to protect the client in situations of imminent SDV. Moreover, in some US states, a statutory waiver of confidential information exists for situations in which a patient makes serious threats self-harm (Simon & Schuman, 2007). In the context of neurodisability, if the severity of cognitive impairments has limited the capacity of the client to understand why such a course of action has been taken, then the clinician may contact the client's substitute or proxy decision-maker about the need to break confidentiality. Apart from breaking confidentiality to inform family or close others about elevated risk of suicide, the Health Insurance Portability and Accountability Act (HIPAA) of 1996 allows clinicians who are treating the same patient to communicate without expressed permission from the patient (Simon, 2012) thus enabling better coordination of care when more than one agency is involved.

On the other hand, although clinicians do not have a duty to warn relatives, they do have some discretion about the circumstances under which they might pursue this path. The determination from the highly referenced case of *Tarasoff v Board of Regents of the University of California* in 1976 suggests that clinicians have a duty to disclose the contents of a confidential communication and warn relatives in the case of potential violence. However, subsequent case law refined the application of "*Tarasoff* warnings" to situations of potential violence endangering others and not to potential acts of SDV or property damage (Bongar, 2002). However, the decision to disclose the content of confidential communication if there is an impending risk of SDV is still an option for clinicians, particularly in outpatient settings (Fremouw, de Perczel, & Ellis, 1990).

A list of practical clinical considerations that will help to minimize risk in managing suicidal clients can be found in Box 13.1 (adapted from Simpson [2001] and Berman [2006]). This chapter provides an introduction to a number of the key concepts that clinicians will need to be aware of when working with suicidal clients.

BOX 13.1
STRATEGIES FOR GOOD CLINICAL PRACTICE THAT ALSO MINIMIZE
LEGAL RISK

Clinician Management
- Consider limiting the number of at-risk clients managed at any one time.
- Within available resources, prioritize the provision of necessary support to the client.
- If unable to provide the degree of support judged necessary to maintain the client's safety, examine options to (1) refer the client or (2) increase additional supports acceptable to the client.
- Document risk assessment and intervention procedures in sufficient detail and in real time.

Clinical Management
- Consent and seek permission to consult with others and then do so.
- Inform the client regarding the limitations to confidentiality.
- Seek to establish and maintain a strong therapeutic alliance with the client.
- Validate the client's experience of pain and normalize his or her expression of suicidal distress.
- Undertake a multidimensional risk assessment and document results.
- Organize psychiatric assessments and liaison.
- Monitor mental health status.
- Support all elements of the treatment plan.
- Repeat the suicide risk assessment as often as clinical imperatives require.
- Make all assessments and treatment plan decisions via face-to-face consultations.
- Do not assume that client denial of current suicide ideation is an accurate summation of the level of suicide risk.
- Collaborate as appropriate.
- Do not use "no-suicide" contracts.
- Make reasonable efforts to obtain and/or review medical records.
- Monitor and reduce lethality of the client's environment.

Adapted from Berman (2006); Simpson (2001).

More detailed information about these issues can be obtained from the references cited in this chapter.

APPLICATION TO NEURODISABILITY

As outlined in earlier chapters, there is limited evidence to support standards of practice in the assessment and treatment of suicide among clients with neurodisability. Therefore, to optimize risk management, Berman (2006) and Simon (2012) recommend that clinicians need to demonstrate that they have made use of published practice guidelines on suicide prevention, professional codes of ethics, organizational policy and procedures, and legal precedent, in addition to any guidance provided by senior/supervisory staff. These sources can be supplemented by any practice recommendations relating to neurodisability-specific treatment approaches to the management of mental health issues (although these are rare), the research on suicidal thoughts and behaviors after neurodisability (albeit also rare), and the practice recommendations arising from this research, with the qualification that many of these recommendations are still tentative and have a limited underlying evidence-base. Finally, Berman (2006) points out that although practice guidelines do not define standards of care, they do provide a guide as to what would be considered reasonable and prudent assessment and treatment responses.

Wish to Hasten Death or End One's Life

Decisions regarding death and dying are informed by individual, social, and societal beliefs and values (Seymour, Janssens, & Broeckaert, 2007). As such, delivery of care to those living with intractable or terminal conditions, which includes those with neurodisabilities such ALS or Huntington's disease (HD), is "predicated on a variety of clinical, ethical, and sociocultural assumptions" as well as on "legal codes governing end of life care" (Seymour et al., 2007, p. 1680). Beliefs and values regarding the wish to hasten death and euthanasia or physician-assisted suicide have been highlighted in the ongoing conversation between patients, medical professionals, caregivers, families, and the public at large regarding end-of-life decision-making. Contributing to current challenges is the confusion regarding similarities and differences between terms associated with hastened death (Table 13.1).

As expected, most peer-reviewed research regarding the wish to hasten death or physician-assisted suicide has been conducted in or regarding places where such actions are legally sanctioned. In a systematic review of euthanasia and assisted suicide

TABLE 13.1

Terms associated with the wish to end one's life

Term	Definition
Euthanasia	Euthanasia and is defined as a doctor intentionally ending a person's life by the administration of drugs at that person's voluntary and competent request (Materstvedt et al., 2003).
Palliative sedation	Sedation used to engender unconsciousness until death occurs among dying individuals experiencing symptoms (e.g., delirium, agitation, extreme dyspnea) that are refractory and unresponsive to conventional treatments (Seymore et al., 2003).
Physician-assisted suicide	A doctor intentionally helping a person to end their life by providing drugs for self-administration at that person's voluntary and competent request. (Materstvedt et al., 2003).
Wish to hasten death	A reaction to suffering in the context of a life-threatening condition from which the patient can see no way out other than to accelerate his or her death. This wish may be expressed spontaneously or after being asked, but it must be distinguished from the acceptance of impending death or from a wish to die naturally, although preferably soon. The wish to hasten death may arise in response to one or more factors, including physical symptoms (either present or foreseen), psychological distress (e.g., depression, hopelessness, fears, etc.), existential suffering (e.g., loss of meaning in life), or social aspects (e.g., feeling that one is a burden) (Balaguer et al., 2016).

in selected European countries and US states Steck, Matthias, Maessen, Reisch, and Zwahlen (2013) reported that among all deaths the percentage of physician-assisted suicide ranged from 0.1% to 0.2% in the United States to 1.8%–2.9% in Luxembourg and the Netherlands. Steck et al. (2013) also highlight legal frameworks in countries where assisted dying is legal (e.g., Netherlands: "Euthanasia law since April 2002; physician-assisted suicide and euthanasia are not punishable if provided by a physician who has met the requirements of due care" [p. 939]; Oregon; "The Oregon Dignity Act, enabled in October of 1997, legalizes physician-assisted suicide, but not euthanasia" [p. 939]). Jankowski and Campo-Engelstein (2013) suggest that a person's right to refuse life-sustaining treatment is a "fundamental expression of patient autonomy" which also poses ethical dilemmas for practitioners and health-care systems. They extend this argument in a discussion regarding suicide in the context of terminal illness and in doing so highlight challenges related to suicide prevention among those with neurodisabilities who are interested in exploring assisted suicide. In specific, this may require providers to clarify and operationalize, per existing legal guidelines, under which circumstances the desire for death would be suicidal or hastened death. For example, according to Dutch law "One of the mandatory conditions . . . for performing physician-assisted suicide is that the patient requesting physician-assisted suicide is suffering unbearably and the outlook is hopeless" (Maessen et al., 2010).

Veldink, Wokke, van der Wal, Vianney de Jong, and van den Berg (2002) explored end-of-life decision-making among those with ALS by asking physicians about their patients who had died between 1994 and 1999. Results suggested that 20% of patients with ALS in the Netherlands died as a result of euthanasia or physician-assisted suicide. According to their medical providers, patients for whom religion was important were less likely hasten death. Moreover, disability was more severe (i.e., loss of function in arms) among those who died in this manner. Ganzini, Silveira, and Johnston (2002) surveyed caregivers of decedents with ALS and found that one-third of those with the condition discussed the desire for assisted suicide in the last month of their life. As the disease progressed, hopelessness and interest in hastened death predicted the desire for assisted suicide. Other contributing factors included greater distress at the thought of being a burden and more insomnia, pain, and discomfort. Although research in this area has suggested that those with ALS who chose hastened death were more depressed, Albert et al. (2005) caution against this and highlight that individuals in their sample were more likely to meet criteria for depressive disorder secondary to the fact that they more frequently reported that "they would be better off dead" (p. 72). The authors highlight challenges associated with differentiating depression and "existential suffering" among those with end-stage disease.

RESPONDING TO CLIENT REQUESTS TO DIE

A range of healthcare staff (e.g., psychologists, social workers, nurses) who do not play the central medical management role in end-of-life care may still be called on to undertake assessment or counseling as part of the clinical management and decision-making process. Regardless of personal beliefs or values in relation to end-of-life decision-making, healthcare professionals need to be prepared to respond "professionally" and "compassionately" to patient statements regarding the desire to die (Hudson et al., 2006). Moreover, as new and more efficacious treatments are identified, conditions that had more frequently been discussed in relation to a wish to end one's life may no longer be considered intractable or terminal (e.g., MS);

thereby requiring patients, family members, and care providers to rethink long-term prognoses and patient desires vis á vis the condition.

In terms of approach, being aware of any national practice guidelines relating to patients with particular medical conditions (e.g., ALS) or the position of professional associations in relation to assisted suicide is an important first step. Knowledge regarding the legal status of assisted suicide in the jurisdiction within which one practices is critical. Currently, physician-assisted suicide is legal in four European counties (the Netherlands, Belgium, Luxembourg, Switzerland) and a number of US states (i.e., Oregon, Washington, Montana, Vermont, Colorado, California).

In a resolution on assisted suicide, the American Psychological Association (2016) has recently undertaken to better prepare the profession to deal with the matter of assisted suicide (http://www.apa.org/about/policy/assisted-suicide.aspx). The APA outlined a number of areas for psychologists to focus on in their practice with people who have raised the issue of assisted suicide (Box 13.2). Furthermore, the resolution calls for further research and training to better equip psychologists in addressing assisted suicide. This emphasis on training and research also applies to every other health profession working in the field of assisted suicide.

Hudson and colleagues (2006) argue that providers must seek to understand the meaning behind patient's statements of a wish to die in order to respond. In specific, they suggest an approach in which professionals (1) "explore issues underpinning the statement," (2) "identify the critical clinical issues," and (3) "discuss the interpersonal factors involved" (p. 706). The authors also highlight the importance of the professional "being alert to their own response" (p. 706). Further specific guidance is provided regarding strategies to manage clinical interactions regarding the wish for death, as well as recommended phrases and questions to respond to such statements (for further information, see Hudson et al., 2006). As legal, ethical, and medical issues related to the wish to die continue to unfold, providers working with those with neurodisability must continue to identify professional guidance and best practices regarding how to meet the needs of those living with intractable and terminal illness.

Conclusion

Though the chances of clinicians facing legal action as the results of a suicide are statistically remote, pursuing good practice by acting in a competent and professional manner and undertaking contemporaneous documentation while consulting with peers or supervisors will help minimize any risk of litigation. This can reassure clinicians to engage with clients with neurodisability who are experiencing suicidal distress. While there is a significant body of literature addressing these legal issues,

---

BOX 13.2
POSITION OF THE AMERICAN PSYCHOLOGICAL ASSOCIATION ON
ASSISTED SUICIDE

- Advocate for quality end-of-life care for all individuals; and
- Promote policies that reduce suffering that could lead to requests for assisted suicide; and
- Inform oneself about criminal and civil laws that have bearing on assisted suicide in the states in which they practice; and
- Recognize the powerful influence psychologists may have with clients who are considering assisted suicide; and
- Identify factors leading to assisted suicide requests (including clinical depression, levels of pain and suffering, adequacy of comfort care, and other internal and external variables) and fully explore alternative interventions (including hospice/palliative care and other end-of-life options such as voluntarily stopping eating and drinking) for clients considering assisted suicide; and
- Be aware of personal views about assisted suicide, including recognizing possible biases about entitlement to resources based on disability status, age, sex, sexual orientation, or ethnicity of the client requesting assisted suicide; and
- Be especially sensitive to the social and cultural biases which may result in some groups and individuals being perceived by others, and/or being encouraged to perceive themselves, as more expendable and less deserving of continued life (e.g., people with disabilities, women, older adults, people of color, gay men, lesbians, bisexual people, transgendered individuals, and persons who are poor).

---

pathways to navigate the ethical issues relating to the wish to hasten death are still at a much earlier point of development. In the field of neurodisability, they have been most commonly explored in relation to progressive conditions, most notably ALS, but may also have application to the most aggressive forms of MS and HD.

Implications for Clinicians

1. It is important that practitioners do not resort to "defensive approaches" to clinical practice in seeking to minimize the risk of litigation; good clinical practice is the best defence against litigation.
2. In the absence of neurodisability-specific guidelines, clinicians need to demonstrate that they have made use of generic published practice guidelines on suicide prevention, professional codes of ethics, organizational policy and

procedures, and legal precedent, in addition to any guidance provided by senior/supervisory staff in the assessment and management of suicide.

3. Contemporaneous and clear (not shorthand) documentation of the assessment and treatment of suicidal clients is a critical component of risk management.

4. Regardless of personal beliefs or values in relation to the wish to hasten death, palliative sedation, or physician-assisted suicide, healthcare professionals need to be prepared to respond "professionally" and "compassionately" to patient statements regarding the wish to die.

5. In response to a client raising the issue of the wish to hasten death, it is important to explore the range of factors (e.g., clinical depression, presence of pain, lack of treatment, cultural and social biases that might lead individuals to believe they are a burden) that might underlie the clients' state of mind and to carefully explore the range of alternatives (including, if legal, physician-assisted death) with the client.

References

Albert, S. M., Rabkin, J. G., Del Bene, M. L., Tider, T., O'Sullivan, I., Rowland, L. P., & Mitsumoto, H. (2005). Wish to die in end-stage ALS. *Neurology, 65*(1), 68–74.

American Psychological Association. *Ethical principles and codes of practice*. Retrieved from http://www.apa.org/ethics/code/index.aspx

American Psychological Association. (2016). *Resolution on assisted suicide*. Retrieved from http://www.apa.org/about/policy/assisted-suicide.aspx

Appelbaum, P. S., & Gutheil, T. G. (2000). *Clinical handbook of psychiatry and the law* (3rd ed.). Philadelphia, PA: Lippincott, Williams & Wilkins.

Berman, A. L. (2006). Risk management with suicidal patients. *Journal of Clinical Psychology: In Session, 62*, 171–184.

Balaguer, A., Monforte-Royo, C., Porta-Sales, J., Alonso-Babarro, A., Altisent, R., Aradilla-Herrero, A., . . . Voltz, R. (2016). An international consensus definition of the wish to hasten death and its related factors. *PLoS ONE 11*(1), e0146184. doi:10.1371/journal. pone.0146184

Bongar, B. (2002). *The suicidal patient: Clinical and legal standards of care* (2nd ed.). Washington, DC: American Psychological Association.

Fremouw, W. J., de Perczel, M., & Ellis, T. E. (1990). *Suicide risk: Assessment and response guidelines*. New York: Pergamon Press.

Ganzini, L., Silveira, M. J., & Johnston, W. S. (2002). Predictors and correlates of interest in assisted suicide in the final month of life among ALS patients in Oregon and Washington. *Journal of Pain and Symptom Management, 24*(3), 312–317.

Gutheil, T. G. (1999). Liability issues and liability prevention in suicide. In D. G. Jacobs (Ed.), *The Harvard Medical School guide to suicide assessment and intervention* (pp. 561–578). San Francisco: Jossey-Bass.

Hudson, P. L., Schofield, P., Kelly, B., Hudson, R., O'Connor, M., Kristjanson, L. J., . . . Aranda, S. (2006). Responding to desire to die statements from patients with advanced disease: Recommendations for health professionals. *Palliative Medicine, 20*(7), 703–710.

Jacobs, D., & Brewer, M. (2004). APA practice guideline provides recommendations for assessing and treating patients with suicidal behaviors. *Psychiatric Annals, 34*(5), 373–380.

Jankowski, J., & Campo-Engelstein, L. (2013). Suicide in the context of terminal illness. *The American Journal of Bioethics, 13*(3), 13–14.

Maessen, M., Veldink, J. H., van den Berg, L. H., Schouten, H. J., van der Wal, G., & Onwuteaka-Philipsen, B. D. (2010). Requests for euthanasia: Origin of suffering in ALS, heart failure, and cancer patients. *Journal of Neurology, 257*(7), 1192–1198. doi:10.1007/s00415-010-5474-y

Malone, K. M., Szanto, K., Corbitt, E. M., & Mann, J. J. (1995). Clinical assessment versus research methods in the assessment of suicidal behavior. *American Journal of Psychiatry, 152*, 1601–1607.

Materstvedt, L. J., Clark, D., Ellershaw, J., Forde, R., Gravgaard, A. M. B., Muller-Busch, H. C., . . . Rapin, C. H. (2003). Euthanasia and physician-assisted suicide: A view from an EAPC Ethics Task Force. *Palliative Medicine, 17*(2), 97–101.

Peters, P. G. Jr. (2000). The quite demise of deference to custom: Malpractice law at the millennium. *Washington Lee Law Review, 57*, 163–205.

Robertson, J. D. (1988). *Psychiatric malpractice: Liability of mental health professionals*. New York: Wiley.

Sadoff, R. L. (1975). *Forensic psychiatry: A practical guide for lawyers and psychiatrists*. Springfield, IL: Charles C. Thomas.

Seymour, J. E., Janssens, R., & Broeckaert, B. (2007). Relieving suffering at the end of life: practitioners' perspectives on palliative sedation from three European countries. *Social Science & Medicine, 64*(8), 1679–1691.

Simon, R. I. (1988). *Concise guide to clinical psychiatry and the law*. Washington, DC: American Psychiatric Press.

Simon, R. I. (1992). *Concise guide to psychiatry and the law for clinicians*. Washington, DC: American Psychiatric Press.

Simon, R. I. (2004). *Assessing and managing suicide risk: Guidelines for clinically based risk management*. Washington, DC: American Psychiatric Association.

Simon, R. I. (2012). Suicide risk assessment: Gateway to treatment and management. In R. I. Simon & R. E. Hales (Eds.), *The American Psychiatric Publishing textbook of suicide assessment* (pp. 3–28). Washington, DC: American Psychiatric Publishing.

Simon, R. I., & Schuman, D. W. (2009). Therapeutic risk management of clinical-legal dilemmas: should it be a core competency? *Journal of the American Academy of Psychiatry and the Law, 37*, 155–161.

Simpson, G. (2001). Suicide prevention after traumatic brain injury: A resource manual. Sydney, Australia: South Western Sydney Area Health Service, Brain Injury Rehabilitation Unit.

Simpson G. K., & Tate, R. L. (2005). Clinical features of suicide attempts after TBI. *The Journal of Nervous and Mental Disease, 193*, 680–685.

Steck, N., Matthias, E., Maessen, M., Reisch, T., & Zwahlen, M. (2013). Euthanasia and assisted suicide in selected European countries and US states: Systematic literature review. *Medical Care, 51*(10), 938–943.

US Department of Health and Human Services (USDHHS), Office of the Surgeon General, & National Action Alliance for Suicide Prevention. (2012). *2012 National strategy for suicide prevention: Goals and objectives for action.* Washington, DC: HHS.

Veldink, J. H., Wokke, J. H., van der Wal, G., Vianney de Jong, J. M. B., & van den Berg, L. H. (2002). Euthanasia and physician-assisted suicide among patients with amyotrophic lateral sclerosis in the Netherlands. *New England Journal of Medicine, 346*(21), 1638–1644.

14 Conclusions

THIS BOOK REPRESENTS a departure from previous publications on suicide and suicide prevention among people with health conditions. It is the first to specifically target neurodisability. Previous books have examined suicide in the context of diseases and chronic illnesses more generally and touch on different types of neurodisability; however, neurodisability is unique in that it comprises a group of conditions caused by injury or disease processes directly affecting the central nervous system. Not only do these conditions have a primary impact on cognition, behavior, motor-sensory function, and emotions, there are also a number of related consequences: the effects of these impairments on psychological adjustment, the capacity to participate in treatment, the idiosyncratic presentation of mental health problems such as depression, and the profile and risk factors for suicidal thoughts and behaviors. By concentrating the focus on neurodisability, we hope to have highlighted these key areas as they pertain to suicide risk.

Second, the book has taken a thematic approach, rather than following the practice of previous books that have organized each chapter on a diagnostic basis. The thematic approach provided a unique opportunity to identify key similarities and differences rooted in underlying neuropathology. Moreover, impairments associated with these conditions increase or decrease the observed prevalence, predictors, and clinical presentations of suicidal thoughts and behaviors across different types of neurodisability. This is extremely important in the context of mixed neurological practices, such as neurology clinics, and in inpatient or outpatient neurorehabilitation. In short, we believe that this broadening focus may help clinicians and researchers translate observations among those living with one type of neurodisability to other groups with neurodisability. It also helps to highlight gaps in clinical knowledge and research because areas that have received attention for one group may have been completely neglected in another (e.g., while there is published research into suicide attempts in traumatic brain injury [TBI], similar research is has not been reported in spinal cord injury [SCI]).

Furthermore, across the diagnostic groups that were the subject of this book, the majority of research has been conducted in the areas of prevalence and predictors of suicidal thoughts and behaviors, with virtual silence in the areas of assessment, intervention, and prevention. By aggregating the scant work that has been done across the varied areas of clinical practice, we hope that it is now possible to outline a far more comprehensive approach to suicide prevention after neurodisability than would have been achieved if fragmented by diagnostic group. The significant focus on TBI throughout the book reflects the expertise and background of the two authors, but also reflects the reality that this is the group for whom the greater part of the research has been done to date.

The book also highlighted how the preponderance of the research and the clinical constructs that have driven the research are based around responding on an individual level to clients displaying suicidal thoughts and behaviors. This is in keeping with the clinical characterization of suicide introduced in Chapter 1; that suicide post-neurodisability is the "endpoint of an unsuccessful adaptation process" (Achte, Lonnqvist, & Hillborm, 1971). Although the individual challenges with adaptation to neurodisability are a key to suicide risk, the book has also tried to broaden this focus to capture the complex contextual factors that need to be considered in formulating approaches to suicide prevention among those with neurodisability. This expanding of perspective takes on greater importance because, over the past 15 years (1999–2014), the total suicide rate in the United States, inclusive of those with and without neurodisability, has increased by 24%, from 10.5 to 13.0 per 100,000 (NIMH, 2017). In fact, in 2015, suicide was the tenth leading cause of death in the United States, with 44,000 people dying secondary to self-directed violence (NIMH, 2017). While suicide is an individual act, rates of suicide often reflect underlying macro-level socioeconomic and cultural effects.

In concert with this broader viewpoint, authors of the World Health Organization (2014) report titled *Preventing Suicide: A Global Imperative*, highlight the importance of suicide prevention efforts "including collaborations between health and non-health sectors at governmental and non-governmental level" (p. 72). They also emphasize the utility of early and effective interventions. These themes, which are echoed throughout this book, suggest the need to rethink suicide as also being an "endpoint" of societal challenges in providing those with and without disabilities strategies and opportunities to develop reasons for living.

One example is the case of TBI sustained during military duty. Secondary to advances in battlefield medical responses, aeromedical evacuations, and the widespread use of body armor, military personnel who served in the Iraq and Afghanistan conflicts survived complex injuries that might have killed those serving in previous conflicts (Bailey, Morrison, & Rasmussen, 2013). Although we have made significant advances in term of saving lives on the battlefield, military personnel with polytrauma (a history of TBI plus injury to at least one other bodily system) have "complex rehabilitation needs" associated with a history of TBI, pain, and co-occurring psychiatric conditions (e.g., posttraumatic stress disorder) that pose significant challenges to veterans trying to return to civilian life (Institute of Medicine, 2014). Similarly, medical science has markedly increased life expectancy for spinal cord injury (SCI), multiple sclerosis (MS), and other types of neurodisability, thus presenting the challenge of survival and longer term social integration and acceptance.

Among this cohort and for others living with neurodisabilities, a public health approach is paramount. This includes activities targeting prevention or providing early interventions for secondary health conditions (e.g., depression) which are prevalent among those with disability and are also risk factors for suicide (Field & Jette, 2007). Although the rates of psychiatric conditions post-neurodisability are well-known, we, as healthcare providers, continue to struggle to facilitate access to mental health services for those who need them. For example, work by Hart et al. (2012) highlighted both the notable rates of major and minor depression among those with TBI 1 and 2 years post-injury, with some individuals developing new-onset depression in year 1 or 2, and others reporting an increase in depressive symptoms from year 1 to year 2, thereby highlighting the need for increased efforts to monitor for depression even among those who do not report symptoms at the time of discharge from acute rehabilitation.

Moreover, additional efforts are needed to provide opportunities for those with neurodisability to return to age-appropriate vocational and avocational activities. Across a wide range of cohorts, work and/or volunteering have been repeatedly identified as reasons for living, yet many with neurodisability are not provided with the support they need to engage in such activities. For example, according to work by Daniel, Wolf, Busch, and McKevitt (2009), among patients in the United Kingdom post-stroke and younger than 65, only 44% of these individuals returned to work. Though traditional outcomes often associated with the "success" of return to work programs include the ability to maintain employment, the addition of psychological outcomes may provide support for the development of and funding for long-term multidisciplinary programs.

Within the chapters of this book we have also emphasized the importance of employing evidence-based screening, assessment, and intervention strategies for those living with neurodisability. Secondary to the limited work that has been done in the area of suicide prevention specifically pertaining to those with neurodisability, this often requires borrowing and adapting evidence-based practices developed for members of the general population. Within this context, the book has sought to interweave theoretical developments, research, and practice within the broader suicide prevention literature with the latest research in suicide prevention in the neurorehabilitation literature.

While this strategy is an important starting point, we want to emphasize the need for the development, as well as dissemination, of psychometrically sound screening and assessment methods that take into account specific factors known to drive increased risk among those with neurodisability. Also of note, there are important differences between the neurodisabilities discussed within this book and how they impact functioning. Moreover, whereas there continues to be some progress in terms of the development of evidence-based suicide prevention interventions for those with neurodisability (e.g., Window to Hope), even when such treatments have been developed and tested, resources necessary to move them into the field in a manner that could benefit those living with such disabilities remain limited (Brenner et al., 2018). It is likely that novel dissemination efforts (e.g., telehealth, web-based formats) will be needed to meet the needs of individuals living with such disabilities. Further research in critical clinical areas such as safety planning, more effective treatments for mental health, and means for building protective factors (such as resilience and self-efficacy) is also needed.

It is our hope that this book provides the foundational information needed to provide the most effective care to those with neurodisability. We hope it will enable staff to engage with clients experiencing suicidal distress with greater knowledge and confidence. Suicidality is not something to avoid, and, given the fact that a very small number of people eventually do take their own lives, we can be confident that in the great majority of cases it will be possible to work with people to reduce their level of suicidal distress. At the same time, we recognize that significant continued efforts are needed in both the areas of clinical practice and research, with the overall goal of decreasing suicidal thoughts and behavior among these high-risk cohorts.

References

Achte, K. A., Lonnqvist, J., & Hillbom, E. (1971). Suicides following war brain-injuries. *Acta Psychiatrica Scandinavica*, Supplement 225.

Bailey, C. J. A., Morrison, M. J. J., & Rasmussen, C. T. E. (2013). Military trauma system in Afghanistan: Lessons for civil systems? *Current Opinion in Critical Care, 19*(6), 569–577. doi:10.1097/mcc.0000000000000037

Brenner, L. A., Forster, J. E., Hoffberg, A. S., Matarazzo, B. B., Hostetter, T. A., Signoracci, G., & Simpson, G. K. (2018). Window to hope: A randomized controlled trial of a psychological intervention for the treatment of hopelessness among veterans with moderate to severe traumatic brain injury. *The Journal of Head Trauma Rehabilitation, 33*(2), E64–E73.

Daniel, K., Wolfe, C. D., Busch, M. A., & McKevitt, C. (2009). What are the social consequences of stroke for working-aged adults?: A systematic review. *Stroke, 40*(6), e431–e440.

Field, M. J., & Jette, A. M. (2007). The future of disability in America. Washington, DC: National Academies Press.

Hart, T., Hoffman, J. M., Pretz, C., Kennedy, R., Clark, A. N., & Brenner, L. A. (2012). A Longitudinal study of major and minor depression following traumatic brain injury. *Archives of Physical Medicine and Rehabilitation, 93*(8), 1343–1349. doi:10.1016/j.apmr.2012.03.036

Institute of Medicine. (2014). *Returning home from Iraq and Afghanistan: Preliminary assessment of readjustment needs of veterans, service members, and their families.* Washington, DC: National Academies Press.

National Institute of Mental Health (NIMH). (2017, November). *Suicide* [Statistics concerning suicide in the United States of America]. Retrieved from https://www.nimh.nih.gov/health/statistics/suicide.shtmlpart_154968

World Health Organization. (2014). *Preventing suicide: A global imperative.* Retrieved from http://www.who.int/mental_health/suicide-prevention/world_report_2014/en/

Snapshots for Each Disability Group

Cerebrovascular Accident (CVA)

Suicide:

Risk of suicide 1.88 (SMR, males) and 1.78 (SMR, females) times greater than general population.[6] Risk 2.8 times greater (OR) than matched controls.[7] Rate of 83 per 100,000, double the general population.[6]

Suicide attempt:

No data for people with CVA.

Suicide ideation (SI):

15.2% cumulative lifetime SI frequency among stroke survivors, 2.07 times greater (OR) than for the general population.[1] Smaller center-based studies have reported SI rates between 6% and 14%.[3,4]

Risk factors: (Sex, age, clinical group.)

(i) Males with CVA almost twice the risk of suicide compared to females with CVA (1.91).[6]
(ii) Males and females both at elevated risk of suicide compared to general population before 59 years.[5,6] Elevated risk of suicide compared to general population disappears after 80 years of age.[5,6] People with CVA aged <79 years elevated suicide risk compared to people with CVA >80 years. (iii) Risk of suicide (SMR) elevated for all clinical groups (SAH 1.83, ICH 2.60, ischemic stroke 1.77, undefined CVA 1.79).[6]

Clinical features:

Limited information. Two early case reports.[2]

Key references:

1. Fuller-Thomson, E., Tulipano, M. J., & Song, M. (2012). The association between depression, suicidal ideation and stroke in a population-based sample. *International Journal of Stroke, 7*, 188–194.

2. Garden, F. H., Garrison, S. J., & Jain, A. (1990). Assessing suicide risk in stroke patients: Review of two cases. *Archives of Physical Medicine and Rehabilitation, 71*, 1003–1005.

3. Kishi, Y., Robinson, R. G., & Kosier, J. T. (1996). Suicidal plans in patients with stroke: Comparison between acute-onset and delayed-onset suicidal plans, *International Psychogeriatrics, 8*, 623–634.

4. Pohjasvaara, T., Vataja, R., Leppävuori, A., Kaste, M., & Erkinjuntti, T. (2001). Suicidal ideas in stroke patients 3 and 15 months after stroke. *Cerebrovascular Disease, 12*, 21–26.

5. Stenager, E. N., Madsen, C., Stenager, E., & Boldsen, J. (1998). Suicide in patients with stroke: Epidemiological study. *British Medical Journal, 316*, 1206.

6. Teasdale, T. W., & Engberg, A. W. (2001). Suicide after stroke: A population study. *Journal of Epidemiology and Community Health, 55*, 863–866.

7. Waern, M., Rubenowitz, E., Runeson, B., Skoog, I., Wilhelmson, K., & Allebeck, P. (2002) Burden of illness and suicide in elderly people: Case control study. *British Journal of Medicine, 324*, 1355–1358.

Spinal Cord Injury (SCI)

Suicide:

Risk of suicide between 3.0 and 5.7 times greater (SMR) than general population.[2,4,6,8,10] Rates of 59.2 or 62.5 per 100,000 for all SCI compared to 12per 100,000 in the general population.[3,9] Rate of 54.3 per 100,000 (paraplegia) and 64.5 per 100,000 (quadriplegia).[3]

Suicide attempt:

Sparse data for SCI. Among 42 people who died by suicide, 14.3% (6/42) made post-injury attempts.[3]

Suicide ideation (SI):

No studies have specifically investigated SI after SCI. In a study into depression among the 16 US Model Systems SCI units, 15.4% of 849 respondents endorsed the SI item on the Patient Health Questionnaire-9.[1]

Risk factors: (Sex, age, clinical group, time post-onset.)

(i) Males and females both at elevated risk of suicide compared to general population.[1] (ii) Elevated risk of suicide up to 54 years of age.[4,10] (iii) Risk of suicide elevated for all clinical groups (tetraplegia complete and incomplete, SMR range 3.4–7.8,[4,6,10] paraplegia complete and incomplete, SMR range 4.2–7.6[4,6]). (iv) Elevated rate of suicide up to 5 years post-onset, SMR range 5.3–6.9.[4,10]

Clinical features:

Given the similar rates of suicide among people with paraplegia and tetraplegia, there is limited evidence supporting the concern about suicide through self-neglect due to an inability to actively end life.[6,10] Three studies have found that 1.6%,[7] 2.0%,[11] and 3.0%,[6] respectively, of SCIs were the result of a suicide attempt. Limited follow-up evidence to determine post-SCI suicide risk for these cases. No data for any suicidal thoughts and behaviors among people with nontraumatic causes of SCI.

Key references:

1. Bombadier, C. H., Richards, J. S., Krause, J. S., Tulsky, D., & Tate, D. G. (2004). Symptoms of major depression in people with spinal cord injury: Implications for screening. *Archives of Physical Medicine and Rehabilitation, 85*, 1749–1756.

2. Cao, Y., Massaro, J. F., Krause, J. S., Chen, Y., & Devivo, M. J. (2014). Suicide mortality after spinal cord injury in the United States: injury cohorts analysis. *Archives of Physical Medicine and Rehabilitation, 95*, 230–235.

3. Charlifue S. W., & Gerhart, K. A. (1991). Behavioral and demographic predictors of suicide after traumatic spinal cord injury. *Archives of Physical Medicine and Rehabilitation, 72*, 488–492.

4. DeVivo, M. J., Black, K. J., Richards, J. S., & Stover, S. L. (1991). Suicide following spinal cord injury. *Paraplegia, 29*, 620–627.

5. Harris, E. C., Barraclough, B. M., Grundy, D. J., Bamford, E. S., & Inskip, H. M. (1996). Attempted suicide and completed suicide in traumatic spinal cord injury: Case reports. *Spinal Cord, 34*, 752–753.

6. Hartkopp, A., Brønnum-Hansen, H., Seidenschnur, A.-M., & Biering-Sørensen, F. (1997). Survival and cause of death after traumatic spinal cord injury: A long-term epidemiological survey from Denmark. *Spinal Cord, 35*, 76–85.

7. Kennedy, P., Rogers, B., Speer, S., & Frankel, H. (1999). Spinal cord injuries and attempted suicide: A retrospective review. *Spinal Cord, 37*, 847–852.

8. Lidal, I. B., Snekkevik, H., Aamodt, G., Hjeltnes, N., Stanghelle, J. K., & Biering-Sørensen, F. (2007). Mortality after spinal cord injury in Norway. *Journal of Rehabilitation Medicine, 39*, 145–151.

9. Savic, G., DeVivo, M. J., Frankel, H. L., Jamous, M. A., Soni, B. M., & Charlifue, S. (2017). Long-term survival after traumatic spinal cord injury: A 70-year British study. *Spinal Cord, 55*, 651.

10. Soden, R. J., Walsh, J., Middleton, J. W., Craven, M. L., Rutkowski, S. B., & Yeo, J. D. (2000). Causes of death after spinal cord injury. *Spinal Cord, 38*, 604–610.

11. Stanford, R. E., Soden, R., Bartrop, R., Mikk, M., & Taylor, T. K. F. (2007). Spinal cord and related injuries after attempted suicide: Psychiatric diagnosis and long-term follow-up. *Spinal Cord, 45*, 437–443.

Traumatic Brain Injury (TBI)

Suicide:

Risk of suicide between 1.4 and 4.05 greater (SMRs, AOR) for people with TBI compared to the general population.[2,4,6–8, 10–12,15, 23,25] The range of increased risk encompasses both mild and moderate to severe injuries, as well as civilian and military/veteran cohorts.

Suicide attempt:

Adolescents with TBI 3.1 times (OR) to have made SA within previous 12 months compared to general population. Still significant after controlling for sex, education, and emotional distress (AOR 2.9).[13] Adults with TBI had 8.1% lifetime history of suicide attempts compared to 1.9% in general population (AOR 2.4).[18] In center-based studies, post-injury rate of 17.4%[20] and 27.3% among military veterans with inpatient psychiatric admission.[9]

Suicide ideation (SI):

SI significantly higher after TBI compared to general population.[1] Adolescents with TBI significantly more likely to report SI in the last 12 months compared to the general population (AOR 1.68).[1] Center-based studies have reported a cumulative rate of SI up to 25% within the first year post-injury, almost 7 times greater than rates in general population,[14] and rates of 16–30% in chronic groups.[17,19,24]

Risk factors: (Sex, age, clinical group, substance abuse.)

(i) Males and females both at elevated risk of suicide compared to general population.[23] (ii) Elevated risk of suicide for all age groups from <21 yrs to >60 yrs compared to general population.[23] (iii) Elevated risk for both "severe" (lesion) and concussion groups compared to general population; "severe" injury group (lesion) has significantly elevated SMR compared to the concussion group (HR 1.9[23] (iv) People with TBI plus substance misuse have higher risk for suicide compared to people with substance misuse alone.[6] (v) People with TBI and mental health conditions have higher risk for suicide compared to people with mental health conditions alone.[6]

Clinical features:

People with TBI more likely to die by non-violent means (e.g., gas, self-poisoning) than violent means in comparison to the general population.[16] Up to a third of people with TBI left suicide notes.[22] Between 0.8%[23] and 1.4%[3,16] of people sustain their TBI through a SA. Two studies have provided data on clinical features of SAs after TBI.[9,20] In both studies, self-poisoning was the most frequent method, and approximately half of clients made more than one SA. Approximately two-thirds of clients required medical treatment for injuries arising from the SA.

Intervention:

Validated psychological (cognitive-behavior therapy) intervention for treatment of moderate-severe hopelessness among civilians[21] and veterans[5] with chronic moderate to severe TBI.

Key references:

1. Anstey, K., Butterworth, P., Jorm, A. F., Chistensen, H., Rodgers, B., Windsor, T. D. (2004). A population survey found an association between self-reports of traumatic brain injury and increased psychiatric symptoms. *Journal of Clinical Epidemiology, 57,* 1202–1209.
2. Bethune, A., Da Costa, L., van Niftrik, C. H. B., & Feinstein, A. (2017). Suicidal ideation after mild traumatic brain injury: A consecutive Canadian sample. *Archives of Suicide Research, 21*(3), 392–402.

3. Brenner, L. A., Carlson, N. E., Harrison-Felix, C., Ashman, T., Hammond, F., Hirschberg, R. E. (2009). Self-inflicted traumatic brain injury: Characteristics and outcome. *Brain Injury, 23*, 991–998.

4. Brenner, L. A., Ignacio, R. V., & Blow, F. C. (2011). Suicide and traumatic brain injury among individuals seeking Veterans Health Administration Services. *Journal of Head Trauma Rehabilitation, 26*, 257–264.

5. Brenner, L. A., Forster, J. E., Hoffberg, A. S., Matarazzo, B. B., Hostetter, T. A., Signoracci, G., & Simpson, G. K. (2018). Window to hope: A randomized controlled trial of a psychological intervention for the treatment of hopelessness among veterans with moderate to severe TBI. *Journal of Head Trauma Rehabilitation, 33*, E64–E73. doi: 10.1097/HTR.000000000000351

6. Fazel, S., Wolf, A., Pllas, D., Lichtenstein, P., & Långström, N. (2014). Suicide, fatal injuries, and other causes of premature mortality in patients with traumatic injury: A 41-year Swedish population study. *JAMA Psychiatry, 71*, 326–333.

7. Fralick, M., Thiruchelvam, D., Tien, H. C., & Redelmeier, D. A. (2016). Risk of suicide after a concussion. *Canadian Medical Association Journal, 188*, 497–504.

8. Fralick, M., Sy, E., Hassan, A., Burke, M. J., Mostofsky, E., & Karsies, T. (2018). Association of concussion with the risk of suicide: a systematic review and meta-analysis. *JAMA Neurology.* doi:10.1001/jamaneurol.2018.3487

9. Gutierrez, P., Brenner, L. A., & Huggins, J. A. (2008). A preliminary investigation of suicidality hospitalized veterans with traumatic brain injury. *Archives of Suicide Research, 12*, 336–343.

10. Harris, C., & Barraclough, B. (1997). Suicide as an outcome for mental disorders. *British Journal of Psychiatry, 170*, 205–228.

11. Harrison-Felix, C., Whiteneck, G. G., Jha, A., DeVivo, M. J., Hammond, F. M., & Hart, D. M. (2009). Mortality over four decades after traumatic brain injury rehabilitation: A retrospective cohort study. *Archives of Physical Medicine and Rehabilitation, 90*, 1506–1513.

12. Harrison-Felix, C., Kreider, S. E., Arango-Lasprilla, J. C., Brown, A. W., Dijkers, M. P., Hammond, F. M., . . . Zasler, N. D. (2012). Life expectancy following rehabilitation: a NIDRR traumatic brain injury model systems study. *The Journal of Head Trauma Rehabilitation, 27*, E69–E80.

13. Ilie, G., Mann, R. E., Boak, A., Adlaf, E. M., Hamilton, H., Asbridge, M., . . . Cusimano, M. D. (2014). Suicidality, bullying and other conduct and mental health correlates of traumatic brain injury in adolescents. *PloS one, 9*, e94936.

14. Mackelprang, J. L., Bombardier, C. H., Fann, J. R., Temkin, N. R., Barber, J. K., & Dikmen, S. S. (2014). Rates and predictors of suicidal ideation during the first year after traumatic brain injury. *American Journal of Public Health, 104*, e100–e107.

15. Madsen, T., Erlangsen, A., Orlovska, S., Mofaddy, R., Nordentoft, M., & Benros, M. E. (2018). Association between traumatic brain injury and risk of suicide. *JAMA, 320*, 580–588.

16. Mainio, A., Kyllonen, T., Viilo, K., Hakko, H., Sarkioja,T., & Rasanen, P. (2007). Traumatic brain injury, psychiatric disorders and suicide: A population-based study of suicide victims during the years 1988–2004 in Northern Finland. *Brain Injury, 21*, 851–855.

17. Seel, R. T., & Kreutzer, J. S. (2003). Depression assessment after traumatic brain injury: An empirically based classification method. *Archives of Physical Medicine and Rehabilitation, 84,* 1621–1628.

18. Silver, J. M., Kramer, R., Greenwald, S., & Weissman, M. (2001). The association between head injuries and psychiatric disorders: Findings from the New Haven NIMH Epidemiologic Catchment Area Study. *Brain Injury, 15,* 935–945.

19. Simpson, G. K., & Tate, R. L. (2002). Suicidality after traumatic brain injury: Demographic, injury and clinical correlates. *Psychological Medicine, 32,* 687–697.

20. Simpson, G. K., & Tate, R. L. (2005). Clinical features of suicide attempts after TBI. *The Journal of Nervous and Mental Disease, 193,* 680–685.

21. Simpson, G. K., Tate, R. L.,Whiting, D. L., & Cotter, R. E. (2011). Suicide prevention after traumatic brain injury: A randomized controlled trial of a program for the psychological treatment of hopelessness. *Journal of Head Trauma Rehabilitation, 26,* 290–300.

22. Tate, R. L., Simpson, G. K., Flanagan, S., & Coffey, M. (1997). Completed suicide after traumatic brain injury. *Journal of Head Trauma Rehabilitation, 12,* 16–28.

23. Teasdale, T. W., & Engberg, A. W. (2001). Suicide after traumatic brain injury: A population study. *Journal of Neurology, Neurosurgery and Psychiatry, 71,* 436–440.

24. Tsaousides, T., Cantor, J. B., & Gordon, W. A. (2011). Suicidal ideation following traumatic brain injury: Prevalence rates and correlates in adults living in the community. *Journal of Head Trauma Rehabilitation, 26,* 265–275.

25. Ventura, T., Harrison-Felix, C., Carlson, N., DiGuiseppi, C., Gabella, B., Brown, A., . . . Whiteneck, G. (2010). Mortality after discharge from acute care hospitalization with traumatic brain injury: A population-based study. *Archives of Physical Medicine and Rehabilitation, 91,* 20–29.

Amyotrophic Lateral Sclerosis (ALS)

Suicide:

Risk of suicide 5.80 (SMR) times greater than general population.[3]

Suicide attempt:

No data for people with ALS.

Suicide ideation (SI):

Two small center-based studies found 28% rate of SI[5] and SI was higher among people with ALS in comparison to people living with cancer.[2]

Risk factors: (Sex, age, education, time post-onset, marital status.)

(i) Males (SMR 4.7) and females (SMR 10.9) with ALS both at elevated risk compared to general population[3]. (ii) Age of onset before 70 years has elevated risk in comparison to general population, but not for age of onset after 70 years.[3] (iii) Elevated risk of suicide for people at all education levels (Primary school vs high school or more).[3] (iv) People with ALS at elevated risk of suicide compared to the general population in first three years post-onset (SMR 11.3, <1 yr; SMR 5.5, 1–3 yrs) but not after 3 years.3 (v) People who are married/cohabiting at significant risk (SMR 7.50) compared to general population.[3]

Clinical features:

Reliable levels of suicide and SI hard to determine because of the focus on wish to end life[1,4,6] confounds assessment of SI.

Key references:

1. Albert, S. M., Rabkin, J. G., Del, Bene, M. L., Tider, T., O'Sullivan, I., Rowland, M. P., et al. (2005). Wish to die in end-stage ALS. *Neurology, 65*, 68–74.

2. Clarke, D.M., McLeod, J.E., Smith, G.C., Trauer, T., & Kissane, D. W. (2005). A comparison of psychosocial and physical functioning in patients with motor neurone disease and metastatic cancer. *Journal of Palliative Care, 21*, 173–179.

3. Fang, F., Valdimarsdóttir, U., Fürst, C. J., Hultman, C., Fall, K., Sparén, P., & Ye, W. (2008). Suicide among patients with amyotrophic lateral sclerosis. *Brain, 131*, 2729–2733.

4. Ganzini, L., Silveira, M. J., & Johnston, W. S. (2002). Predictors and correlates of interest in assisted suicide in the final month of life among ALS patients in Oregon and Washington. *Journal of Pain and Symptom Management, 24*, 312–317.

5. Palmieri, A., Sorarù, G., Albertini, E., Semenza, C., Vottero-Ris, F., D'Ascenzo, C., et al. (2010). Psychopathological features and suicidal ideation in amyotrophic lateral sclerosis patients. *Neurological Sciences, 31*, 735–740.

6. Veldink, J. H., Wokke, J. H., van der Wal, G., Vianney de Jong, J. M. B., &, van den Berg, L. H. (2002). Euthanasia and physician-assisted suicide among patients with amyotrophic lateral sclerosis in the Netherlands. *New England Journal of Medicine, 346*, 1638–1644.

Epilepsy

Suicide: Suicide risk after epilepsy is 3.30 times greater than for the general population, based on 74 studies.[1] Risk still elevated (AOR 1.99) after being adjusted for socioeconomic factors and excluding people with a history of psychiatric disease.[2] Risk was elevated for temporal lobe epilepsy (SMR 6.57), incident/newly diagnosed epilepsy in the community (SMR 2.13), prevalent populations in the community (SMR 4.64), and in tertiary care clinics (SMR 2.28) and epilepsy institutions (SMR 4.64).[1]

Suicide attempt: Epilepsy associated with elevated risk of SA (OR 4.4) among people with SI or a suicide plan after adjusting for demographic, disease, and other mental health variables.[7] A total of 4.8% of patients reported a history of at least one SA among a series of 145 consecutive admissions of people with idiopathic generalized epilepsy attending a tertiary epilepsy clinic.[3]

Suicide ideation (SI): People with epilepsy report a lifetime history of SI at an elevated rate compared to the general population (OR 2.2).[7,8] A single-center study found a 12.2% rate of current SI (17/139).[5]

Risk factors: (Sex, surgery, time post-onset, comorbid psychopathology.)

(i) Males (AOR 9.86) and females (AOR 23.6) with epilepsy and comorbid psychiatric conditions at elevated risk compared to general population.[2] (ii) People undergoing temporal lobe excision (SMR 13.9) or other epilepsy surgery (SMR 6.37) were at elevated risk in comparison to the general population.[2] (iii) Risk was highest early post-onset (0–6 mths AOR 5.35; 6–12 mths AOR 2.20; ≥1 yr AOR 1.79).[2] (iv) Risk was much higher post-onset for epilepsy with comorbid psychopathology (0–6 mths AOR 29.2; 6–12 mths AOR 24.7; ≥1 yr AOR 12.40).[2]

Clinical features:

Means of suicide included self-poisoning (26.9%, 7/26) with 10/26 (38.4%) dying from violent means (e. g., gunshot, hanging, jump, cutting).[6] People with epilepsy admitted to hospital due to SA used the same means as the general population.[4]

Key references:

1. Bell, G. S., Gaitatzis, A., Bell, C. L., Johnson, A. L., & Sander, J. W. (2009). Suicide in people with epilepsy: How great is the risk? *Epilepsia, 50,* 1933–1942.

2. Christensen, J., Vestergaard, M., Mortensen, P., Sidenius, P., & Agerbo, E. (2007). Epilepsy and risk of suicide: A population-based case-control study. *Lancet Neurology, 6,* 693–698.

3. Hara, E., Akanuma, N., Adachi, N., Hara, K., & Koutroumanidis, M. (2009). Suicide attempts in adult patients with idiopathic generalized epilepsy. *Psychiatry and Clinical Neurosciences, 63,* 225–229.

4. Hawton, K., Fagg, J., Marsack, P. (1980). Association between epilepsy and attempted suicide. *Journal of Neurology, Neurosurgery and Psychiatry, 43,* 168–170.

5. Jones, J. E., Hermann, B. P., Barry, J. J., Gilliam, F. G., Kanner, A. M., & Meador, K. J. (2003). Rates and risk factors for suicide, suicidal ideation and suicide attempts in chronic epilepsy. *Epilepsy and Behavior, 4,* S31–S38.

6. Nilsson, L., Ahlbom, A., Farahmand, B. Y., Åsberg, M., & Tomson, T. (2002). Risk factors for suicide in epilepsy: A case control study. *Epilepsia, 43,* 644–651.

7. Scott, K. M., Hwang, I., Chiu, W.-T., Kessler, R. C., Sampson, N. A., Angermeyer, M., et al. (2010). Chronic physical conditions and their association with first onset of suicidal behavior in the world mental health surveys. *Psychosomatic Medicine, 72,* 712–719.

8. Tellez-Zenteno, J. F., Patten, S. B., Jetté, N., Williams, J., & Wiebe, S. (2007). Psychiatric comorbidity in epilepsy: A population-based analysis. *Epilepsia, 48,* 2336–2344.

Huntington's Disease (HD)

Suicide:

Risk of suicide 2.90 (SMR) times greater than general population based on meta-analysis.[3]

Suicide attempt:

The HD study group found a 9.5% lifetime rate of SAs among 1,941 participants.[6]

Suicide ideation (SI):

The HD study group found a 26.5% lifetime rate of SI among 1,941 participants.[6] An earlier study from the same database found an overall rate of 17.5%, but only 1.3% had a suicide plan.[5]

Risk factors:

To the best of our knowledge there are no data on RFs for suicide, SAs or SI.

Clinical features:

Methods of suicide differed after HD compared to the general population (significantly fewer hangings in HD group compared to general population)[2] and 11% of people left a suicide note.[4] One study has collected data on SAs after direct testing for the mutation was available (though some participating centers were still reported patients who had undertaken a linkage analysis). Among the 21 individuals who made SAs, 17 had the mutation or were at increased risk. Ten attempts occurred within 6 months of the receipt of the results, with 15/21 attempts occurring within the first year. At the time of the attempts, 10 were asymptomatic, with another eight either possibly or probably affected and only three having a confirmed diagnosis, suggesting that the receipt of the results rather than HD symptom onset was the decisive trigger for the SA in a majority of cases.[1]

Key references:

1. Almqvist, E. W., Bloch, M., Brinkman, R., Craufurd, D., Hayden, M. R., on behalf of an international Huntington disease collaborative group. (1999). A worldwide assessment of the frequency of suicide, suicide attempts or psychiatric hospitalization after predictive testing for Huntington disease. *American Journal of Human Genetics, 64*, 1293–1304.
2. Baliko, L., Csala, B., & Czopf, J. (2004). Suicide in Hungarian Huntington's disease patients. *Neuroepidemiology, 23*, 258–260.
3. Harris, C., & Barraclough, B. (1997). Suicide as an outcome for mental disorders. *British Journal of Psychiatry, 170*, 205–228.
4. Lipe, H., Schultz, A., & Bird, T. D. (1993). Risk factors for suicide in Huntingtons disease: A retrospective case controlled study. *American Journal of Medical Genetics, 48*, 231–233.
5. Paulsen, J. S., Ferneyhough, Hoth, K., Nehl, C., Stierman, L., & The Huntington Study Group. (2005). Critical periods of suicide risk in Huntington's disease. *American Journal of Psychiatry, 162*, 725–731.
6. Wetzel, H. H., Gehl, C. R., Dellefave-Castillo, L., Schiffman, J. F., Shannon, K. M., Paulsen, J. S., and The Huntington Study Group. (2011). Suicidal ideation in Huntington disease: The role of comorbidity. *Psychiatry Research, 188*, 372–376.

Multiple Sclerosis (MS)

Suicide:

Risk of suicide between 1.83 and 2.36 (SMR) times greater than general population.[2,5,6,8]

Suicide attempt:

The only population-based study found no evidence of elevated rates of SA.[10] One center-based study found people with MS had three times the number of hospital admissions for SAs than the general population.[4] Two other center-based studies reported lifetime rates of SAs of 6.4%[3] and 12%.[7]

Suicide ideation (SI):

Limited information about SI. In the US, 29.4% (131/445) of military veterans reported SI over the previous 2 weeks, using the SI item on the Patient Health Questionnaire-9.[11] Single-center study found lifetime SI rate of 28.6% (40/140).[3]

Risk factors: (Sex, age, time of risk post-diagnosis.)

(i, ii) Males and females under 40 years at the time of diagnosis are at elevated risk of suicide compared to the general population.[5,8] Females from 40 to 60 years at the time of diagnosis are still at elevated risk of suicide.[5] After 60 the rate is no different to the general population. (iii) Evidence for elevated risk of suicide in the first 5 years post-diagnosis but not longer.[5] No breakdown of suicide risk by clinical group (relapsing remitting, primary progressive, secondary progressive, progressive relapsing).

Clinical features:

Most common means of suicide was gunshot, poisoning and hanging[1,9] with 38% leaving a note.[9] Most common method of SA was overdose (64%) followed by stabbing, gunshot, and ingestion with about half (54%, 12/22) having made a threat of suicide prior to the attempt.[1]

Key references:

1. Berman, A. L., & Samuel, L. (1993). Suicide among people with multiple sclerosis. *Journal of NeuroRehabilitation, 7*, 53–62.

2. Brønnum-Hansen, H., Stenager, E., Stenager, E. N., & Koch-Henriksen, N. (2005). Suicide among Danes with multiple sclerosis. *Journal of Neurology, Neurosurgery and Psychiatry, 76*, 1457–1459.

3. Feinstein, A. (2002). An examination of suicidal intent in patients with multiple sclerosis. *Neurology, 59*, 674–678.

4. Fisk, J. D., Morehouse, S. A., Brown, M. G., Skedgel, C., & Murray, T. J. (1998). Hospital-based psychiatric service utilization and morbidity in multiple sclerosis. *Canadian Journal of Neurological Science, 25*, 230–235.

5. Fredrikson, S., Cheng, Q., Jiang, G. -X., & Wasserman, D. (2003). Elevated suicide risk among patients with multiple sclerosis in Sweden. *Neuroepidemiology, 22*, 146–152.

6. Harris, C., & Barraclough, B. (1997). Suicide as an outcome for mental disorders. *British Journal of Psychiatry, 170*, 205–228.

7. Minden, S. L., Orav, J., & Reich, P. (1987). Depression in multiple sclerosis. *General Hospital Psychiatry, 9*, 426–434.

8. Stenager, E. S., Stenager, E., Koch-Henriksen, N., Brønnum-Hansen, H., Hyllested, K., Jensen, K., et al. (1992). Suicide and multiple sclerosis: An epidemiological investigation. *Journal of Neurology, Neurosurgery and Psychiatry, 55*, 542–545.

9. Stenager, E. N., Koch-Henrikson, N., & Stenager, E. (1996). Risk factors for suicide in multiple sclerosis. *Psychotherapy and Psychosomatics, 65*, 86–90.

10. Stenager, E. S., Jensen, B., Stenager, M., Stenager, K., & Stenager, E. (2011). Suicide attempts in multiple sclerosis. *Multiple Sclerosis Journal, 17*, 1265–1268.

11. Turner, A. P., Williams, R. M., Bowen, J. D., Kivlahan, D. R., & Haselkorn, J. K. (2006). Suicidal ideation in multiple sclerosis. *Archives of Physical Medicine and Rehabilitation, 87*, 1073–1078.

Parkinson's Disease (PD)

Suicide:

Little evidence of elevated suicide risk among people with PD.[1-3,7,10] One single-center study did find elevated risk (SMR 5.2) but with only 2 suicides among a series of 102 patients.[4] However, people with PD who have undergone deep brain stimulation are at elevated risk.[11]

Suicide attempt:

There is limited data about SA after PD.[8,9]

Suicide ideation (SI):

Current level of SI was 7–11% with SI/death ideation 14.4–30%.[4-6,8]

Key references:

1. Gale, C. R., Braidwood, E. A., Winter, P. D., & Martyn, C. N. (1999). Mortality from Parkinson's disease and other causes in men who were prisoners of war in the Far East. *Lancet, 354*, 2116–2118.

2. Harris, C., & Barraclough, B. (1997). Suicide as an outcome for mental disorders. *British Journal of Psychiatry, 170*, 205–228.

3. Juurlink, D., Herrmann, N., Szalai, J. P., Kopp, A., & Redelmeier, D. A. (2004). Medical illness and the risk of suicide in the elderly. *Archives of Internal Medicine, 164*, 1179–1184.

4. Kostić, V. S., Pekmezović, T., Tomić, A., Ječmenica-Lukić, M., Stojković, T., Špica, V., et al. (2010). Suicide and suicidal ideation. *Journal of the Neurological Sciences, 289*, 40–43.

5. Kummer, A., Cardoso, F., & Teixeira, A. L. (2009). Suicidal ideation in Parkinson's disease. *CNS Spectrum, 14*, 431–436.

6. Leentjens, A. F. G., Marinus, J., Van, Hilten, J. J., Lousberg, R., & Verhey, F. R. J. (2003). The contribution of somatic symptoms to the diagnosis of depressive disorder in Parkinson's disease: A discriminant analytic approach. *Journal of Neuropsychiatry and Clinical Neurosciences, 15*, 74–77.

7. Myslobodsky, M., Lalonde, F. M., & Hicks, L. (2001). Are patients with Parkinson's disease suicidal? *Journal of Geriatric Psychiatry and Neurology, 14*, 120–124.

8. Nazem, S., Siderowf, A. D., Duda, J. E., Brown, G. K., Have, T. T., Stern, M. B., et al. (2008). Suicidal and death ideation in Parkinson's Disease. *Movement Disorders, 23*, 1573–1579.

9. Soulas, T., Gurruchaga, J.-M., Palfi, S., Cesaro, P., Nguyen, J.-P., & Fénelon, G. (2008). Attempted and completed suicides after subthalamic nucleus stimulation for Parkinson's disease. *Journal of Neurology, Neurosurgery and Psychiatry, 79*, 952–954.

10. Stenager, E. N., Wermuth, L., Stenager, E., & Boldsen, J. (1992). Suicide in patients with Parkinson's disease: An epidemiological study. *Acta Psychiatrica Scandinavica, 90*, 70–72.

11. Voon, V., Krack, P., Lang, A. E., Lozano, A. M., Dujardin, K., Schüpbach, M., . . . Speelman, J. D. (2008). A multicentre study on suicide outcomes following subthalamic stimulation for Parkinson's disease. *Brain, 131*, 2720–2728.

AOR, adjusted odds ratio; OR, Odds ratio; HR, hazard ratio; SA, suicide attempt; SI, suicidal ideation; SMR; standard mortality rate.

Cross-Cultural E-Resources

American Psychological Association. Guidelines on multicultural education, training, research, practice, and organizational change for psychologists. http://www.apa.org/pi/multiculturalguidelines/formats.html

Hogg Foundation for Mental Health. Cultural competency: A practical guide for mental health service providers. http://www.hogg.utexas.edu/PDF/Saldana.pdf

National Center for Cultural Competence. http://www11.georgetown.edu/research/gucchd/nccc/

National Mental Health Association (now Mental Health America). Cultural and linguistic competency in mental health systems. http://www1.nmha.org/position/ps38.cfm

New York City Department of Health and Mental Hygiene. Cultural competence websites—mental health. http://www.nyc.gov/html/doh/downloads/pdf/qi/qi-ccpriorityresources.pdf

Rainbow Heights. Guidelines for effective and culturally competent treatment with lesbian, gay, bisexual, and transgender people living with mental illness: Excerpted from Rosenberg, S., Rosenberg, J., Huygen, C., & Klein, E. (2005). No need to hide: Out of the closet and mentally ill, Best practices in mental health. *An International Journal, 1,* 72–85. http://www.rainbowheights.org/Guidelines.htm

Substance Abuse and Mental Health Services Administration. Factsheets on specific races and ethnicities. http://mentalhealth.samhsa.gov/cre/factsheet.asp

Substance Abuse and Mental Health Services Administration. Culturally specific mental health resources. http://mentalhealth.samhsa.gov/cre/resources.asp

Cultural Competence in Mental Health. (n.d.). UPenn Collaborative on Community Integration: A Rehabilitation Research & Training Center Promoting Community Integration of Individuals with Psychiatric Disabilities. www.upennrrtc.org

Index